COLORED INSANE

RACE, INEQUALITY, AND HEALTH

RACE, INEQUALITY, AND HEALTH

Edited by Samuel Kelton Roberts Jr. and Michael Yudell

The Race, Inequality, and Health series explores how forms of racialization have created a wide range of phenomena, from producing inequities in health and healthcare to inspiring social movements around health. The goal of this series is to publish field-defining works across history, the social sciences, the biological sciences, and public health that deepen our understanding of how claims about race and race difference have affected health and society.

Jonathan Kahn, *The Uses of Diversity: How Race Has Become Entangled in Law, Politics, and Biology*

Eram Alam, Dorothy Roberts, and Natalie Shibley, editors, *Ordering the Human: The Global Spread of Racial Science*

Sebastián Gil-Riaño, *The Remnants of Race Science: UNESCO and Economic Development in the Global South*

Rob DeSalle and Ian Tattersall, *Troublesome Science: The Misuse of Genetics and Genomics in Understanding Race*

Michael Yudell, *Race Unmasked: Biology and Race in the Twentieth Century*

COLORED INSANE

SLAVERY, ASYLUMS, AND MENTAL ILLNESS IN THE NINETEENTH CENTURY

DIANA MARTHA LOUIS

Columbia University Press
New York

Columbia University Press
Publishers Since 1893
New York   Chichester, West Sussex

Copyright © 2025 Columbia University Press
All rights reserved

Cataloging-in-Publication Data is available from the Library of Congress.
ISBN 9780231212861 (hardback)
ISBN 9780231212878 (trade paperback)
ISBN 9780231559607 (ebook)
LCCN 2025018748

Cover image: Jacob Lawrence, *Forward*, 1967. North Carolina Museum of Art, Raleigh, Purchased with funds from the State of North Carolina, 70.8.1.

GPSR Authorized Representative: Easy Access System Europe, Mustamäe tee 50, 10621 Tallinn, Estonia, gpsr.requests@easproject.com

CONTENTS

INTRODUCTION 1

1. ANTEBELLUM PSYCHIATRIC AND MEDICAL DISCOURSES ON THE BLACK BODYMIND 19

2. MENTAL DISABILITY AND THE INTELLECTUAL THOUGHT OF JAMES McCUNE SMITH 46

3. PSYCHOLOGICAL COSTS OF BLACK WOMEN'S ENSLAVEMENT IN HARRIET JACOBS'S *INCIDENTS IN THE LIFE OF A SLAVE GIRL* (1861) 88

4. HARRIET TUBMAN AND NINETEENTH-CENTURY CONCEPTIONS OF MENTAL DISABILITY 111

5. BLACK WOMEN'S PSYCHIATRIC INCARCERATION AT GEORGIA LUNATIC ASYLUM IN THE NINETEENTH CENTURY 140

6. CHARLES CHESNUTT AND MENTAL DISABILITY
IN THE AGE OF BLACK FREEDOM   171

CODA   199

Acknowledgments 209
Notes 213
Bibliography 271
Index 295

COLORED INSANE

INTRODUCTION

The year 1850 was a terrifying one for free and fugitive Black people in the North. American slavery apologists tightly gripped the reins of an economic system that depended on human bondage. The US Congress passed the draconian Fugitive Slave Act of 1850, widening the reach of slavery beyond the borders of the South and requiring northern state and local governments to assist in the hunt, capture, and reenslavement of Black bodyminds. Harriet Jacobs, a woman who went to great lengths to free herself and her children at the expense of her body and mind, found herself among those at risk. She penned a narrative about her life wherein she bore witness to her emotional experiences and personal reactions to her terrible circumstances in slavery and freedom. Through her words, she made plain the suffering and resistance that were at once visible and invisible, specific and universal, individual and communal. She painted a grim picture of life under the new law; New York was no longer a safe haven for Blacks as slave catchers prowled the streets. The law wreaked havoc on Black people's minds. Amid the "reign of terror," Jacobs imparted, there was widespread "incessant fear," "distress," "consternation," and "anguish."[1]

After scanning the newspaper to make sure there were no southerners at hotels in town, she ventured out to run errands for her employer. As she scurried through the streets, she ran into Luke, a fellow fugitive slave she had known in slavery. She recounted Luke's story; he, like her, had survived torturous physical and sexual abuse at the hands of a despotic slave master. When she set her eyes upon Luke, she was filled with joy: "I always rejoiced to see or hear of any one who had escaped from the black pit."[2] She chose for her readers the image of a "black pit" to describe a system they had likely never seen yet sought to understand. The black pit was both a physical place—a hole in the ground inescapable without aid—and a psychological state, one into which she and Luke sank deeply under the weight of despair. The imagery of a pit also signifies extreme darkness that invariably mutes one sense, sight, and amplifies others, like sound and touch. In this highly sensitized space, the voices and touch of loved ones become all the more dear and sustaining. Having experienced the horrors of this physically confining and mentally depleting pit, Jacobs and Luke found in each other a fellow traveler, the gift of being seen, and the comfort each imparted to the other.

This reading of Jacobs turns our attention to the psychological economy of slavery. It forces us to consider how she and the countless others for whom she spoke engaged deeply with contentious conversations of the time about mental disability and mental suffering. Jacobs shows one facet of an untold story about cultural discourses of race, gender, and mental disability in the nineteenth century. Her writings bring into view concerns about freedom, slavery, psychiatric treatment, healing, and social mobility that emerge from a literary and cultural study of mental disability in the Black experience. Focusing on the nineteenth century, *Colored Insane* pursues a number of intellectual questions: How have Black people articulated the psychological impact of slavery and subsequent forms of violence? How did American cultural perceptions of insanity shape Blacks' embodied experiences of mental disability within asylums? How did Black people conceptualize individual and communal notions of mental health? *Colored Insane* pursues these questions by exploring conceptualizations and experiences of Black mental disability from the inside: from the perspective of leading figures and advocates for the care of the "colored insane" and from the vantage points of Black Americans. This book investigates how Black mental disability was theorized by a diverse group of elite white men and women, including mental asylum superintendents and mental health reformers, and how these mental health reformers mobilized their beliefs in their efforts to treat Blacks with mental disabilities, then referred to as the "colored insane." *Colored Insane* argues that nineteenth-century psychiatric discourses made Black Americans "mad" both by constructing disorders according to prevailing notions of race, class, gender, and insanity and by inflicting real psychological harm within asylums, plantations, jails, and society writ large. However, as *Colored Insane* contends, medical and psychiatric discourses that inscribed meaning on the Black bodymind did not go unchallenged. *Colored Insane* centers Black perspectives on mental suffering and mental disability from a multivocal group of Black figures, including the medically trained James McCune Smith, the self-liberated women Harriet Jacobs and Harriet Tubman, and the premier Black intellectual Charles Chesnutt. Together, these figures constitute a Black American counter-discourse on mental disability that challenged medicalized views of Black people's mental and physical health and embodied or conceptualized alternative visions of the Black bodymind. These writers and thinkers generated more vibrant, complex, and fully human portraits of the Black bodymind.

Colored Insane examines singular sites, people, cultural developments, literary works, and specific groups, such as Black women in mental hospitals, that illuminate the battle over conceptualizations of the Black bodymind. It is anchored in the cultural histories of two of America's prototypical institutions of physical and social confinement—slavery and asylums. It sheds light on the scientific, medical, and psychiatric discourses that drove both institutions. Presenting responses from Black writers and thinkers, the book highlights the work of the medically trained Black intellectual and writer James McCune Smith, who devoted his life to challenging such proslavery and racist discourses as a medical researcher, physician, and literary writer. He not only pushed back on demeaning representations of Black people but also used his experimental fiction to create images of thriving Black people poised to live full lives unfettered by oppression. During the height of the internal slave trade, which resulted in the proliferation of mental distress caused by family separations, fear of recapture, and racial hostility, Harriet Jacobs wrote in her narrative, *Incidents in the Life of a Slave Girl, Written by Herself* (1861), about the multiple forms of mental suffering she experienced.[3] She was fully aware of the harm being levied against her mental and physical body and shared this devastation with her northern white audience. The larger-than-life figure Harriet Tubman integrated various altered mental states, such as hallucinating and hearing voices, into her life as a fugitive in 1849 and a free woman thereafter. She found in those experiences purpose and power for living a satisfying life despite the pathologizing popular and medical ideas that circulated around her and drew on those experiences when she established the Harriet Tubman Home for Aged and Indigent Negroes in 1908. *Colored Insane* also examines the lives of five ordinary women sent to an infamous southern mental hospital, the Georgia Lunatic Asylum, during the nadir of race relations, a historical moment characterized by race riots, lynching, and legal forms of segregation and disenfranchisement. These women likely suffered from adverse and unwanted mental health conditions and were subject to oppressive intersecting conceptualizations of Black femininity and insanity in postbellum Georgia. From the post-Reconstruction period up to the turn of the twentieth century, Charles Chesnutt's writings, both fiction and nonfiction, offered alternative ideas about the Black bodymind from Black-originated sources of medical knowledge and authority such as Conjure women and Black physicians. Chesnutt's literature not only dismantled racist medicalized norms about the Black body and mind but also presented new visions of health and human unity.

TERMINOLOGY

Studying mental disability among Blacks in the nineteenth century poses many challenges regarding terminology and definitions. Mental disability as a topic of study is hard to pin down because it entails grappling with a subject that operates in the realms of the real and imagined, material and immaterial, permanent and ethereal, literal and figurative, durable and fleeting. The story of Black experiences of mental disability requires an uncomfortable embrace of such slipperiness precisely because in it we find the most significant sites of knowledge about the Black bodymind. I use multiple terms to hold together this dynamic story of Black mental disability that includes nineteenth-century biomedical terms such as "insanity," nineteenth-century lay terms such as "mental suffering" and "madness," and some present-day language such as "mental disability" and "bodymind." As Geoffrey Reaume importantly argues, "No term in the history of madness is neutral—not mental illness, madness, or any other term."[4] The chief aim of this study is to interrogate the meaning of the terms as they were used by various actors in the past because terms do "particular kinds of cultural work in particular contexts," as Margaret Price reminds us.[5]

"Mental illness" is a contemporary biomedical term to describe physiological illnesses often associated with various contemporary diagnostic categories including but not limited to bipolar disorder, depression, anxiety, and schizophrenia. In *Colored Insane*, "mental illness" is not used extensively in the book's analysis. It serves instead as a bridge term to connect present-day understandings of health and illness to the past. Reflecting the failure of language to fully represent various mental health conditions or counteract legacies of stigmatization, a number of terms have emerged to define mental disability, including "neurotypicality," "neurodivergence," "emotional illness," "psychosocial disability," "psychiatric disability," and "cognitive" or "intellectual disability." Rather than using any one of these specific terms, I use "mental illness" as an umbrella term for health concerns related to people's brains, behavior, and emotions. Although modern medicine is still in its relative infancy in terms of knowledge of the brain, I conducted my analysis in its shadow and marshal it when it is useful to explain the past. The book thus works with a broad definition of mental illness, informed by the contemporary understanding that mental health conditions are linked to various factors including culture, biology, environment, society, and individual life experiences. Hence, my analysis pays close attention to historical evidence associated with these arenas as one way to locate issues of mental disability. Although *Colored Insane* is careful not to diagnose Black people in the nineteenth century or impose contemporary taxonomies of disease on them, it purposely sheds light on the ways oppressive conditions created *real* harm, pain, and undesirable physiological changes among Black Americans.

"Mental illness," however, was not a term used in the nineteenth century. What we now broadly understand as mental illness mapped onto several nineteenth-century terms, including "madness," "insanity," "lunacy," and "craziness." The mental conditions that are examined in this book under this banner include various psychotic states that are not limited to diagnostic categories, such as delirium and hallucination, as well as serious addictions and extreme responses to traumatic and emotionally disturbing events. They also include biopsychological conditions that emerge from underlying illnesses, such as syphilitic infections, pellagra, malnutrition, sleep deprivation, or head trauma. Mental disability manifested in many forms but generally pertained to states of mind that required some type of outside intervention from other enslaved people, family members, white plantation owners, public officials, local governing bodies, mainstream physicians and psychiatrists, Conjurers, and homeopathic doctors.

When discussing the nineteenth-century medical diagnostic categories used by psychiatrists and physicians, I use the terms "insanity" and "lunacy" to refer to the copious theorizations about insanity that occurred throughout the nineteenth century and appeared in the form of medicalized sources, including textbooks, journal articles, and addresses. When discussing psychiatric ideas from these sources, I use terms such as "lunatic," "insane," and "mad" interchangeably and as historical markers, not as derogatory idioms meant to typify people with mental health conditions. The most glaring display of the century-long use of the term insanity is evidenced in the name of the main organ of psychiatric conceptualizations, the *American Journal of Insanity*. Begun by a superintendent of Utica State Hospital, Amariah Brigham, in 1844, the journal remained in publication until 1921, at which time it was renamed the *American Journal of Psychiatry*. Although the psychiatric term "insanity" had particular legal consequences in the 1850s (the insane could not vote or hold property), it was often used synonymously with "madness." The latter term was common among the general public and served colloquially as a catch-all for psychological illness.

Modern readers may find nineteenth-century terms to be unsettling, outdated, or pseudoscientific lingo. However, in the nineteenth century, "madness" and "insanity" were not derogatory terms. They were acceptable "scientific" language used by various actors, including Blacks, whites, and the mentally disabled, to describe mental health conditions. In using these terms, I follow the lead of the mad studies scholars Brenda A. LeFrancois, Robert Menzies, and Geoffrey Reaume, who embrace the term "madness" specifically in critical ways: "To work with and within the language of madness is by no means to deny the psychic, spiritual, and material pains and privations endured by countless people with histories of encounters with the psy disciplines. To the contrary, it is to acknowledge and validate these experiences as being authentically human, while at the same time rejecting clinical labels that pathologize and degrade; challenging the reductionistic assumptions and effects of the medical model; locating psychiatry and its human subjects within wider historical, institutional, and cultural contexts."[6] *Colored Insane* engages in deep contextualization to reveal how common terms such as "madness" and "insanity" were used. Even if these were the standard terms in use in the nineteenth century, it is nonetheless the case that the mentally ill were regularly pathologized as "deviant," "deficient," and "inferior," which are all hallmarks of a medical model of disability.[7] People given such labels by doctors, psychiatrists, and state officials such as judges and policemen were seen as existing outside of the parameters of socially accepted ideas about what was and was not "normal."[8] Nineteenth-century language reflects the power of those using these terms, their cultural sensibilities, and technological and taxonomic developments. Even so, medicalized terms are woefully insufficient for capturing the multiperspectivity and complexity of perspectives on Black mental disability, which sometimes existed outside mainstream medical worlds in the nineteenth century.

"Mental suffering" was a nineteenth-century colloquial term used by the non–medically trained public. It was chosen by a newspaper writer to describe the sexualized violence that Harriet Jacobs experienced at the hands of her nefarious slave master.[9] Mental suffering captures various types of emotional forms of distress as well as adverse mental and physical health states, injuries, and conditions resulting from physical, sexual, or psychological abuse or incidents. It reflects experiences of mental strain that diverge from an individual's typical or unencumbered state of mind. For example, as Jacobs's *Incidents in the Life of a Slave Girl* reveals, it includes emotional responses to everyday practices during slavery, such as malnourishment, sexualized violence, forced and controlled reproduction, family separation (between plantations and across continents), runaway attempts, witnessing violence, and hazardous labor and living conditions. These common incidents may or may not lead to complete incapacitation. In and of themselves, emotional responses such as sorrow, fear, and anxiety are not necessarily indicative of illness. However, *Colored Insane* does its best to parse out the moments when they may point to psychological disturbance. At other times, mental suffering is interchangeable with what we might now broadly understand as mental illness, then labeled "madness" or "insanity." For instance, mental suffering could take the form of a suicide attempt following an episode of melancholy, which we now consider depression. These distinctions are difficult to measure decisively, of course, but such challenges do not preclude the pursuit of a deeper understanding of how enslaved people experienced the peculiar institution of slavery. Mental suffering is one facet of the contemporary concept of mental disability that emerges from the scholarly field of disability studies.

Colored Insane most often uses the term "mental disability" to refer to people's embodied experiences and social constructions of the body. The feminist disability scholar Elizabeth Donaldson contends that disability-informed understandings of mental health "begin with the premise that mental disability is a neuro-biological disorder and still remain committed to . . . an agenda that fights to dismantle ideologies of oppression."[10] Thus, mental disability often refers to embodied experiences of mental illness, distress, and pain. However, other times the term goes beyond the embodiment of mental disability. A disability framework provides intellectual terrain to consider how cultural institutions are potentially *disabling* even if everyone subject to them is not affected in the same ways. This book is attuned to the disabling features of nineteenth-century society, whether they play out in major systems like slavery or in specific incidents like acts of sexual exploitation, lynching, or a race massacre. More than overt and acute emotional and psychological traumas, this study includes experiences of mental distress that were mundane yet routinely unsettling, like the terrifying uncertainty children felt when being torn from their mothers on an auction block or the incessant fear Black men felt of being killed after bumping shoulders with a white woman on a postbellum sidewalk. *Colored Insane* shuttles between unearthing individual and group embodied experiences of disability and critiquing medicine and psychiatry's pathologizing impetus to identify, measure, and assess what constitutes the "normal" mind and body and subsequently contain, manage, and regulate people accordingly. It thus makes considerable room for the meaning Black figures themselves made around disability. Sometimes that meaning is counteractive to psychiatric definitions and reasonings, and other times, it is connected to their visions of health, freedom, family, religion, and citizenship.

Although new terms have emerged to refer to people who encounter psychiatrists or receive treatment in mental health facilities, including "psychiatric system survivors" and "consumer/survivor/ex-patient (c/s/x)," these are not quite accurate for the nineteenth-century individuals I consider here.[11] In reference to the men and women who were psychiatrically incarcerated, I purposely refrain from using the word "patient," preferring the word "people," so as to untether people from the diagnostic rubrics and medical regimes that sought to objectify them into passive roles and exercise power over their lives.[12]

Perhaps most importantly, I use the term "bodymind" to describe the inextricable ties between the body and the mind. The term is generative for the argument unfolded here because mental embodiment often gets lost or overlooked in discussions of power and the body. First used by disability studies scholar Margaret Price, "bodymind" rejects the dichotomies between the mind and the body that originate in Western Enlightenment thinking and that distort people's actual experiences of pain and suffering.[13] Bodymind is a materialist feminist disability studies concept that replaces the need to repeatedly delineate that a discussion applies to both the body *and* the mind. However, as Price admonishes, the use of the term goes beyond a shorthand to include theorizations of the body; the bodymind is a "sociopolitically constituted and material entity that emerges through both structural (power- and violence-laden) contexts and also individual (specific) experience."[14] This study unearths how Black people's bodyminds were acted upon by medical and psychiatric authorities, with special attention to Black women's experiences within psychiatric spaces of confinement. Nineteenth-century Black writers and figures such as James McCune Smith, Harriet Jacobs, Harriet Tubman, and Charles Chesnutt countered medical and psychiatric traditions that medicalized the Black bodymind as pathological or abnormal and offered their own conceptualizations of the Black bodymind as both vulnerable to American violence and powerful and poised to flourish.

With this dual approach to examining mental disability as both a social construction and an embodied experience, the book's term "colored insane" carries meaning as both a noun and a verb. As a noun, it pinpoints an identity category that holds the material experiences of illness. As a verb, it highlights a process of labeling, imbuing, distorting, or misrepresenting African Americans as mentally ill or deranged. Whether real or imagined, the label "colored insane" or "colored lunatic" justified the treatment and confinement of Black Americans. Archival records of southern asylums show that there were often severe repercussions to being labeled insane. It meant subjection to state-sanctioned disciplinary regimes, such as brazen police officers and unsympathetic judges, and the experiences of harsh treatment modalities in asylums, including taxing labor assignments. In asylums, for example, Black people lived in segregated, dilapidated, and overcrowded dwelling spaces, received little treatment for deadly diseases such as tuberculosis, and were exposed to physical and sexual violence from staff and their white mentally disabled counterparts.

The psychiatric establishment was not the only group to use psychiatric terms—the so-called "colored insane" used them themselves. When they did so, however, it was not simply a reification of race- and gender-based psychiatric formulations; it was a mechanism for rejecting pathologization, expanding the concept of health, and asserting medical authority. *Colored Insane* focuses on these competing and complementary nineteenth-century definitions of Black mental disability—definitions that emerge from a range of actors, including whites, Blacks, physicians, psychiatrists, and the general public.

READING PRACTICES

My reading practice is to simultaneously examine and patch together various types of narratives—slave narratives, novels, short stories, biographies, medical case studies, newspaper articles, life narratives reconstructed from both historical and asylum records, and meta-level cultural narratives about Blackness and mental disability—to create an account of nineteenth-century Black Americans' encounters with psychiatry and their experiences of and thoughts about mental disability. *Colored Insane* navigates this broad landscape using the theoretical lenses of disability theory and black feminist theory, which together reveal a multivalent story about Black people's mental health in the nineteenth century.

Reading various narratives in conjunction creates mutually contingent interventions that are at once historiographical, archival, and methodological. The book thus brings together two sets of previously siloed historical sources, figures, and institutions, all of which invite critical suspicion and interpretation. One set emerges from predominantly white-authored medicalized documents and official records, including census data, army statistics, asylum records, government documents, and family papers. The second is Black-authored and includes medical publications, slave narratives, novels, songs, stories, sketches, and biographies. Whereas many of the white-authored texts are from various kinds of medical professionals, the Black-authored works encompass heterogeneous thinkers, actors, and ordinary people who, when examined together, patch holes in the official records that habitually omit the voices of the so-called "colored insane."

Colored Insane's historiographical intervention is reflected in its use of disability studies to renarrate familiar sources in the history of psychiatry. Nineteenth-century humanistic scholarly studies on mental disability—whether focused on insanity and slavery or histories of psychiatry and asylums—rely primarily on medicalized primary sources, such as census data, army statistics, asylum records, government documents, and family papers. These sources center white voices, such as those of slaveholders, physicians, census takers, jailers, and federal, state, and local legislators. In this study, I unveil how the words of psychiatrists, physicians, and mental health reformers function on two levels, with one being a surface level to describe people and the other a metadiscourse that occurs on an ideological level. The language and narrative conventions present within official records and medicalized and psychiatric documents reflect broader discourses of racialization, medicalization, and marginalization.

Through its examination of various iterations of such proslavery discourses from the fields of medicine and psychiatry, *Colored Insane* offers an account of the embodied experiences of mental disability in antebellum society. In most antebellum cities and towns, jails served as the primary place of confinement for mentally disabled Blacks. However, many enslaved Blacks were treated on plantations. To depict Black people who were treated outside asylums, I incorporate asylum case narratives from medical and psychiatric journals. Medical journals published during slavery give accounts of the mentally disabled being treated by physicians.

In addition to reading the ideological underpinnings of psychiatric thought before slavery ended, I examine postbellum medicalized records and official documents to make an archival intervention specifically by reconstructing the life narratives of five women who were sent to Georgia Lunatic Asylum at the end of the nineteenth century. Unlike whites with mental disabilities during the nineteenth century, Black Americans did not produce asylum narratives from which we can glean their perspectives. To fill in these gaps using elements of the women's lives, I read medical records and official documents "against the grain." Reading in this way entails paying careful attention to sources' language and context to gain insight into the experiences of those they most silence. Rather than institutions that exercised total power over those they held, a top-down understanding of psychiatric power, nineteenth-century asylums were made up of what Michel Foucault calls various "relations of power." Foucault sees power as not being possessed by any one person but rather characterized by relations of force consisting of maneuvers, strategies, and practices that are not fixed but are always in process and productive.[15] In this formulation, power and resistance exist at the same time and can be altered at any moment. In this study, I understand the interactions between Black people and the institution(s) as a struggle. Taking Foucault's formulation one step further, this study shows that the relations of power in nineteenth-century asylums were not unidirectional between, for example, doctors and people, but multidirectional, between Black people and various actors, including slave masters, hospital attendants, and whites.

Medical sources and official documents reflect the proslavery leanings of mainstream psychiatry and do not include the perspectives of the people to which they refer. Rather than simply noting that silences exist, I seek to unveil how and why silences in medical archives are created and sustained. For instance, archival medical records primarily showcase psychiatric tendencies to police boundaries of normalcy and disability/ability, create gender- and race-based medical science, and/or reinforce stereotypical and controlling images that justify the containment and management of people living at the intersection of multiple systems of oppression. Speculative openness to what is missing and ideological unveiling are perhaps the most promising aspects of disability studies because exposing psychiatry's making and remaking of mental disability leaves room for thinking outside psychiatry and medicine's ideological fictions and intellectual barricades.[16]

To occupy historical worlds that existed outside the confines of Eurocentric traditions of conceptualizing mental disability, *Colored Insane* directs scholarly attention to Black-authored sources that together indirectly speak back to the various silences that exist in medicalized sources and create meaning outside of them. Driven by a Black feminist theoretical imperative that centers Black people in general and Black women in particular (my focus in several chapters), I position literary works as alternative sites of knowledge and valuable sources for alternative conceptual insights on Black mental disability.[17] This book thus turns to an expansive archive to augment our understanding of the modes of representation of Black mental disability that were culturally available. Black conceptualizations appear in the writings of James McCune Smith, the slave narrative of Harriet Jacobs, and the journalism, short stories, and novels of Charles Chesnutt. These works contain ideas about the function, role, and centrality of mental disability in the Black American experience. Harriet Tubman is a unique figure because she was illiterate and did not write her own story; we do, however, know about the stories she told in the Black oral tradition, which reflect her conceptualizations of mental disability and religious expression.

These Black voices always existed, of course, but they have been devalued so much, then and now, that they have been rendered obscure. Nevertheless, Black writings open up distinctive possibilities for meaning that medicalized writings omit entirely. Black writings are "counternarratives" because they are the stories of people whose experiences are not often told. Although Black perspectives are not limited to oppositional thinking, a salient thread reflects the ways Black people directly or indirectly resist racialized and pathologizing psychiatric thought and practice when they encounter it on plantations, within carceral institutions such asylums, and within society writ large. To varying degrees, Black thinkers, actors, and cultural productions directly engage, refute, and provide critical nuance to the ideas, assumptions, and beliefs of prominent figures, reformers, and leaders in the field of psychiatry concerning insanity among Black people.

Historians readily see literary works as valuable sources of evidence. They often use literature to corroborate historical facts, such as the brutality of slavery, and most recently the proliferation of mental disabilities among Black people in the nineteenth century. As a literary critic, I make literature a primary object of analysis and, as such, engage with the field's debates about how we should analyze Black fiction in the nineteenth century. Some scholars call for privileging a work's aesthetic value, whereas others call for elucidating a text's literary merit with the author's contributions to the historical and sociological movements of their time. My work is best aligned with the stance of Jacqueline Goldsby, who contends that "rather than read history *into* [nineteenth-century] literary texts, [we can] read history *out* of them."[18] Reading history out of literary texts means, for me, treating those texts as powerful cultural artifacts in their own right and examining them on their own terms. Black literature made historical contributions to ideological debates, and Black writers intentionally engaged in the battles over providing Blacks with mental health care and contributed to shaping the category of mental disability. Black writings are an indispensable strand of the cultural tapestry of conceptualizations of mental disability. At the convergence of literary artistry and measured engagement with psychiatric discourses, I observe in Black cultural productions intellectual histories of mental disability and new visions of health. Black writings complicate a stale account of mental health in which vulnerable people are powerless and objectified victims of Western medical regimes. Literary and nonfiction writing by or about Blacks created imaginative, mythical, and mysterious worlds in which multiple ideas had room to breathe and inhabitants therein occupied positions of power that their real-life counterparts were denied.

As Charles Chesnutt declared in a speech before a group of dignified Washington, DC, Blacks, "History is instructive, and may warn and admonish; but to this quality literature adds the faculty of persuasion, by which men's hearts are reached, the springs of action touched, and the currents of life directed." He, like other writers, sought to bring about a change in the reader via language.

Unlike the psychiatric establishment, however, postbellum Black authors wrote from a vantage point that was more forthright in its subjectivity and less invested in epistemological omniscience. The evidentiary power of creative writers' works differs markedly from that of case histories, observations, and neurological examinations of psychiatrists. Their painstaking efforts to tell stories about themselves and their characters led to deep contextualization of American life, which granted their readers otherwise dismissed, overlooked, or suppressed insights into the circumstances from which mental disabilities emerged, whether documented by a psychiatrist or not.

Black writers' outlooks were embedded in a keen attentiveness to the social worlds around them and heightened awareness of the popular interests, ideals, symbols, and concerns of the reading public. In the words of

Chesnutt, "Would you know a nation, read its books." Postbellum Black writers spent countless hours reading newspapers, journals, pamphlets, and even anthropological, scientific, and medical writings. They visited the places and sites of atrocities about which they wrote, experienced firsthand cultures of violence, and taught and spoke to people from all corners of society. In their closeness to the people and ideas of their times, they, more than most others, had a handle on the dissemination of psychiatric concepts into the public imagination and at the same time were so sensitive to the machinations of power that they aptly called out the American politics of race that were embedded in psychiatric discourses.

INTERVENTIONS

Colored Insane intervenes in key discussions about the complexities of Black life and health that cut across literary, historical, and cultural studies, including scholarship on slavery and slave narratives, psychiatry and asylums, and disability studies. Since its emergence as an academic field in the 1980s, disability studies has examined the ways in which society has been built for the able-bodied and, to a lesser extent, the able-minded.[19] In 2006, Christopher Bell challenged the field to confront the centrality of whiteness in its theorists, activists, and objects of study.[20] Bell provided some of the earliest, albeit cursory, disability studies readings of various texts in the Black literary tradition. In the last five years, Sami Schalk, Therí A. Pickens, and La Marr Bruce have published major studies on Blackness and disability, the last two on Blackness and madness specifically.[21] These studies consider Black fiction as objects of study, introduce disability as a mode of analysis, and examine the co-constitutive nature of Blackness and madness. *Colored Insane* offers an analysis of Black literary works and figures that serve as antecedents of twentieth-century Black writers, the focus of previous studies. These works are also largely based on literary sources as objects of analysis. Grounded in historical and cultural accounts of Black Americans' embodied experiences of madness and the material conditions of their mental disability, *Colored Insane* offers a more fleshed out study of the history of Black mental disability, both literally and figuratively.

By and large, studies of slavery and slave narratives have been concerned with the various ways that enslaved people resisted or gained resiliency from the horrors of enslavement. Some classic studies nod to the destructive impact of the "peculiar institution" on mental health but do not pursue it in depth.[22] At the turn of the twenty-first century, historians of slavery, such as Nell Irvin Painter and Deborah Gray White, issued direct calls for more research on the psychological costs of enslavement. Referencing sexual violence committed against Black women in particular, White asserted, "If pursued with the rigor that the subject demands, [it] might well de-center lynching as the primary site and preeminent expression of white (sexual) anxiety on the Black body."[23] Studies emerged that focused on the psychological costs and health consequences of slavery and subsequent time periods such as the Civil War, Reconstruction, and post-Reconstruction, including a focus on disability, suicide, and posttraumatic stress disorder.[24] *Colored Insane* answers White's call and advances discussions about the nature of the peculiar institution by attending to beyond-bodily suffering in slavery. It examines the implications of Harriet Tubman's injuries in slavery and examines psychic wounding in Charles Chesnutt's representations of the 1896 Wilmington massacre and coup and post–Civil War lynching and racial violence. Through its discussion of Harriet Jacobs, *Colored Insane* brings attention to Black women's gendered and raced experiences of mental suffering. The book thus contributes to a fuller accounting of the institution's catalog of injuries, its mechanisms for control, and its lasting effect on the bodyminds of Blacks.

The historical landscape regarding the rise and fall of asylums in the United States is well-trodden scholarly ground.[25] Still, here too *Colored Insane* makes a key intervention. Scholarship over the last two decades on insanity, psychiatry, and asylums has focused not only on the structure of individual asylums but also on the relationship between asylums and the broader culture, the impact of particular national and regional contexts, and issues of race and gender.[26] Although these studies provide insightful analyses of the care of the mentally disabled, they primarily focus on whites, and they detail how slaveholders, physicians, census takers, and legislators espoused the belief that slavery protected against mental disability among Blacks. Several recent studies in the history of psychiatry have taken race as a serious category of analysis, considered the politicization of psychiatric and medical theories, explored Black psychiatric incarceration, and recovered the voices and perspectives of Black mentally disabled people and their families.[27] These studies, mostly historical, are foundational to our understanding of the conditions of institutionalized Black psychiatric treatment, the racist underpinnings of American psychiatric administration and care, and significantly, the role of slavery in the development of American psychiatry. They leave much room, however, for deeper explorations of specific groups, such as Black women, and of Black people's intellectual traditions of theorizing about race and insanity during the expansion of modern psychiatry and fall of the asylum movement. *Colored Insane* is the first study to focus on Black women's experiences in an asylum and, further, the first to examine Black intellectual counter-discourses in earnest.

Colored Insane examines the serious counter-discourses on race, insanity, and mental disability of extraordinary Black figures alongside the experiences of ordinary people with mental disabilities.[28] The book begins with a discussion of medical and psychiatric discourses that were prevalent during the nineteenth century. It explores the various sites at which Black people with mental disabilities were treated, with some consideration of Black healing traditions. It also describes the genesis of proslavery psychiatry. The book then dives into Black counter-discourses through an in-depth analysis of the writings and speeches of James McCune Smith. In this study, Smith emerges as one of the major figures to conceptualize Black bodyminds in the midst of scientific, medical, and psychiatric discourses on mental disability.[29] He also purposely generated images of Black people that were a part of new visions of Blacks as fully knowledgeable about their own bodyminds and capable of creating futures in which they could thrive.

Although Smith's was a formidable medical voice, the narratives of former slaves were much more widely consumed by the general public and contained some of the most vivid representations of the harm Black bodyminds experienced in slavery. Harriet Jacobs's slave narrative was written outside the sphere of medicine yet powerfully challenges the reigning idea that slavery was good for Black people's mental health. After Jacobs, the book turns to the life of another woman who escaped from slavery, Harriet Tubman. Tubman is a key figure for locating counter-discourses to medical and psychiatric understandings of the bodymind. Tubman used the aspects of her life that were deemed "crazy" to benefit herself and those she helped on the Underground Railroad, during the Civil War, in her home, and in her caregiving institution.

Tubman's small-scale efforts to care for the poor, elderly, and those with physical and mental disability stand in stark contrast to Black women who found themselves inside one of the largest mental asylums in the South. Chapter 5 traces the lives of five ordinary women, Viney W., Jane G., Olivia W., Alice M., and Amanda C., whose lives were heavily constrained by psychiatric and cultural ideas about insanity, race, and gender. Although they bore psychiatric diagnostic labels such as "lunatic," the broader context of their lives was ignored. The works of Charles Chesnutt provide a fuller picture of the lives of postbellum Blacks. Beyond contextualizing Black life, he offered alternative visions of Black bodyminds and the future of America. Chesnutt is now seen as a prominent figure in the Black literary canon; however, little work examines the significance of mental disability in his works. A parallel figure to Smith, he also saw himself as intellectually on par with race scientists and medical theorists of the Black bodymind and offered his own pre-eugenicist concept of amalgamation as a solution to the problem of the color line.

Colored Insane troubles the notion that mental disability is taboo or *more* stigmatized in Black communities. It demonstrates that Black people have always thought deeply about mental disability. By centering their voices and stories, this book creates space to consider that Black people were more than the "colored insane." Many were often fully aware of attempts to color them insane. Sometimes they resisted the coloring process, and other times they fell victim to it. Some Black people took the instruments into their own hands and crafted new designs. Others forged their own tools for understanding and tending to mental disabilities. And some of them imagined entirely new worlds in which Black bodyminds were healed and healthy.

1

ANTEBELLUM PSYCHIATRIC AND MEDICAL DISCOURSES ON THE BLACK BODYMIND

This chapter explores the national discourse on Blackness, mental health, and slavery that emerged in the mid-nineteenth-century United States. I contend that proslavery psychiatric and medical discourses pathologized Black bodyminds as innately prone to mental illness, what nineteenth-century psychiatrists called "insanity" or "lunacy." Medicalized proslavery discourses, which had their roots in eighteenth-century scientific-racist conceptions of Black people's supposed inherent mental incapacity and lack of intelligence, also implied that freedom was harmful for Black bodyminds. Going further, psychiatrists and physicians argued that only the institution of slavery protected Blacks from impending mental disorder. Popular discourses about race and Blackness were pulled into the administration of asylums that were seen as the premier sites for treating mental disabilities. Race shaped the poor treatment of the few mentally disabled Blacks who were granted access to asylums and hospital wards and their treatment on plantations. These discourses discursively created the "colored insane," even while institutions like slavery in the South and racial discrimination in the North created the circumstances that were injurious to Black mental and physical health. A product of the cultural worlds in which they emerged, racialized medical discourses reinforced and helped create a social order that relied on human bondage. Especially important in this study of Black mental disability, Black intellectuals, writers, and other figures contended with these ideas throughout the nineteenth century. I begin the chapter with a discussion of the rise of psychiatry and asylums and then examine how discourses about the Black bodymind influenced the early mental healthcare of Blacks. I then consider Black mental disability in light of conceptions about Conjure. I pivot to a discussion of the genesis of proslavery psychiatric discourses, which crystallized around the time of the monumental 1840 census. This was not only the first census in the nation to collect data on mental disability but also medicalized the Black bodymind on a national stage. I end the chapter with a discussion of the overlapping discourses about the Black bodymind in the field of medicine.

At the turn of the nineteenth century, psychiatrists developed a revolutionary model for treating mental disability called the "moral treatment" or "moral therapy," which was practiced with varying degrees of success in a newly invented institution designed meticulously to alleviate mental disorder—the asylum.[1] This psychiatric reform project would be in tatters by the end of the nineteenth century from chronic underfunding and overcrowding, but it began with a spirit of optimism, transforming both how people with mental conditions were seen by society and how they were treated. It represented a movement toward a generally therapeutic institutional environment more than specific practices. Early psychiatrists did not have clear, precise, or universally agreed-upon definitions of insanity.[2] When the field emerged, there were a number of poorly defined and liberally applied terms in use, including "melancholia," "maniac," "madness," "hysteria," "epilepsy," and "dementia," all of which were identified by symptoms such as delusions, hallucinations, involuntary convulsions, violent behaviors, distorted or confused thinking, and suicidal ideation.[3]

Although debates over terminology were never fully resolved, even late into the century, early nineteenth-century psychiatrists shared a new sentiment about the general etiology and curability of mental illness. Supported by the elite and upper classes, they sought to relegate to the past archaic treatments such as exorcism, bleeding, leeching, and confinement of the mentally ill. "Moral," as they understood it, was not synonymous with our contemporary concepts of "good" and "evil" or the process of policing social ethics. Although psychiatrists were interested in shaping culturally acceptable behaviors to some extent, "moral" in this period maps onto what we now see as the social and psychological factors of mental health conditions.

Moral treatment was based on the premise that there was a God-derived order for how humans should behave and live; people with mental disabilities could be cured only if they were returned to that order. The historian Nancy Tomes describes the concept of moral as it was understood by nineteenth-century psychiatrists: "[Moral] encompassed the mind, emotions, and soul, which existed independent of the physical body, yet could be influenced by the manipulation of sensory and emotional impressions. Thus, moral treatment aimed to alleviate the psychological causes of mental disease by radically changing the individual's environment and daily regimen."[4] Moral therapy consisted of regulating people's activities—eating, sleeping, leisure, labor, behavior, and religious practices—to restore their minds. The figure most iconic for ushering in this new approach was the French physician and "alienist" (as turn-of-the-nineteenth-century psychiatrists were also called) Philippe Pinel. He favored eliminating harsh treatments, such as physical restraints, cold baths, purgatives, and emetics. Pinel published widely read textbooks on understanding and curing mental ailments. An English Quaker, William Tuke, did much to perfect the key element of the moral treatment: confinement within institutions designed to promote healing. Tuke famously opened the York retreat in 1796, which was run on the principle that people should be treated kindly, treatments should be gentle, and people should be free to move about airy halls while engaging in desirable activities such as sewing and knitting. The York retreat served as a global model for how institutions for the mentally ill should be run.

Embracing the "moral" model was easier for psychiatrists in the United States, who could build their institutions from scratch, rather than repurposing other hospitals, like those previously dedicated to leprosy. Benjamin Rush, the father of American psychiatry and a signer of the Declaration of Independence, made the first significant contribution to the care of mentally disabled people in the United States. In 1751, Rush succeeded in allocating a separate mental ward for the treatment of the mentally disabled in the famous Pennsylvania Hospital. His *Medical Inquiries and Observations Upon Diseases of the Mind* (1812) was the first US textbook on mental illnesses. It was published in 1812, reprinted through 1835 (five editions), and served as the major textbook in the field for almost fifty years.

The construction of US asylums began slowly, with only a few spaces for the mentally disabled, but it picked up. About seventy asylums had opened by 1875, and by the 1890s, every state in the country had at least one major asylum. Philadelphia Quakers were the first to establish a hospital built solely to implement the moral treatment program in the United States, the Friends Asylum, which opened in 1814. McLean Hospital, built outside Boston by Massachusetts General Hospital, had opened a few years earlier in 1811. Eastern Lunatic Asylum in Virginia, one of the only institutions that accepted Black people (albeit briefly), opened in 1824. By 1830, a few dozen hospitals had been built across the country. In 1840, the Pennsylvania Hospital, led by the revered Thomas Kirkbride, created the architectural and programmatic blueprint for hospitals across the nation, known then as the "Kirkbride Plan." In 1844, a group of thirteen asylum superintendents started the first medical organization in the country (three years before the start of the American Medical Association), the Association of Medical Superintendents of American Institutions for the Insane (AMSAII), which later became the American Psychiatric Association. The *American Journal of Insanity* became the organ of this new body; its first editor, Amariah Brigham, was the superintendent of New York State Asylum in Utica.

Early American psychiatrists devoted considerable energy to constructing and perfecting asylums. These institutions, they agreed, should be located in the rural countryside, away from the supposed mental strain of cities and stressful environments of individuals' family homes. Because the asylum was seen as the most important contributor to curability, every aspect of its building was designed to alleviate insanity—from the structure of buildings, to the superintendent's paternalistic image, to the rigorous enforcement of healthy daily living.

Benjamin Rush, along with physicians, non-medically trained reformers such as Dorothea Dix, and members of the AMSAII, enacted their programs of mental healthcare against the backdrop of American slavery.[5] Most eighteenth-century proslavery advocates argued that slavery was a necessary evil. Yet, after the War of 1812, the country experienced a cotton boom. As a result, thousands of enslaved people were sold into the southern states, and by 1850, 1.8 million Black slaves (of 3.2 million) were picking cotton. The Indian Removal Act, which forcibly removed Indigenous communities from their lands, led to the expansion of slavery, bolstering cotton production. At the same time, in the North, slavery was gradually ending.[6] State-level freedom mandates and fugitive slaves posed particular problems for slavery advocates. Northern laws and free Blacks belied their arguments about Black mental and physical capacity, threatening the viability of the southern economic system. In this cultural climate, national debates about insanity interlaced the institutions of slavery and asylums. Ideas about the "colored insane" justified asylum keepers' approaches to treating Blacks who were labeled "insane" in asylums.[7] Psychiatric ideas in turn legitimized slavery. The social climate was ripe for defenses of slavery; religious, scientific, and legal arguments had already been made—psychiatric discourses were a welcomed newcomer to the struggle over Black bodyminds.

In the first few decades of the nineteenth century, American psychiatrists spilled little ink theorizing about race and insanity. They mostly borrowed their conceptions from ideas about Black people developed through the lens of scientific racism in the nascent field of anthropology, which had its roots in Enlightenment-era concepts of Black mental and physical capacity. Most notably in the American context, this discursive field includes the influential thought of Thomas Jefferson.[8] His remarks in *Notes on the State of Virginia* (1781) fall in line with these ideas about Black cognitive capacity and preparedness for full citizenship. In *Notes*, Jefferson contends that Black Americans were likely inferior to the whites in the endowments both of body and mind." In the same essay, Jefferson supports this argument with infamous claims about the work of Black writers: "Religion indeed [had] produced a Phyllis Whately [sic]; but it could not produce a poet. The compositions published under her name are below the dignity of criticism . . . Ignatius Sancho [had] approached nearer to merit in composition; yet his letters do more honor to the heart than the head."[9] Jefferson's ideas supported arguments for the inherent inferiority of Blacks.[10] Such thinking about Black mental capacity was echoed by anthropologists, craniologists, and phrenologists. It had incredible staying power throughout the nineteenth century as a justification for slavery. It also formed a basis for denying Blacks entry into asylums or subjecting them to segregated care.[11]

REGIMES OF CARE FOR THE "COLORED INSANE" BEFORE EMANCIPATION

Records on the care of Blacks with mental disabilities before emancipation are extremely limited. As I discuss in chapter 4, the end of slavery was the turning point for Black asylum care; after that, institutions across the country opened their doors to Black patients. Before emancipation, however, only a small number of Black Americans were treated in asylums.[12] In 1745, the state of South Carolina passed its first law pertaining to the care of the mentally disabled, resulting from a case in which an enslaver could not afford to care for a "lunatic slave" named Kate who had murdered a child.[13] The state assembly passed an act indicating that each of the colony's parishes was responsible for the management of slaves whose owners were unable to care for them. Ironically, however, the South Carolina Lunatic Asylum, founded in 1821, did not accept Black people until the 1840s; only a few dozen Blacks were admitted before the Civil War.

For state hospitals that accepted slaves, the national trend was the construction of separate, usually unequal, living quarters or wards for the small numbers admitted. This was the case at the Worcester Hospital in Massachusetts, St. Elizabeth's Hospital in Washington, DC, California State Asylum, and most of Ohio's hospitals.[14] Eastern Lunatic Asylum (ELA) in Virginia was an exception because it admitted free Black patients from the start and enslaved people from 1846 to 1854.[15] ELA was run for two decades (1840–1861) by John Minson Galt, a medical school graduate who held proslavery views. Galt advocated for the admission of enslaved Blacks, whom he accepted from both Virginia and neighboring North Carolina. Between 1773 and 1861, roughly 7 percent of the population at the hospital were free Blacks and 3.6 percent were enslaved. Enslaved Blacks were only granted legal access to ELA by an act of the state legislature in 1846, after Galt agreed that it would be the sole institution in the state to accept slaves, whose care would be provided for at the expense of their enslavers.[16]

Some enslaved "colored insane" would enter the hospital as a result of a direct request to superintendents for hospital admission by their owners. One slave master wrote to Galt in 1846 about a nineteen-year-old enslaved woman who became "so much deranged" that he believed the asylum was her only option. Out of desperation, he sent her to the Medical College, but the institution refused to treat cases of mental disability. Still they agreed to hold her temporarily until the slaveholder could make other arrangements. He expressed to Galt that he believed the ELA provided "proper treatment" and could therefore cure her "without much difficulty."[17] He added his thoughts on the cause of her insanity, which aligned with gender-based psychiatric ideas that tied mental disease to the female reproductive system—especially women's menstrual cycles. Her "derangement," he concluded, "no doubt proceeded from an obstruction of the monthly courses," which he claimed had happened on an earlier occasion.[18] But even with broader access, enslaved Blacks were relegated to second-class status because white in-state people had priority in the admission process. The Virginia legislature solidified this racial hierarchy in an 1846 statute: "No insane slave shall be received or retained in said asylum to the exclusion of any insane white person being a resident of the state."[19] To comply with the law, ELA's board of directors expelled all slaves and nonstate whites.

St. Elizabeth's Hospital in Washington DC, one of the few federal hospitals, accepted mentally disabled Black people as early as 1855. Proud of its accommodations for Black people, the board boasted that it was the "first and only" hospital "to provide suitable care of the African when afflicted with insanity."[20] Despite these expressions of benevolence, race still shaped the experiences of Blacks at the hospital. On the one hand, the institution focused on the care and rehabilitation of white mentally disabled people at the expense of Blacks, while on the other, it constructed Black minds as abnormal and racially distinct, a sentiment that cut across time and endured after slavery into the twentieth century. From the field's early days, psychiatry viewed Black people as primitive and childlike and embraced the imperative to transform Black bodyminds into objects of labor, preventing any more thorough theorization about the origins of Black mental disability. Conceptions of race had an adverse effect on the Black patient population, as Martin Summers contends; there was "a great deal of ambiguity, ambivalence, and antipathy when it came to treating mentally ill Black people."[21]

Yet the vast majority of the "colored insane," free or enslaved, did not receive treatment in asylums.[22] If they encountered a man of medicine, it was usually a general practitioner sought out by family members or slave masters. Psychiatrists did not make house calls. They were preoccupied with the maintenance of steadily expanding institutions while facing dwindling financial support from state legislatures and declining numbers of paying people. In most cases, mentally disabled enslaved people were treated on plantations with the goal of a speedy return to work. Furthermore, plantation owners were reluctant to label their enslaved as mentally disabled because it would diminish their sale price on the slave market. The historian Elodie Edwards-Grossi argues that it was not in the best economic interest of planters to pathologize their labor source: "The enslavers did not call upon doctors to treat the madness of enslaved people because they considered the cost too high. This partly explains the absence of any systemic pathologization of Blacks suffering from mental afflictions in the antebellum medical literature."[23] With no incentive to assign the label of insanity to their enslaved population, planters dealt with mental disability when necessary. If a mentally disabled person could contribute in some way to the plantation economy and was not troublesome, planters made use of them to the extent they could. Slaveholders varied in their responses to these situations, ranging from harsh, punitive punishments such as binding and beatings to various degrees of sympathy.[24] If treatment was sought by an enslaver, most often a local doctor was called. Like psychiatrists, physicians held the general belief that mental disability was primarily a result of abnormalities of the brain, possibly brought about by excess excitement.[25] If enslaved people sought out a healer on their own accord to help their loved ones, they turned to African healing practitioners because they saw mental disability as evidence of conjuration.[26]

Institutionalized mentally disabled enslaved people generally experienced segregated and comparatively poor accommodations in asylums. This was in part a function of their being housed in separate structures, reflecting the relationship of asylum practices with broader racial politics and public concern about interracial mixing. Although Galt, for example, was in favor of the unpopular idea of interracial asylums, he conceded the issue of segregated wards and buildings. Both he and Charles Nichols of St. Elizabeth's Hospital believed that separate quarters were in the best interests of white people in the asylum, who were their primary focus. Martin Summers discusses the racial implications of psychiatrists' history of centering the care of white people: "What a history of Saint Elizabeth's reveals is the ways in which the American psychiatric profession engaged in an (often) unarticulated project that conceptualized the white psyche as the norm. This not only meant that the white sufferer of mental illness occupied center stage in the psychiatric profession's consciousness. . . . It also meant that the psychiatric profession's routine manufacturing of racial difference constructed the black psyche as alien and fundamentally abnormal."[27] Although white medical interests and Black othering were the driving forces and outcomes of the practice, segregation was also instituted to maintain peace at the hospital. However, there is some evidence that racial tensions often erupted nonetheless. For example, sometimes whites wandered into Black quarters and assaulted Black people. White people also often looked upon Black people in the same light as servants. As a result, violent racially charged fights occurred at hospitals.

Despite their routine denial of admission, many Blacks, out of care, fear, or desperation, wanted an opportunity for their kin to receive care. In an 1852 article in *Frederick Douglass' Paper*, Douglass considers the case of a Black woman who was denied admittance into the Lunatic Asylum of Indianapolis. He states, "A colored insane person can disturb a whole neighborhood just as well as if he or she were white, saying nothing of their common appeals to humanity."[28] His sentiments could be read as a legitimization of asylums or as implicit antagonism toward Black women. However, his frame of reference was more likely the real psychological costs of enslavement and racial hostilities. Hence, his sentiments probably indicate an effort to ensure that Blacks were granted equal access to psychiatric facilities rather than support for the asylum as a paternalistic or even reconfining institution.[29] The emphasis on justice also appeared in an 1866 article in the *Christian Recorder*, the focus of which was a Black woman who sought admission into Long View Lunatic Asylum but was "refused on the ground that there was no separate ward for her."[30]

There are no verifiable records of the numbers of Blacks with mental disabilities before emancipation.[31] The popular abolitionist T. D. Weld presented figures about disabilities among slaves in *American Slavery as It Is: Testimony of a Thousand Witnesses* (1839). It was a meticulous compilation of the stories of enslaved and formerly enslaved people, alongside accounts of slave owners, regarding the daily conditions of enslaved people across several states and years. Although he admitted the impossibility of estimating the actual numbers, Weld claimed that there were at least 100,000 enslaved people who fit the category of the "old, the worn out, the incurably diseased, maimed and deformed, idiots, feeble infants, [and] incorrigible."[32] Regarding insanity in particular, he was left only to guess at the number of instances, using proportional data from northern states and an 1838 Chatham County Georgia census. Writing before the 1840 census, when, as I will discuss, data on insanity would first be collected on the population at large, Weld conceded that there was no way to know whether insanity was more prevalent among the enslaved. Nevertheless, he argued that, based on slavery's brutality, there probably was more insanity among the enslaved, writing that "the dreadful physical violence to which the slaves are subjected, and the constant sunderings of their tenderest ties, might lead us to suppose that it would be more."[33]

CONJURE CULTURE AND MENTAL DISABILITY

Although some mentally disabled antebellum Blacks were treated by a psychiatrist or physician when they exhibited mental health symptoms, many looked to their own sacred traditions and respected Black healers, such as root workers and Conjure men and women, for insight into the origins of their affliction and relief. Because of their powers to both heal and harm, these individuals were respected and sometimes feared by both Black and white people. In Black sacred epistemes, insanity was the manifestation of supernatural power rather than a signifier of somatic illness alone. Antebellum Conjure doctors believed that addressing supernatural problems with solely natural means was futile. Conjure doctors had an alternative set of assumptions and epistemological orientations that had explicit conceptualizations about mental disability. The historian of medicine Sharla Fett explains that, in contrast to white medical doctors, Black people had a relational vision of health that tied an individual's illness to conflicts in communal relationships and encounters within the "enchanted universe."[34] Although Conjure is most often associated with Black religious practice, especially sorcery, witchcraft, or occultism, it played a dominant role in the medical treatment of physical and mental ailments. Emphasizing the integral role of healing in Black religious cultures, Theophus Smith argues that Conjure culture encompassed a "pharmacopeic tradition of practices." By this, Smith means that Conjure men and women were seen as experts or "doctors" in folk pharmaceutical medicines, mostly in the form of plants, roots, herbs, and charms, but also via spells and spiritual intercession. Conjure doctors used many of the same skills and sources of knowledge as other healers who specialized in the "doctoring arts," such as midwives, root workers, and herbalists.[35] Significantly, and distinct from psychiatric explanations for the etiology of disease that tried to bracket religion and spirituality, Conjure doctors believed that the "magical" or "supernatural" was germane to irregularities or disturbances appearing in the "natural" body.[36]

Many Black Americans maintained that encounters with natural entities that had significant power in the spiritual world could have grave consequences for an individual's mental health. One such creature that was imbued with spiritual power was the moonack. Moonacks lurked in the forests and could be found in hollow trees or caves. If an unsuspecting person came across the mythical animal, believers held that they were "doomed," destined for psychological impairment or illness. After encountering the moonack, a person's "reason [is] impaired until he becomes a madman, or is carried off by some lingering malady." Encountering this animal was particularly dire because there was no known cure for the impending insanity, nor any identifiable method of preventing death. Even if someone tried to conceal the encounter, their fate was sealed: "Old-knowing negroes [would] shake their heads despondingly and say, 'He's gwine to die: he's seed de moonack.'"[37]

Although nothing could be done for a person who encountered a moonack, Conjure doctors did have methods for treating insanity when the source was interpersonal social conflict. Indeed, many Black people thought signs of insanity were indications that a person had been "conjured," "tricked," or "fixed" by another member of the community. A range of methods could be the origin of Conjure—from the manipulation of inanimate objects, such as dolls, to being "poisoned" by something they consumed or contaminated by a substance, such as a powder they touched. The former bondsman Fred Jones remarked, "Wenebuh a pusson go crazy, wut is dat but cunjuh?"[38] His rhetorical question reflected the widespread assumption that in the case of a sickness, especially regarding mental health, Conjure was a prime suspect. Conjure was often seen as the culprit in unexplained disease or when someone did not respond to medical treatment. Thus, Conjure was seen as both a possible cause of mental disability and a possible cure. One Black woman, who had convulsions, abdominal pain, and unexplained swelling of the stomach long after the birth of her second child, believed that she was "bewitched" because no medicine from mainstream doctors helped her.[39] Although she was able to work for decades with the condition, she was never cured and died suddenly of convulsions at the age of sixty.

A range of afflictions would alert a family member that Conjure could be behind changes in their relative's changed mental or emotional state, including "mental confusion, impeded judgment, and outright insanity."[40] Robert Pinckney remembered that a spell was the cause of his brother's change in mental state and eventual death: "Muh own brudduh wuz conjuhed. He hab a spell put on um. He hab fits all duh time—hydrophobical fits—act lak he crazy."[41] Because they believed Conjure was the culprit in many cases of insanity, family members often turned to Conjure doctors to help their loved ones. Much to the chagrin of his sister's slave master, who thought him "an internal fool" for seeking out a Conjure doctor, Free Billy procured the services of Old Sancho to help cure his "deranged" sister Nancy, who had been sick for two years and "[would] not speak to anyone."[42] Like other Black people, Free Billy believed that Conjure doctors' spiritual intercession was necessary to prevent permanent insanity or death.[43] As one Conjure doctor in North Carolina warned, without intervention the conjured person "either goes crazy or dies."[44]

Similar to asylum superintendents, Conjure doctors approached mental disability with both direct and indirect treatments. Superintendents in asylums used a range of practices to combat mental disability that included immediate attention to symptoms such as restraints, bleeding, or cold baths and indirect approaches that regulated behavior and environment. Conjure doctors also had indirect approaches, but their guiding philosophy on the origin of disease made for very different treatment methods than those of white doctors and psychiatrists. Conjure doctors would not seek to treat the symptoms of insanity directly. Rather, they would identify the source of the problem in the spiritual realm. They first had to pinpoint the source of the conflict, then determine if they were powerful enough to counter the magic at work, and finally decide whether there would be some form of retaliation.[45] Once these factors were established, Conjure doctors would initiate their dual powers of healing and harming on behalf of the individual.

Although many Black people put a great deal of faith in Conjure doctors to cure insanity, physicians and psychiatrists were skeptical at best and dismissive at worst, both of the belief in Conjure and of the related practices of Black doctoring arts. In addition to inventing drapetomania, the runaway slave disease, as I discuss later, Samuel Cartwright made broad arguments about disease among Black people. He was aware of the common belief that sickness was a sign of spiritual power for many in the Black community and saw this belief as the true sickness. He claims, "The patients themselves believe that they are poisoned; they are right, but it is not the body, but the mind that is poisoned."[46] Cartwright saw these beliefs as deadly, arguing that Black people needed to be treated in light of such "ethnological peculiarities" or death was the sure outcome.[47] He argued that the belief in Conjure was so powerful that enslaved people who thought they were conjured often died without showing any signs of physical illness.[48]

Cartwright was not alone in this assumption about the perceived superstitious nature of Black people. Dr. W. S. Forwood wrote in the widely circulated, proslavery southern magazine *De Bow's Review* that because a delusional belief in witches, sorcerers, and spells so dominated Black peoples' "imagination," doctors should play into the idea that they were combating the "evil influence" to cure people.[49] Dr. A. P. Merrill claimed that Black people's belief in the supernatural and divine providence in matters of health generally predisposed them to sickness because it tended to "depress their vital energies."[50] White skepticism endured well after the Civil War. For example, Dr. Ambrose McCoy argued in the *Louisville Medical News* journal that the belief that one has been conjured was an "imaginary affection" that existed extensively among Blacks in the South, who he believed were the "most ignorant and most superstitious of all mankind."[51]

THE NEXUS OF SCIENTIFIC RACISM AND PROSLAVERY PSYCHIATRY

Black experiences of mental disability were also shaped by national cultural discourses on race and insanity, which I argue constituted "proslavery psychiatry." This is neither language used at the time nor a term used in extant scholarship, but I marshal it to categorize the dominant nineteenth-century national discourse on mental disability. Proslavery psychiatry arguments comprised two separate yet cross-fertilizing spheres of thought that coalesced around the 1840 census.[52] One sphere included mainstream psychiatrists, superintendents, and asylum reformers who did not have a proslavery agenda but sometimes inadvertently reinforced proslavery discourses; this group included Dorothea Dix, Samuel Woodward, Edward Jarvis, Isaac Ray, Amariah Brigham, and John Minson Galt. The second sphere was composed of psychiatrists, politicians, and physicians who used explicit proslavery arguments in their contributions to mainstream discourses about insanity, including Cartwright, George Fitzhugh, C. B. Hayden, and Secretary of State John Calhoun. The unifying idea of proslavery psychiatry writ large was that insanity was more prevalent among Blacks in the North than Blacks in the South because Blacks were physiologically and intellectually suited for the conditions of slavery.

Political and medical actors went to great lengths to compare free and enslaved people. Both groups drew upon the 1840 census to make claims that Black bodyminds had distinct features that made them prone to insanity. Because the 1840 census was the first to collect data concerning the incidence of mental disability in the United States, it launched Black mental disability as a national concern and point of political contestation, thus spurring the first serious consideration of race and mental disability nationally and even globally.[53]

According to the census's findings, the total number of those reported to be "insane and feeble-minded" in the United States was more than 17,000, of whom nearly 3,000 were Black. The ratio of insanity among northern whites was 1:995. For southern whites, the ratio was 1:945. There were 2.7 million Blacks in the South, of whom 1,734 were reported to be "insane or retarded," a ratio of 1:1,558. But in the free states, about 1,200 Blacks out of 171,894 were reported to be "insane or retarded," a ratio of 1:144.[54] The figures, if accurate, indicate that the incidence of mental disability was eleven times higher among free Blacks than among Blacks in the South and six times higher than among whites. The census did not distinguish between free and enslaved Blacks in the South.

Edward Jarvis, a nineteenth-century physician and social statistician, refuted these findings because he discovered significant errors in the 1840 census figures. For example, he showed that there were more instances of insanity among whites than were reported. There were also major tabulation errors. He also noticed, for example, that 133 Black insane paupers were purported to live in Worcester, Massachusetts, even though the total Black population was listed as 151. Notwithstanding the fact that the accuracy of the census findings was contested within two years of their release, proslavery activists and medical doctors seized on them to comment on the relationship between slavery and mental disability.[55] The implications of the study were grave for Black Americans. As Sander Gilman explains, "The anti-abolitionist forces were thus provided with major scientific evidence that blacks were congenitally unfit for freedom." These census data, as well as data from later censuses, fueled claims about race and insanity into the late nineteenth and early twentieth centuries.[56]

Mainstream psychiatrists and asylum reformers used the faulty census results to support, sometimes inadvertently, proslavery claims and aims. In part, they relied on the census because they were following the trend in the developing field of medicine, which favored quantitative methodologies for determining the individual and social causes of disease.[57] Midcentury psychiatrists, who numbered only a couple dozen asylum doctors, worked from the premise that human beings were governed by immutable principles for healthy living such as good hygiene and diet. They believed that these laws, like the scientific laws of gravity, offered guidelines for healthy social behavior. If they were violated, mental disability could result. Midcentury psychiatrists also believed mental instability could emerge from situational causes, such as financial troubles or bereavement. A person could become mentally disabled as a result of physical abnormalities in the brain as well. Thus, treatment for mental disability included drugs, tonics, bleeding, and laxatives, but such measures were coupled with moral therapies.[58] Their environmental arguments were accompanied by the unchallenged pre–Civil War contention that mental disability, although somatic in some cases, ultimately had its roots in the accelerated course of civilization or an unhealthy social order.[59]

When Jarvis called attention to the technical errors in the collection of the census data, he also forwarded his own analysis on race and insanity. In his 1842 article, "Statistics of Insanity in the United States," Jarvis argued that the higher incidence of insanity among free Blacks in general was unsurprising.[60] However, his claims differed from those of proslavery advocates.[61] Jarvis's ideas about Blacks were connected to his general thoughts about mental disability. He attributed the higher rates of mental disability in the North to southern enslaved Blacks' supposedly lower "state of civilization." He held that higher states of civilization generated greater mental activity and, therefore, more opportunities for derangement. Furthermore, Jarvis believed that free Blacks had more instances of mental disability because they occupied a "false social position" in the North.[62]

Jarvis's conclusions about civilization were representative of one key thread of mainstream global psychiatric thought during the period. Prominent mental health reformer Dorothea Dix and asylum superintendents Woodward and Galt, among others, believed the United States to be an ideal case for observing the increase in insanity that accompanied the increasing pressures of an advancing civilization.[63] For them, this was most likely a result of the dominance of Jacksonian democracy, characterized by the expansion of big business and commercial enterprise.[64] Psychiatrists surmised that Jacksonian democracy promoted more financial, and therefore mental, instability in the lives of ordinary people. They also believed that industrialization, revolution, immigration, democratization, and urbanization heightened access to social vices and stimulated greater intellectual activity—what we now might call "stressors"—which were mentally destabilizing.[65] The supposed link between mental disability and civilization appeared in Dix's claim that there were "comparatively very few" instances of mental disability in the southern states, which were populated mostly by "Blacks and Indians."[66]

Although most nineteenth-century psychiatrists thought that mental disability in the entire population was linked to the progression of civilization, they relied on racial doctrines to explain certain results of the 1840 US census. Dix and others essentially blended their mainstream psychiatric thought with mainstream American racial attitudes, thus reinforcing proslavery claims. For example, Galt reasoned that the higher rates of insanity among Blacks were "perhaps owing not only to the less degree of mental cultivation, but much also to the absence of all cares for the future, the great depressing influence with the whites."[67] Galt's perspective represented the general consensus among superintendents of asylums throughout the country. When it came to the institutionalized care of the Black mentally disabled, psychiatrists drew more on social and cultural constructions of race entrenched in the American practice of slavery than on any kind of empirical scientific research.[68]

The statistical census data collected on the occurrence of mental disability in Blacks had particular significance for slavery apologists and the abolitionist struggle. A vocal advocate of slavery, Calhoun seized the opportunity to use the statistics.[69] Writing to the British ambassador, Calhoun contends: "The census and other authentic documents show that, in all instances in which the States have changed the former relation between the two races, the condition of the African, instead of being improved, has become worse. They have invariably sunk into vice and pauperism, accompanied by the bodily and mental afflictions incident thereto—deafness, blindness, insanity, and idiocy—to a degree without example; while, in all other States which have retained the ancient relation between them, they have improved greatly in every respect—in number, comfort, intelligence, and morals."[70] Calhoun's assertions about the suitability of Blacks to slavery and the census findings legitimized medical claims about Blackness and madness. Calhoun's use of statistical data represented a trend by southern whites to defend the institution of slavery using "naturalists, physicians, and preachers."[71] Adding to this arsenal, C. B. Hayden's interpretation of the census data supported the correlation between freedom and mental disability.[72] In his 1844 article, "On the Distribution of Insanity in the United States," he explains the higher rates of mental disability among Blacks in free states: "[In] the non-slave-holding states, the blacks are in a condition of social helotage, constituting the pauper caste and the heirs of all the ills which poverty entails upon its subjects. The negro of the South, on the contrary, cares not for the morrow, well knowing, that another will provide what he shall eat, what he shall drink, and wherewithal he shall be clothed; his simple mode of life secures him health, and in the winter of life he crowns 'a youth of labor, with an age of ease.'"[73]

After the release of the census, Jarvis called for more research on the census and on possible correlations between race and mental disability. His call was answered by an editorial in the *Southern Literary Messenger* in 1843 entitled "Reflections on the Census of 1840." In it, the editors argued that Black mental disability increased according to a Black person's time in freedom, associated mental disability with northern exposure to "vicious habits" and "uncontrolled passions," and warned against interracial marriage (because it supposedly caused the onset of disease and premature death). The Black community was outraged by these sentiments; Black leaders held public gatherings to address the claims.[74] Physician James McCune Smith wrote his own response denouncing the commentary, "Freedom and Slavery for Afric-Americans (1844)," which I discuss in chapter 2. This article was part of his robust response to scientific and medical notions of Black mental disability.

A decade after the census, the discussion of mental disability and Blackness that it sparked continued to fuel proslavery debates, which were glaringly evident in the works, professional endeavors, and personal associations of the American physician and proslavery advocate Cartwright.[75] In his 1851 "Report on the Diseases and Physical Peculiarities of the Negro Race," Cartwright drew on the census results and the research they generated to make claims about mental disability among Black Americans. With this article, he joins the chorus of proponents of southern slavery: "The laws of his nature, are in perfect unison with slavery, and in entire discordance with liberty. . . . [Slavery improves Blacks] in body, mind and morals. . . . [Liberty is] not only unsuitable to the negro race, but actually poisonous to its happiness."[76] Cartwright's article warrants attention because many of its themes and arguments had implications beyond slavery.[77] Remnants of his stance on Black mental disability and freedom and the supposedly mentally protective aspects of slavery resurface in the perspectives of psychiatrists, including T. O. Powell, the superintendent of Georgia Lunatic Asylum, which I discuss in chapter 5.

Cartwright's "Report" presents the results of an investigation he conducted with three other doctors concerning the distinct diseases and physical conditions of Black Americans, work he hoped would contribute to the growing body of research on what was called the "science and mental progress" of southern Blacks.[78] It insisted that the differences in disease between whites and Blacks were rooted in the "deep, durable and indelible" anatomical and physiological distinctions between the races. Cartwright posited that the origins of mental disability in Blacks were not located in the social or cultural world but rather were inherent in the body. Moreover, he attributed the differences between Blacks and whites to "unalterable physiological laws." Like Thomas Jefferson, Cartwright compared Blacks to apes, saying that they shared a smaller "field of vision," which allowed them to "exclud[e] the sun's rays." Also like the statesman, the doctor contended that this distinction could be observed in Black cultural life; when considering music, for example, Cartwright contended that they had "melody, but no harmony."[79]

Cartwright further claimed that an irregularity in Black peoples' brains had halted the development of their civilization on the African continent. This stunted development, he argued, effectively makes "the people of Africa unable to take care of themselves."[80] Here Cartwright and other like-minded slavery advocates diverged from mainstream psychiatry, which viewed the "primitive civilization" of Africans as favorable for mental health.[81] Cartwright's frame of reference on the matter was older scientific-racist discourses, not mainstream psychiatry, which explains why he concluded that, if left alone, American Blacks were naturally inclined to return to a backward and barbaric state. These "unalterable physiological laws," according to Cartwright, were responsible for the "mental debasement" in Black Americans that made them unfit for liberty.[82]

In Cartwright's formulation, slavery was not only more suitable than freedom for Blacks but also a necessary form of treatment for their mental debasement. As he contends, forced labor and exercise have the effect of "vitalizing the blood more perfectly than is done when they [Blacks] are left free to indulge in idleness." Cartwright's discussion of idleness supported his claim that physiologically and anatomically, Blacks revealed that they were not only like apes but also like white children. He advises on the best course of action given this conclusion: "Like children, they require government in every thing; food, clothing, exercise, sleep—all require to be prescribed by rule, or they will run into excesses."[83] Cartwright's comparison of slaves to children is of particular interest to historians of psychiatry. Scholars have noted that mentally disabled people were also treated like children in need of constant instruction. Like slaves, the mentally disabled had no right to property (including themselves). Although this comparison between the mentally disabled and the slave is partially accurate, it is also problematic because unlike children or "lunatics," slaves were not given the opportunity to grow up or be cured. The vehement slavery apologist George Fitzhugh unwittingly makes this clear in his paternalistic proslavery tract:

> Children cannot be governed by mere law; first, because they do not understand it, and secondly because they are so much under the influence

of impulse, passion and appetite, that they want sufficient self-control to be deterred or governed by the distant and doubtful penalties of the law. They must be constantly controlled by parents or guardians, whose will and orders shall stand in the place of law for them. Very wicked men must be put into penitentiaries; lunatics into asylums, and the most wild of them into straight jackets [sic], just as the most wicked of the sane are manacled with irons; and idiots must have committees to govern and take care of them. Now, it is clear the Athenian democracy would not suit a negro nation, nor will the government of mere law suffice for the individual negro. He is but a grown up child, and must be governed as a child, not as a lunatic or criminal.[84]

Fitzhugh's statement reflects the reigning ideology among slavery advocates that Black inferiority was immutable and therefore should govern every aspect of their lives. His statement rejects the possible overlap between the slave and the mentally disabled. In other words, he did not—perhaps could not—imagine a mentally disabled enslaved person.

At the behest of his peers, Cartwright became keenly interested in the occurrence of mental disability among slaves. Cartwright presented two diseases in particular that relate specifically to the mental health of Blacks—"drapetomania" and "dysaesthesia aethiopis." He argued that drapetomania was a mental disease that caused slaves to run away. This illness, which caused Blacks to "abscond from service," as Cartwright described it, was preventable and curable.[85] He claimed that most incidences of mental disability appeared when masters treated their slaves either as equals or too cruelly. In his formulation, the disease could be prevented by whites ensuring that Blacks remained in a proper position of submission to whites. He contended that when slaves were not in awe of their masters, they became "rude and ungovernable and [would] run away."[86] He posited that Blacks could also be prevented from running away if whites refrained from abusing their God-given right to govern Blacks by being neglectful and condescending. Instead, he argued, whites should provide for all their slaves' needs and be kind, protective, and gracious toward them.

Like drapetomania, Cartwright argued that dysaesthesia aethiopis was a mental disability specific to Blacks but that it manifested differently in slaves than in free Blacks.[87] He described the disease as different from all other mental diseases because it appeared physically on the body as skin lesions that are "thick and harsh to the touch." Unlike drapetomania, he contended, dysaesthesia aethiopis was not particular to slaves but rather "more prevalent among free negroes living in clusters by themselves." He thought that enslaved Blacks only showed evidence of the disease when they lived as "free negroes" with control over their own "diet, drink, [and] exercise"; he further surmised that most free Blacks, all of whom lacked white guardianship, had the disease. He reasoned that the afflicted were "apt to do much mischief" but not intentionally. Their supposed mischief was primarily caused by "stupidity of mind and insensibility of the nerves" and "idleness," which he linked to lung function, blood deterioration, unclean skin, and an inactive liver, among other things. He noted that in the case of blood illnesses, Blacks were not unique. Cartwright considered blood deterioration a major contributing factor to contraction of disease for all races: "That the blood, when rendered impure and carbonaceous from any cause, as from idleness, filthy habits, unwholesome food or alcoholic drinks, affects the mind, is not only known to physicians, but was known to the Bard of Avon when he penned the lines—'We are not ourselves when Nature, being oppressed, commands the mind to suffer with the body.' "[88] Of course, the latter portion of the quote is compelling because it suggests that prolific literary writers had special insights about the nature of mental and bodily suffering. Their insights, he believed, could support or even stand in for scientific inquiry. Cartwright's use of Shakespeare was akin to asylum superintendents looking to literature for inspiration and scientific theories.[89]

The use of Shakespeare was not the only aspect that linked Cartwright to asylum superintendents. Cartwright's disease categories offer an example of the intersection between polemics and medicine. These ideas about Black insanity continued to have traction after slavery ended. As historian Herbert Gutman contends, "Neither the Civil War nor the Thirteenth Amendment emancipated northern whites from ideological currents that assigned inferior status to nineteenth-century blacks, women, and working-class men."[90] How Black people were defined after slavery continued to be informed by racialized psychiatric thought. Whites' ideas about Black women in particular also relied on slavery-era stereotypes about Black femininity.⁹¹ As I show in the second half of this book, these ideas reverberated into postemancipation asylums in light of the changing economic, political, and cultural developments and interests that animated the period.⁹²

MEDICAL PERSPECTIVES ON MENTAL DISABILITY

Physicians, some of whom were also slaveholders, also had race-based theories about Black bodyminds. Even before contestations over slavery in the US context, physicians were assigning meaning to Blackness, as Rana Hogarth writes: "The racial idioms that [physicians] deployed in their discussions of black people's bodies formed the corpus of medical knowledge that buttressed their credibility among other practitioners, planters, medical officers, and the lay public." Their meaning making was applied to both physical and mental disease.⁹³ Furthermore physicians' ideas were in step with the psychiatric beliefs about Black people's propensity for mental disability and the conjecture that freedom was especially injurious to Black mental health. The fields of both medicine and psychiatry engaged in what Ellen Samuels calls "bio-certification." By this, Samuels means that nineteenth-century institutions of medicine, science, and psychiatry used their medical training, population statistics, journal articles, case studies, conferences, and public publications to tie constructions of normalcy, which existed simultaneously along racial, gender, and disability lines, to objective science. These fields produced "fantasies of identification" that saw social identities as "fixed, legible, and categorizable."⁹⁴ As joint participants in the project of creating social identities, medicine and psychiatry shared similar beliefs about the body and health. For example, nineteenth-century physicians shared with psychiatrists basic assumptions about the somatic origins of mental disease and the role of heredity in its manifestation. Generally, the medical field's conceptualizations about mental health posed few serious challenges to psychiatric beliefs about the etiology of mental disability; most often, they amplified them.

Most physicians believed that mental disabilities arose from somatic causes such as malfunctions in the nervous system or physical problems in the brain. Physicians sometimes used the term "brain disease" to describe mental health conditions. The physician W. Camp explained that "insanity is far more a bodily disease than has hitherto been considered; and in cases of this malady there is mostly, if not always, impairment of the proper healthy cerebral structure."[95] Physicians also believed heredity played a role in a person's predisposition to insanity. When discussing the case of a white woman who was said to have endured "frequent hysterical attacks," James Green speculated about whether her condition had been passed down: "All the female members of this lady's family have been troubled in a similar way."[96] Physicians' materialist explanations for mental disability led to their pursuit of "heroic medicine" solutions over "moral therapy." Physicians did not see the orderly environment and kind treatment in asylums as harmful but believed such measures were no replacement for strong narcotics, purges, blistering, and bloodletting, even if their treatments yielded no better results. Despite this significant difference in treatment modalities, psychiatrists' and physicians' logics about mental disability among the "colored insane" converged.

Physicians were not only aware that there was a tie between the body and the mind but also eager to understand how race, gender, and geographic location, such as the South, informed the nature of the connection. As the historians Marli Weiner and Mazie Hough put it, physicians and laypeople alike "were intent on understanding the ways in which body influenced mind and mind influenced body. . . . Only by examining their patients' bodies and their minds in the context of their race, sex, and place could physicians hope to cure their ills."[97] When it came to Black bodyminds, southern physicians started from the assumption of anatomical distinctions between Blacks and whites.

Racist presuppositions meant that physicians' references to Black bodies always already referred to Black people's entire physiological constitution, which they took for granted as being composed of the body and mind, even if they sometimes separated "mind" and "body." Mid-nineteenth-century physicians' use of terminology that separates the Black body and mind is a rhetorical display of the seriousness with which they took mental health concerns. The mind included both specific mental health ailments that emerged such as insanity and Black people's general cognitive capacity or intellectual aptitude. Discourses about the interconnection between mental and physical characteristics of Black bodyminds surfaced in an essay by the physician A. P. Merrill entitled "An Essay on Some of the Distinctive Peculiarities of the Negro Race."[98] Merrill referenced debates in the fields of science and ethnology about the evolution of the human species and the origins of various racial groups.[99] He presented the field of medicine as outside the debate, agreeing only about supposed undeniable "facts." Chief among the "facts" that Merrill and other southern physicians embraced was the existence of "physical and mental peculiarities, which are found to differ in different races."[100]

Psychiatrists also relied on arguments about Black anatomical differences. In 1839, Amariah Brigham, the first editor of the *American Journal of Insanity* and founding member of the first professional organization of psychiatrists, interviewed members of *La Amistad* slave ship rebellion who visited a Connecticut mental asylum.[101] The rebellion's leader Joseph Cinqué remarked that he had only seen one case of insanity akin to those in the Hartford asylum.[102] This confirmed Brigham's widely held psychiatric belief that less civilized people, including Indigenous Americans, were less prone to mental illness. This presupposition made Brigham less apt to challenge the belief that slavery protected Blacks from the mental stressors of living in civilized American society. As did many others at the time, he accepted the race-science claim that Black bodyminds were fundamentally different at the anatomical level. A year after interviewing Cinqué, Brigham took up race scientists' obsession with collecting and analyzing cranial measurements. Using his small collection of statistical data, he "confirmed" the popular belief that the "negro brain," like that of the "idiot" with "low mental powers," was smaller than that of whites. He reasoned that Black brains were smaller because, unlike Europeans, Black people had not had centuries of exposure to "a greater amount of mental culture" and thus had not continued to grow or develop.[103]

Yet, although psychiatrists borrowed the inclinations of race scientists, their beliefs did not translate into race-specific mental health treatments.[104] For physicians like Merrill, however, the mental and physical differences of Black Americans did have therapeutic implications. As Merrill explains, the "negro constitution" warranted specific "habits of life in health" and different "remedial measures in sickness." Among the necessary race-based therapeutics were, he argued, certain climatic and dietary needs. Southern climates, he held, were better than northern ones for Black people in the United States. To offset the deleterious effects of the cold in areas closer to the North, he counseled giving Black people oily diets that could be derived from the "fattest pork." Failing to tend to these peculiarities, Merrill argues, would be disastrous for enslaved Black people's productivity as laborers and their mental and physical health, longevity, and vitality: "Without a full abundance of [an oily diet], the negro not only cannot become an effective laborer in cold climates, but must necessarily suffer in his bodily and mental health, become short-lived, imbecile, and unprolific."[105] Merrill's discussion of enslaved people's diet makes clear the fact that their health was not just a practical matter of disease management but also an economic consideration. Medical discourses provided justifications for the capitalist enterprise of enslaving millions of Black people. Merrill's environmental argument about the protective nature of slavery for Black mental health exemplifies this twofold nature of medical discourses.

Physicians aligned with psychiatrists in the belief that there was a strong correlation between an individual's engagement in social vices and health conditions. Although gambling and illicit sex were viewed very negatively, one of the prime social vices that medical professionals warned against was alcohol abuse. The founding of the American Temperance Union in 1826 reflected an intense national push to curtail drinking in the general population—it was taken up vigorously by the men of medicine. Where this danger is concerned, Merrill celebrates that enslaved Blacks are saved from the health risks associated with pathological drinking because of slavery: "Drunkenness, therefore, is a vice which is almost unknown among slaves; and it is, perhaps as much due to the restraints imposed upon them in this respect . . . that their lives and the vigor of their bodily and mental constitutions, are so well preserved."[106] Psychiatrists were also intensely focused on the negative effects of excessive drinking on mental health, and their institutions were critical to the social response to the issue. The venerable Samuel Woodward, superintendent of the Worcester State Hospital in Massachusetts, saw a parallel between insanity and alcohol abuse. He argued that both had somatic etiologies that resulted in behaviors and inclinations outside of an individual's will or control. Woodward joined Philadelphia physicians and temperance advocates to open institutions specifically for treating "inebriates." No boom in inebriate institutions materialized, but asylum superintendents reported that the rising cases of mental disability caused by intemperance were met with varying degrees of success in treatment.[107]

Merrill's discussion of the relationship of enslaved people to alcohol is crucial to understanding the aim of his essay as a whole. The threat to enslaved people exposed to alcoholic drinks is not just that they might be subject to insanity, Merrill maintains, but that it also precludes their ability to develop intellectually and morally. In sum, alcohol would lead eventually to racial extinction: "Were the slaves of the southern states to be emancipated upon the grounds they now occupy, and permitted to indulge without restraint in the use of alcoholic drinks, all hope of such [intellectual and moral] improvement in the race, in our country, would at once be at an end; and, instead . . . there would undoubtedly be a rapid diminution of them, until extinction, as with some of the Indian tribes."[108] Even though he pushes aside race-science arguments at the outset of his article about the development of racial groups, he returns to them in his suggestion that slavery is important for the evolution of Black people. Without the supposedly sanitizing effect of slavery, he reasons, Black people as a race would die off.

Although he makes much of the connections between slavery and Black health, there remains an open question in Merrill's article: If the institution of slavery is so protective for Black bodyminds and their offspring, how does slavery affect the health of white enslavers? He acknowledges that slavery as an institution is rife with what he called "egregious abuses." "It must not be denied," he writes, "that it is a system which leads to egregious abuses. Of these we are not the apologist. To his own master let every slaveholder render up his account."[109] Merrill suggested that unnamed wrongs committed by slave owners evoked in them uneasiness on a deeper, perhaps spiritual level about the justness of chattel slavery. The mental health implications of carrying out violence against enslaved people was equally unacknowledged in the field of psychiatry. Benjamin Rush wrote that derangement was characterized by "every departure of the mind in its perceptions, judgments, and reasonings, from its natural and habitual order; accompanied with corresponding actions."[110] Even Rush's antislavery commitments did not cause him to consider how his conceptualization of mental disease was complicated when the natural social order in which one existed could be defined as deranged.[111] For Merrill, with his deep investment in the idea that slavery is a source of "improvement" and "elevation" for enslaved people, it is unimaginable that the system's "egregious abuses" might be hazardous to Black people's health.

Medicalized ideas about the Black bodymind did not go unchallenged. In the next chapter, I discuss a Black intellectual response from James McCune Smith. One of the most educated men of his time, white or Black, Smith used his elite medical training and intellectual prowess to treat Blacks with mental and physical disabilities, combat proslavery discourses, and carve out space for a complex, vibrant, and flourishing Black bodymind.

2

MENTAL DISABILITY AND THE INTELLECTUAL THOUGHT OF JAMES McCUNE SMITH

Throughout the civilized world, the statement has gone forward, that . . . slavery is more than tenfold more favorable to mental health than freedom.

—EDWARD JARVIS, "INSANITY AMONG THE COLORED POPULATION OF THE FREE STATES" (1844)

It is a prevalent opinion that emancipation has made the free blacks deaf, dumb, blind, idiots, insane. . . . Freedom has not made us mad; it has strengthened our minds by throwing us upon our own resources and has bound us to American institutions with a tenacity which nothing but death can overcome.

—JAMES McCUNE SMITH, "FREEDOM AND SLAVERY FOR AFRIC-AMERICANS" (1844)

The sixth US census, taken in 1840, once again brought the issue of slavery to the forefront.[1] In the United States, as across Europe, there was growing national sentiment for using social statistics not just for legislative purposes but also to understand social problems. Scientists and physicians began to favor quantitative measures to ascertain what they believed to be the divine order of nature, the individual, and society—particularly as it concerned sickness and disease. Several new categories appeared on the 1840 census, providing information on literacy rates, educational institutions, and, most relevant for this book, "insane and mentally retarded" people under state-funded care. These statistics about the occurrence of mental disability, which psychiatrists in the nineteenth century called "insanity," were collected along racial lines.[2] The census discovered that there were more Black individuals deemed "insane" in the North than the South. This conclusion spurred a debate about Black people's physical and mental capacity that extended well into the twentieth century.[3]

Although the veracity of the census findings would be challenged within two years of their release, both proslavery activists and medical doctors seized this moment to theorize about the relationship between slavery and insanity among Black Americans.[4] They concluded that slavery protected Blacks against mental disability.[5]

This argument was made dozens of times in several popular newspapers and medical journals in the United States and was republished throughout Europe. Drawing on his own training in medicine and science, James McCune Smith, a Black intellectual, was uniquely qualified to refute the false correlation between Black freedom and insanity.

The struggle over the parameters of mental disability among Blacks in the wake of the 1840 census compelled Smith to intervene. He wrote several articles, beginning with an essay in the *New York Tribune* titled "Freedom and Slavery for Afric-Americans" (1844) that was later reprinted in *The Liberator* and the *National Anti-Slavery Standard*, both auxiliaries of the American Anti-Slavery Society. The article's only header, "Vital Statistics," aligns with his priority: to dispute the statistical facts concerning Black mental capacity. To make his case, Smith references an article by the Harvard-educated social statistician and physician Edward Jarvis, published one month before, in which Jarvis debunks the accuracy of the census data. To bolster Jarvis's claims, Smith includes a numerical chart from the 1840 census, which enumerates the "total inhabitants" and "coloured insane" in Maine. The chart shows that there were more Black people counted as insane than there were Black residents within the locality—nineteen and one, respectively. After a tongue-in-cheek dismissal of the figures—"To make 19 crazy men out of one man, is pretty fair calculation even for 'down east'"—Smith takes direct aim at physicians' and politicians' claim that freedom caused insanity among Blacks. "Freedom has not made us mad," he proclaims, "it has strengthened our minds by throwing us upon our own resources, and has bound us to American institutions with a tenacity which nothing but death can overcome."[6] His assertion undercuts the organizing logic that the risk of insanity increases among Blacks precisely because they live in the North, free from the constraints of slavery. Smith's study went to the heart of this recurrent theme in scientific, medical, and psychiatric writings about Black mental and physical health in the nineteenth century.

Chapter 1 discussed ideas about the "colored insane" and how they manifested in various spaces of confinement in which psychiatrists treated enslaved Blacks with real or imagined mental disabilities. In this chapter, I turn to the medical writings, official reports, and literary works that James McCune Smith (figure 2.1) published to generate counterdiscourses to the proslavery arguments that dominated the fields of science, medicine, and psychiatry. Smith, the most vocal Black intellectual in the debates about Black mental health during the nineteenth century, was also the first Black man to earn a medical degree in the United States.[7] Smith has received increased attention in studies on Black intellectuals in antebellum America, including, more recently, histories of medicine.[8] These medical and historical studies have returned Smith to his place as one of the most important Black intellectuals in the struggle for the abolition of slavery and as a sophisticated social scientist, medical researcher, and practitioner, a crucial precursor to the venerable social scientist and writer W. E. B. Du Bois and the Black intellectual Charles Chesnutt.[9]

This chapter brings to the fore Smith's commentary on mental disability among Blacks composed during his lifetime. It not only considers Smith's medical and scientific writings but also sheds light on his literary works as alternative sites of knowledge production regarding the nineteenth-century Black condition as well as the various meanings assigned to Blacks' physical and mental health. Smith debunked racist medicalized ideologies about Black bodyminds, contended that the cultural machinations of slavery and racial prejudice were the real source of harm to Blacks, and presented images of Blacks as healthful and fully capable of tending to their own mental and physical health needs. Writing as a personified counternarrative to assertions of Black mental deficiency, Smith rebutted racist medical, psychiatric, and scientific discourses. He also offered nuanced accounts of Black humanity through portraits of Black mental acuity and emotional and psychological depth that escape

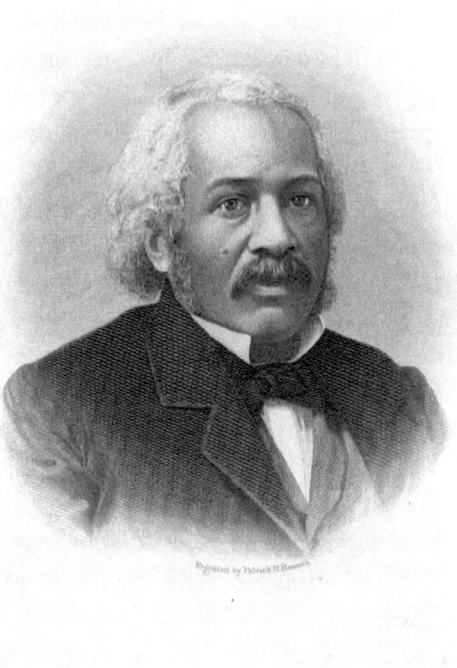

FIGURE 2.1 Engraving of James McCune Smith by Patrick H. Reason. New York Historical Society.

the one-dimensional, impersonal, and often objectified depictions of Black people in medical writings.

Although they each appealed to a distinct readership, Smith's scientific publications, abolitionist writings, and literary creations were separate enterprises. In all his writings, Smith simultaneously upheld and built upon the knowledge produced by the scientific and medical world, including the subfield of psychiatry. Customarily, scholarship about the nineteenth century has emphasized specific political struggles and social movements such as abolition, temperance, and suffrage. However, abolitionists were deeply and just as intensely engaged in other arenas of social change. They were equally zealous about reform movements for social institutions, social groups (such as the disabled or socially deviant young women), and individuals, especially concerning issues related to education, criminality, and health. They also responded to vociferous proslavery apologists who defended biased conclusions perpetuated by the medical, psychiatric, and scientific establishment. Britt Rusert argues that the work of early practitioners like James McCune Smith can be understood as "fugitive science," in which thinkers "repeatedly questioned the very definition of science, radically expanding its borders while presenting themselves as vital scientific agents who had the power to manipulate and experiment with the objects of the natural world."[10] Smith positioned himself as a medical authority using the power of observation and statistics to make declarations about Black people's health and illnesses. Unlike the blunt link between enslavement and good health that physicians and psychiatrists promulgated, Smith argued that Blacks' mental health was multifactorial—dependent on biological and physiological processes, environmental context, and social position, all working in tandem to affect individual health conditions for better or worse. Smith's work epitomizes this complicated engagement with medicine, clearly reflected in the fact that it was as political as it was scientific.

Smith's view of abolition and medicine as mutually constitutive reflected his understanding that the world of medicine was a battlefield, one with a topography configured by one of the greatest political struggles of the nineteenth century—that over the abolition of slavery. As a result, his medical writings aligned with his political convictions, and his political and literary writings relied on esteemed research publications. He used statistical data to appeal to a medical establishment that prized evidence of this kind. Smith was acutely aware that the battle for control over Black people's bodies was simultaneously a battle for control over their health and, profoundly, their mental health. His literary writings bore witness to the complexity of Black people and offered a vantage point on the Black condition elided in most medical writings. In such works, Smith unveiled Black people's aspirations for good mental and physical health. He stressed their desires to live full and meaningful lives outside the specter of white cultural measurements and assessments of their worth. He shined light on Black people's resiliency in the midst of ongoing challenges to their well-being. His works offer counternarratives to the distorting white supremacist concepts of race and health that prevailed in medical, scientific, and psychiatric traditions of knowing, and they also show that Black people were active participants in defining their own lives and creating their own visions of physical and mental health.

BACKGROUND ON JAMES McCUNE SMITH

James McCune Smith's commitment to advancing modern medical practice was matched only by his dedication to the fight against slavery. He was born enslaved in New York and freed at the age of fourteen on the state's emancipation day in 1827.[11] As a youth, he attended African Free Schools that the New York Manumission Society created, where he excelled in a range of topics in arts and sciences, including penmanship, spelling, poetry, grammar, astronomy, and geography. Smith is best known for writing the introduction to his close friend Frederick Douglass's book *My Bondage and My Freedom* (1855); however, in the nineteenth century, he was a prominent figure in his own right. Smith was a remarkable person—the son of a former slave, a master essayist, a gifted literary writer, a superb researcher, and a respected physician.

Among both Blacks and whites, he was one of the most highly educated people in the nation. He was denied entry into both Columbia University and Geneva Medical College because of his race but was accepted by the University of Glasgow in Scotland, where he earned a BA in 1835, an MA in 1836, and an MD in 1837. Fluent in seven languages, including Greek, Hebrew, and Latin, he authored over one hundred articles in ethnology, geography, medicine, and literature. After completing his medical degree, he opened a joint medical practice and pharmacy on 55 West Broadway in New York City. In the evenings, he taught both Black and white students math, geography, and literacy. Although Smith drifted into relative obscurity after his death, recent scholarly attention to his life and works highlights his singular place in Black history.[12] Henry Louis Gates aptly summarizes Smith's historical significance: "[W]e might think of James McCune Smith as the African American tradition's first man of letters, its first intellectual, and its first professional writer."[13] Smith's experimental essays, "The Heads of Colored People," were ahead of their time in their representations of dignified Black working-class life and labor that stressed a steadfast pursuit of the American dream. The essays rejected dominant modes of depicting Black people during the period: accounts of Black enslavement, portraits that supported middle-class respectability politics, and writing in the popular literary modes of sentimentality and romanticism.[14]

Smith's commitments reflected his fervent abolitionism. When studying for his medical degree, he joined the Glasgow Emancipation Society, where he was among abolitionists in Scotland and England. Upon returning to the United States, Smith promptly joined the American Anti-Slavery Society. He was an outspoken public figure for the cause of abolition, giving lectures including "Destiny of the People of Color," "Freedom and Slavery for Africans," and "A Lecture on the Haitian Revolution, with a Note on Toussaint L'Ouverture." He worked against the most devastating legal blow to abolition, the 1850 Fugitive Slave Law, and helped people gain safe passage on the Underground Railroad. About Smith, Douglass professed, "No man in this country more thoroughly understands the whole struggle between freedom and slavery, than does Dr. Smith, and his heart is as broad as his understanding."[15] The two worked together in several capacities, including the formation of the National Council of Colored People in Rochester, New York, which sought to expand educational opportunities for Black people across the nation.

Smith contributed extensively to the debates and issues most germane to the Black public, as evidenced by his numerous writings in Black press outlets. He financially supported and contributed to the Black newspaper *The Weekly Anglo-African*, which opposed the American Colonization Society's idea of Blacks emigrating back to Africa. He edited and wrote for the *Anglo-African Magazine*, where his contributions showcased his standpoint as a social scientist.[16] He also was an editor at *The Colored American*, a Black newspaper, and was a regular contributor to Frederick Douglass's paper under the pseudonym "Communipaw."[17] Along with James C. Pennington and others, he established the Legal Rights Association in New York, which worked against segregation in New York.

Smith was a devoutly religious man who believed that the true practice of Christianity necessitated the pursuit of racial equality. He was among the most radical of abolitionists and aligned with the National Liberty Party, which advocated for immediate, as opposed to gradual, emancipation. More importantly, unlike the Garrisonians, he was not wedded to nonviolence. Although he did not believe in retribution or revenge against slaveholders, he was in favor of "righteous violence," like his friends, the wealthy abolitionist Gerrit Smith and the well-known crusader John Brown.[18] Nevertheless, Smith's abolitionist efforts most often took the form of political speeches and writings that appeared in various outlets, including *Frederick Douglass' Paper*, the *Liberator*, and the *National Anti-Slavery Standard*. In addition to his more polemical writings about slavery and racial equality in newspapers, Smith stands out in the story this book tells about Black mental disability because of the persistent challenges he made to racist conceptions of Black bodyminds through his pioneering research and medical case studies, publications in medical and scientific journals, commentaries on popular medical and scientific theories such as phrenology, analyses of white physicians' reports, and experimental essays.

Perhaps Smith's fiercest counternarratives to racist medicalized discourses about Black bodyminds sprang from his work caring for sick patients, both white and Black. He opened his medical practice and pharmacy in 1837, and a decade later, he accepted the post of chief physician at the Colored Orphan Asylum, where he tended to the healthcare needs of Black children for nearly twenty years until his death. This important position did not prevent him from continuing his work on behalf of enslaved and free Black Americans throughout the country.

STATISTICAL COUNTERNARRATIVES

Smith's main arsenal in the fight against racist scientific and medical arguments was his training in medicine, science, and notably statistics while in Scotland and Paris in the 1830s. As a medical doctor and scientist, he deeply believed in the power of mainstream medicine and inquiry to explain and uncover medical and social phenomena. Consider the following statement Smith makes in a written cross-examination of white physicians' medical reports of the Colored Orphan Asylum (discussed more later), where he uses poetic language to express his faith in science as an objective realm of knowledge creation and his anguish over its misuse in cultural battles over race: "And we have hoped for much from Science; born in penury, nursed by persecution, we have fondly dreamed that she would ever rear her head far above the buzz of popular applause, or the clash of conflicting opinion in the moral world; it is therefore almost with the anguish that springs from a blasted hope that we view this first, however flimsy, attempt to demean her to the contemptible office of ministering to public prejudices."[19] Committed to the notion that science could unveil universal truths about society and health, Smith believed that most of the medical and scientific thought that perpetuated ideas of Black inferiority were based on flawed research. With passion and conviction, Smith set out to correct the record in his writings using accurately and rigorously collected data.

Smith published a series of articles refuting John C. Calhoun's statements about higher rates of vice, poverty, and "bodily and mental" afflictions among free Blacks in the *New York Daily Tribune*, a white newspaper that had one of the broadest readerships in the world at the time. In these articles, he outlined several imperatives for the national government. In addition to a reexamination of the 1840 census, Smith called on the US Senate to collect annual data on "sanitary" or health conditions, births, deaths, and marriages. He also argued that the upcoming 1850 census should include literacy rates among enslaved people, free Blacks, and whites. At the same time, Smith published Calhoun's claims, debunking them point by point in his signature cross-examination style. As he does elsewhere, in the *Tribune*, Smith declares that the 1840 census statistics on the "insane, blind, deaf, and dumb" are faulty, showing that in multiple states, including Maine, New Hampshire, Vermont, Massachusetts, New York, Pennsylvania, Ohio, Indiana, Illinois, Michigan, and Iowa, the census data reveal an "excess of colored insane over colored residents." Furthermore, accurate statistics, Smith argues, do not demonstrate disproportionate rates of mental disability among Blacks compared to whites: "The proportion of the insane among the free colored is not greater than among the white population of the free States."[20]

Smith understood that psychiatrists were the main medical authority on Black mental disability, and therefore, his *Tribune* pieces cite the rates of psychiatric institutionalization of Blacks in the North to demonstrate the small numbers being treated in asylums. He draws on the work of Dr. J. Ray, the physician at the Lunatic Asylum of the State of Maine, who indicated that there were fewer than five "colored lunatics" in the entire state. He also referenced statistics from New York City's Blackwell Island asylum, which recorded only seventeen "colored insane" in the county where it was located. He argued that that figure reflected the fact that only one out of every one thousand Blacks in the county had mental disabilities. He asserted the same relatively small proportion of Blacks had mental disabilities within Philadelphia's free Black population.

Smith also refuted Calhoun's claims about diminishing intellectual capacity in free northern Blacks. Smith stressed that Blacks in the North were taking advantage of educational opportunities and some were being educated at white schools, including Oberlin Western Theological Seminary and Dartmouth College. He also argued that the North had higher Black literacy rates than the South and seven Black newspapers that reflected a sizable, and growing, reading population. Smith noted, too, that southern literacy rates should be understood as dependent on southern laws that banned enslaved people from learning to read under the penalty of death.

The final element of health Smith addressed was the acquisition of good morals. During the nineteenth century, morality was fundamentally connected to health. Doctors believed that poor morals could lead to bad habits that in turn fueled mental strain. Practicing religion, as Smith pointed out, was one way for people in the nineteenth century to perfect their morality. He presented statistics to demonstrate that Blacks were attending church at high rates across various denominations, including Independent Methodists, Baptist Association, Methodist, Baptist, Presbyterian and Congregational, Episcopal, and Lutheran. Listing the actual church denominations was especially important because psychiatrists were publicly wary of evangelical traditions that they believed stirred up "mental excitement," a commonly listed cause of insanity, a topic I discuss in chapter 4.

Two years after the publication of "Freedom and Slavery for African-Americans" and "Facts Concerning Free Negroes," Smith released a masterful statistical study in *Hunts Merchant's Magazine* to develop his point in a more sustained fashion. In addition to challenging the 1840 census for failing to correct for age and annual mortality rates, the study argued that free Blacks in the North actually "improved in longevity" because they were not subject to the conditions created by "the system of slavery."[21] Smith framed the work as an inquiry into the impact of geography and climate on longevity, referencing a large catalog of life insurance and census data to support his conclusions. The overarching claim in the publication is that the northern climate is more favorable than that of southern states in general. In addition, he asserted that the impact of climate on southern Black peoples' longevity was further eroded by slavery. In his estimation, the adverse conditions that are built into the system of slavery, what he called "depressing circumstances," curtailed Black health and longevity.[22]

Chief among the environmental conditions he outlined was the requirement to perform strenuous labor under high temperatures in the open air, which subjected enslaved people to extreme heat and malaria. Following this line of argumentation, he concluded that without slavery, southern Blacks would have longevity rates exceeding those of southern whites. In making this claim, Smith drew on his belief in the inherent biological makeup of people of color globally. In line with many scientists of the day, Smith writes that "the negro, and the dark races of mankind" have better longevity at high temperatures.[23] Following the logical implications of this widespread belief, he contends that, without slavery, southern Blacks would outlive southern whites. His boldest claim, however, is that the longevity rates of southern Blacks could match those of northern whites were their conditions improved. Smith asserted that if Blacks were given a "standard of civilization" of a "high grade," the playing field would be leveled. This claim was a direct response to various scientific racist schools of thought, from early Jeffersonian speculations to phrenology to polygenesis, about the inherent biological inferiority of Black Americans.[24] Quality of life being equal, Smith saw no reason for Blacks in the North not to attain the same longevity as their white counterparts. Smith's statistical writings were on the intellectual front lines in the battle against negative conceptions of the Black bodymind. He knew that there was a growing respect for numbers and figures, so he demonstrated his mastery of them to oppose the dominant constructions of Black people as mentally and physically prone to disease. He generated his own discourse about Black bodyminds that he did not merely believe was scientifically true but that he observed firsthand in his medical practice, where he treated people with physical and mental ailments.

JAMES McCUNE SMITH'S MEDICAL CASE STUDIES

Importantly, some of Smith's medical assessments do not acknowledge race-based medicine. Instead, his case studies foreground what he saw as the highest standards of medical research. However, he was not allowed to present the findings of his first medical case study because of his race. The New York Medical and Surgical Society was prepared to miss out on medical knowledge that could advance the field because they believed Smith's presentation would have disturbed the "harmony" of the newly formed institution. But Dr. Watson, a white physician who consulted with Smith on the case, read it in his place. The report, "Case of Ptyalism with Fatal Termination," was about a woman with tongue swelling so severe she was unable to speak; it also caused gingivitis, gastrointestinal distress, and a "chronic hacking cough."[25] She had been married for nine years and had one child; she attributed her excessive salivation to pills, possibly calomel or mercury chloride. Smith treated her with the heroic medical techniques favored by most physicians of the time—bleeding, leeches, blistering at the nape of the neck, sulfur, copper, and aluminum on the tongue.[26] Modern medicine suggests that these treatments were harsh and invasive and likely did more harm than good; however, like other practitioners of orthodox medicine, Smith saw them as tools to alleviate her pain. Despite his initial rejection by the New York Medical and Surgical Society, Smith continued to see patients and pursue medical research.

Although Smith was not a psychiatrist, he made daily assessments of the mental and physical health status of his patients, Black and white. In 1844, Smith authored the first case histories published by a Black man, which appeared in the *New York Journal of Medicine*. Entitled "On the Influence of Opium Upon the Catamenial Functions," Smith's article studied five women, four of whom were sex workers, who experienced a cessation of their menstrual cycles upon using opium.[27] Physicians understood regular menstruation as critical to accessing the overall health of a woman so this was an important topic.[28] Against prevailing medical opinion, Smith writes that the return of menses occurred when opium usage stopped. He also contends that "skillfully regulated doses" of opium might be used to help women through "the change of life." He was aware that the "change of life" mostly referred to menopause but could also connote other times connected to a woman's menstrual cycle, like pregnancy or childbirth. Physicians were not the only medical professionals concerned about women's "change of life"; psychiatrists also thought that "the change of life" was an especially vulnerable time during which mental disabilities like hysteria could emerge.[29] Psychiatrists kept records of women's menstrual cycles in asylums as important markers of the progression of mental disease. For example, John Minson Galt was suspicious of women's regular cycles because they were thought to weaken women's physical and mental health. In the early 1840s, Galt recorded the case of a woman named Lucy at his Eastern Lunatic Asylum who was usually rational but became "deranged" when her period commenced, at which point she demonstrated physical assaults of caregivers and emotional instability such as "fits of laughing [that] sometimes terminate[d] in crying."[30] Smith would have been aware of this multifield query about women's menstrual cycles and their health.

Although Smith did not draw causal links between the women's menstrual cycles and their mental health to the same degree psychiatrists did, in his article on opium use, he used his medical position and authority to ascertain that two of the three women's debilitations included psychological ailments. Smith was not unique in his evaluative practice regarding mental health; often people who ended up being treated by psychiatrists were initially seen or treated by physicians. One case in Smith's publication on opium use was of an eighteen-year-old unmarried "colored" woman, E. R., who saw Smith because of an increase in the "quantity and frequency of the catamenia" in the summer of 1841. He describes E. R., who was the only woman of the five who was not a sex worker, in terms of both her physical comportment and her temperament: "She was pale, thin, and of the nervo-sanguine temperament."[31] He also notes that she had a "frequent" but "soft" pulse and that her "head [was] dizzy." The second woman who Smith determined to have mental health symptoms was twenty-four-year-old E. L–d. She came to see Smith because of an excessively heavy menstrual cycle. She had previously been given opiates by a physician in the wake of a drug-induced abortion. From that point on, she was addicted to laudanum, an opiate. Smith's description of her appearance when he encountered her in his office includes both mental and physical characteristics: "Her appearance last April, was as follows: look, stupid; complexion florid; person, fat; bowels, regular; and she ate very little food."[32] In this context, "stupid" refers to her mental health—likely a condition of neurodivergence like Down syndrome—not her intelligence. People described in nineteenth-century diagnoses as "stupid" or "idiots" were often treated in asylums alongside "lunatics" and "epileptics," often in separate wards or buildings. We do not know if E. L–d. went on to be treated in an asylum, but Smith noted that he believed that she might have been sent to Magdalen Asylum at Yorkville, an institution to reform "fallen" women and girls.[33] Smith not only made assessments of people's mental health in his regular practice but also encountered hundreds of children with a range of physical and mental health conditions during his time as the medical director of the Colored Orphan Asylum.

JAMES McCUNE SMITH AND PHRENOLOGY

While Smith worked to generate sound research on Black people and promote solid scientific methods, he also attacked what he saw as faulty scientific fields. Phrenology particularly incensed him because it made the tentacles of scientific and medicalized racism that he opposed vehemently particularly visible.[34] Furthermore, the doctrine had seeped into the consciousness of the most learned members of society. Smith called it out explicitly in his works and combated specific ideas that the discipline promulgated about Black mental and physical capacity, many of which dovetailed with the discourses present within the fields of medicine and psychiatry. In this section, I discuss the influence of phrenology before turning to an analysis of Smith's responses to phrenological claims of Black innate mental and physical inferiority and degeneration in his medical and fictional writings.

Phrenology began with the work of the German neuroanatomist Franz Joseph Gall (1758–1828), who wrote its foundational texts. The practice was popularized by his students Johann Spurzheim and George Combe; the latter was influential in the United States. Although it is relegated to the realm of "pseudoscience" today, phrenology was a serious field of scientific inquiry during its heyday from 1820 to 1850.[35] In 1830, for example, the University of Maryland granted the first degree in the subject.[36] Phrenologists asserted that the mental aptitude, personality traits, morals, and mental health of an individual or racial group (in the case of Black and Indigenous persons) were correlated with separate and independent regions of the brain that they called "faculties" or "organs." However, phrenologists did not agree as to the number of faculties that existed, which ranged from twenty-seven to thirty-five. These faculties corresponded to areas of the brain that led to benevolence, wit, cautiousness, timidity, intelligence, reason, vindictiveness, docility, affection, destructiveness, secretiveness, aggression, and empathy (among others). Phrenologists contended that weaknesses in various regions resulted in criminality, delinquency, or "insanity." Whereas Gall often performed postmortem examinations of skulls to determine the vitality of the facilities, phrenologists who outlived him measured the so-called organs of the brain through external cranial measurements of the bumps, hollows, and contours of people's heads. For the phrenologist, the lack of large bumps in a given region reflected defectiveness in the faculty. Although Gall saw these deficiencies as innate and fixed, Spurzheim and Combe believed that regions could be improved upon. Combe spent considerable energy on developing psychosocial programs that were designed to reform the pupil, criminal, and "insane."[37] Phrenology was not only a scientific discourse but also immensely popular among the public. Various famous figures, such as the abolitionist Lucretia Mott and the major American writers Edgar Allen Poe, Mark Twain, and Herman Melville, welcomed the detailed and intricate examination of their skulls.[38] The practical phrenologists Lorenzo Niles Fowler and Orson Squire Fowler published cheap leaflets with descriptions of the faculties and charts that everyday people could use to get their heads examined.

Psychiatrists found phrenology's principles, if not its methods, critical for understanding mental disease. For example, although Amariah Brigham, like other prominent psychiatrists, did not call himself a phrenologist, he was impressed by European phrenologists' work in neuroanatomy. In 1833, he helped bring Spurzheim's *Observations on the Deranged Manifestations of the Mind* to an American audience, writing an appendix to the volume. He was not convinced by the methods of craniometry for determining pathology but did agree with phrenology's fundamental principle—that mental disease originated in the brain. However, whereas phrenologists held that the brain included multiple organs, psychiatrists saw it as a single organ. Spurzheim's contention that "the brain is the organ of the mind," and "the cause of insanity will be looked for in the brain" correlated with Brigham's position that the brain, not the mind, was the root of mental impairment.[39] Brigham wove this phrenological idea throughout his writings in the *American Journal of Insanity* and elsewhere.[40] The concept became widely accepted in psychiatric circles and a mainstay in psychiatric theories of mental disease. Unlike phrenologists, however, psychiatrists focused their attention more on treatment than on the formulaic assessment of mental disease.

Although some phrenologists measured an individual's innate traits, others used the field to support longer-standing claims about the inferiority of entire racial groups. Charles Caldwell, a student of Benjamin Rush, a physician and slaveholder, is a prime example of the latter. He became acquainted with phrenology during a trip to Paris in the 1820s and, upon returning to the United States, became a homegrown adherent, writing and lecturing extensively on its merits. He also aligned himself with the polygenist Samuel Morton; both maintained that God created Blacks as a separate species, which they believed was evidenced by the supposedly lower volumes of Black skulls.[41] Caldwell contended that European cranial superiority was reflected in the fact that their "entire brain is larger than that of any other race," which then explained their "higher intellectual faculties." Such faculties led to superiority in the arts, sciences, and other spheres of society: "It is in the Caucasian race alone, that we find real human greatness, marked by the omnipotency, and decorated in all the elegancies, of genius... There alone that we find a Homer, a Socrates, an Alexander, an Aristotle, a Cesar, a Cicero, a Bacon, a Shakespeare, a Milton, a Franklin, a Washington, or a Bonaparte. Hanno, Hannibal, and many other great men." Caldwell claimed that Blacks, in contrast, occupied "an intermediate station between the figure of the Caucasian and the Ourangoutang."[42]

Whereas Caldwell used phrenology to justify slavery, abolitionists found in it a tool to oppose human bondage.[43] George Combe, who called enslavement "a cancer in the moral constitution" of Americans, discerned its damaging impact on the skulls of both whites and Blacks in the South. He argued that enslaved people's brains were generally smaller than northern Blacks and that whites showed less developed skulls in the area of conscientiousness, benevolence, acquisitiveness, and self-esteem.[44] Although he openly critiqued American slavery, Combe believed in racial hierarchies. He argued that Africans were easy to enslave because, by nature, they were a "*tame* man, submissive, affectionate, intelligent and docile."[45] Despite his criticism of American slavery, Combe's claims about the superiority of European culture and intellectual capacity parallel the proslavery stances of phrenologists like Caldwell. In *A System of Phrenology*, Combe asserts: "If we glance over the history of Europe, Asia, Africa, and America, we shall find distinct and permanent features of character which strongly indicate natural differences in their mental constitutions.... As far back as history reaches, we find society instituted, arts practised [sic], and literature taking root.... Under the Greek and Roman empires, philosophy, literature, and the fine arts, were sedulously and successfully cultivated."[46]

Other antislavery advocates were critical of the entire doctrine of phrenology as antithetical to the cause of freedom. In his third and final autobiography, *Life and Times of Frederick Douglass*, Douglass notes that he was eager to meet Combe for breakfast while in Europe with William Garrison. The visit satisfied Douglass, who mostly listened as Combe spoke at length. Douglass writes that in meeting Combe, a "very intense desire [was] gratified" for he was an "eminent mental philosopher" with fervent command of the "peculiar mental science" of phrenology.[47] Douglass viewed Combe as more enlightened than blatantly racist phrenologists like Caldwell, noting that Combe's *Constitution of Man* "relieved [his] path of many shadows."[48]

Despite high regard for Combe, Douglass categorically denounced phrenology. In a commencement speech before the Literary Societies of Western Reserve College in 1854, he gave several remarks concerning the prevalent forms of race science at the time, which he summed up as discourses related to "ethnological science, or the natural history of man," which covered the gambit of scientific disciplines that made claims about Blacks, whether using the shape of the head, the volume of the skull, or the angle of the face. He jabbed against phrenology in particular in part because it was an unsystematic study of Black skulls. He argued that for every deficient Black skull phrenologists examined, there were clear examples of the same features among whites. He further insisted that the dataset was essentially biased and incomplete. Douglass scoffed at the fact that the arsenals of phrenological examinations of Blacks excluded the most brilliant of Black minds. His short list of about a dozen out of "hundreds" who could give scientists an "idea of the mental endowments of the negro" includes revered Black men of the time such as Alexander

Crummell, Henry Highland Garnet, Samuel Ward, Martin Delany, and James Pennington.[49]

Beyond these challenges to the faulty science of phrenology, Douglass makes a string of strong declarations that outright reject race science claims as a matter of principle. He attacks both Caldwell's and Combe's claims about fixed racial hierarchies: "Away, therefore, with all the scientific moonshine that would connect men with monkeys . . . making one extreme brother to the ourang-ou-tang [sic], and the other to angels, and all the rests intermediates!"[50] He rehearses what he finds to be unsurprising conclusions within phrenology and other race science fields—that Blacks are mentally and physically diseased according to their rubrics—and he signals the fact that their ideas are synonymous with concepts of race already widely accepted in society: "The European face is drawn in harmony with the highest ideas of beauty, dignity and intellect. . . . The negro on the other hand, appears with features distorted, lips exaggerated; forehead depressed—and the whole expression of the countenance made to harmonize with the popular idea of negro imbecility and degradation." Because race science arguments were more polemical than data driven, Douglass was able to battle the pathologization of the Black bodymind on the same ideological grounds as those professing Black inferiority. Knowing this fact, he declares fiercely and eloquently that Blacks are equal to whites on both a physiological level and a humanistic level. He writes: "Tried by all the usual, and all the *un*usual tests, whether mental, moral, physical, or psycological [sic], the negro is a MAN—considering him as possessing knowledge, or needing knowledge, his elevation or his degradation, his virtues, or his vices—whichever road you take, you reach the same conclusion, the negro is a MAN."[51] Although Douglass's challenge to phrenology was argumentative and based in traditions of reason, he was not speaking as an equal to men of science and medicine.

Although Douglass never sought out a head reading himself, phrenologists could not help but make claims about the most influential Black man of their era. Combe told Mott that Douglass exhibited exceptional intellectual capacity: "Douglas [sic] has an excellent brain. His benevolence and Veneration are both large, & his conscientiousness [is] full while his intellect is vigorous and practical."[52] Later readings of Douglass's head were less generous. In an 1866 article in the *American Phrenological Journal and Life Illustrated*, the editor recognizes Douglass's command of

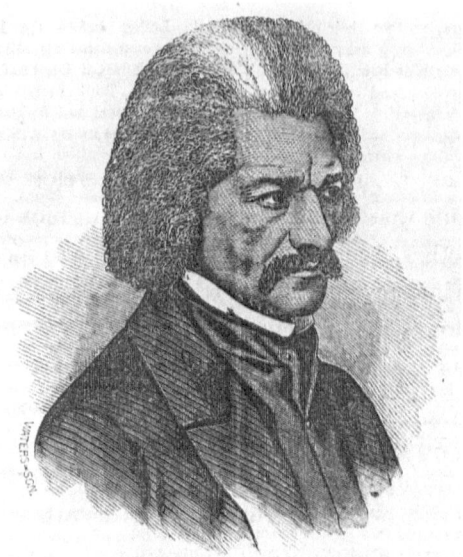

FIGURE 2.2 Portrait of Douglass in the *American Phrenological Journal.*

facts but claims that it does not reach the highest levels of reason characteristic of the venerable intellectual discipline of philosophy: "If his forehead does not indicate the philosopher, it certainly indicates the practical observer and the man of facts" (figure 2.2). Although Douglass's intellect is detectable, the writer opines that it does not reflect an ability for "abstract, metaphysical, or . . . theoretical" thinking.[53] The idea that Blacks fall short of the highest expression of intellect recalls Thomas Jefferson's infamous claim in *Notes on the State of Virginia* that the talented Black poet Phillis Wheatley had a sense of the metaphysical sentiments that religion could stir up in an individual but that she was unable to demonstrate the high level of intellect required to master the metaphysics of poetry.

Unlike Douglass, whose arsenal was limited to rhetorical statements against the faulty claims and practices of phrenology, Smith could draw on his medical practice and research to expose the fallacious racist medical and scientific claims about Black bodyminds made in phrenological discourse. After returning from Glasgow, at the ripe age of twenty-three,

Smith made his debut as a formidable public intellectual, speaking often on phrenology. He gave at least two public lectures about "the fallacy of phrenology," described in a newspaper headline as "Anti Phrenology."[54] Although the lecture transcripts are no longer extant, hints about their content, as well as their reception, appear in several articles in *The Colored American*.[55]

Smith's first lecture was on Friday, September 22, 1837. The audience for the hour-long presentation included both believers in phrenology and skeptics. The editor of the *Colored American* fell into the latter group, calling phrenology's tenets "pretensions" rather than "principles" before proclaiming that the "learned" Smith "uprooted them all." The columnist leveled his own indictment of phrenology, perhaps emboldened by the strong case Smith made the night before, declaring that the head-reading system was "based on assumptions" and had the hallmarks of "witchcraft." The editor's comparison placed phrenology squarely in the realm of metaphysical systems of belief, a stark contrast to the standards of science that Smith favored.[56]

For those in the Black middle class who recognized the reach of phrenology and searched for ways to dissipate it, Smith offered community leaders a singular opportunity. He could battle the ideology of phrenology and, through it, the pervasive assumptions about Black mental and physical inferiority from the privileged domain of science and medicine. In the *Colored American*, the editor highlighted the pressing need for Smith's thoughts on phrenology because the masses, what he calls the "unthinking community," were especially given over to the popular science.[57]

The article also details how the audience was as enamored of Smith's rebuttal as with his captivating oratory style: "Our soul feasted upon the exhibition of thought and learning; his chaste language and discriminating arguments would have done credit to three times his number of years." The editor's praise for Smith serves as an inherent repudiation of phrenology's stance on Blacks' supposed innate lack of intellectual aptitude, especially because the writer's portrait of Smith is one of Black excellence. He praises Smith's educational accomplishments, announces the Black middle class's "patronage" of the talented Smith, and urges "colored youth" to follow his example. He also predicts that Smith is destined to be legendary, not because of the contours of his head but for his masterful scientific aptitude and linguistic artistry: "But give him a chance, and with good health, under God, he will make the moral, literary, and physiological world all his own."[58]

The article published after Smith's second lecture provides more insight into Smith's arguments against phrenology based on physiological issues and comparative analysis. True to his training as a medical scientist, his talk takes the form of a medical school lecture. Like Gall, medical doctors, and psychiatrists, Smith stood before a crowded hall with a set of skulls and a blackboard for "extemporaneous drawings" to help prove his case. The learned men in the room were especially impressed with the fact that Smith made "entirely new" arguments. To be fair, Smith's claims were not particularly novel, although they may have been new to public discourse. Like Brigham and other psychiatrists, Smith thought it impossible to "designate the developements [sic] of the brain, by external convexities upon the skull." Although Brigham may have come to this conclusion from a logical standpoint, Smith did so by demonstrating that there were "no corresponding concavities" on the internal structure of brains that matched the external ones. He also attacked the "arbitrary character of the divisions of the organs" by showing that the natural divisions of the cerebrum did not line up with the "artificial and imaginary separations into distinct organs which phrenology suppose[d]." Although there are no specific examples, the writer claims that Smith proved his point by using "numerous physiological analogies," which might have been to human or animal specimens. Smith argued that phrenological principles did not align with the "organic and functional laws of the animal economy." Smith's emphasis on the laws of nature reflects his medical and scientific training and his fidelity to the new wave of science that sought to discover the laws of nature, which in medicine were often referred to as the "laws of hygiene."[59]

Smith's final charge against phrenology was based less on the actual science than on the mental habits of its adherents. He argued that it was not a coincidence that believers in phrenology tended to be "free thinkers," by which he meant that they were skeptical of religion. Smith, a devout Christian, joined other men of medicine who saw in scientific and medical discoveries examples of God's divine order for the universe.[60] Phrenology posited that some people were born depraved or destructive, a premise that some Christians found troubling; if men were created in God's image, phrenology suggested that God was also depraved and destructive, an ideological concession that not all Christians were willing to make.

Although most of Smith's points were well-taken, some of the learned people in the room took issue with one of his arguments. Like psychiatrists, Smith and his learned peers were unwilling to do away with the phrenological claim that the brain was an organ of the mind. Although in his account of Smith's lecture the editor did not detail the kind of challenge Smith posed to the widely held medical and psychiatric concept, he suggested that Smith simply questioned whether the widely accepted notion could be proven. Despite the importance of his lectures, Smith did not spend all of his time at the podium, seeking to disprove racist perspectives on the Black bodymind. One of his most significant contributions was his long-standing service to children—actual Black bodyminds—at the Colored Orphan Asylum.

COLORED ORPHAN ASYLUM

Smith was the medical director at the Colored Orphan Asylum from 1843 until his death in 1865 (figure 2.3). The orphanage was opened by white Quaker women during a particularly violent time for Blacks in New York City, epitomized by the race riots in the 1830s and the draft riots in 1863, the latter of which targeted the orphanage for destruction.[61] Pushing back against the conservative managers of the orphanage, Black patrons saw it not merely as an institution for caring for children lacking homes or full family support but also as a place of opportunity for educational and moral training for Black children. To the satisfaction of Black citizens, Smith supported this vision of Black uplift through maintaining the physical and mental health of the children who suffered from seasonal, chronic, and epidemic diseases, including whooping cough, colds, influenza, smallpox, tuberculosis, and measles. Although it was not an institution specifically dedicated to the treatment of mental health ailments, Smith as a physician with experience treating all ailments, tended to mental health conditions alongside the physical health complaints of the time. The orphanage, like asylums, prisons, and other reformatory institutions, emphasized good health through regular routine, diet, prayer, religious instruction, outside

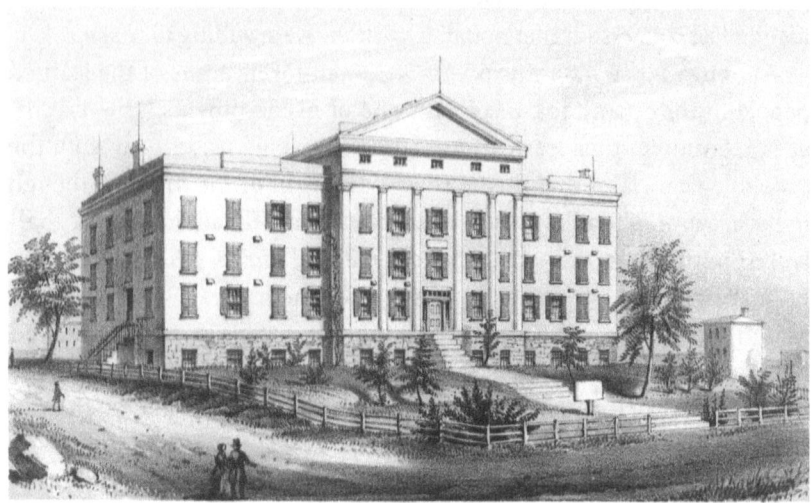

FIGURE 2.3 *Colored Orphan Asylum*, The Miriam and Ira D. Wallach Division of Art, Prints and Photographs: Print Collection, New York Public Library.

recreation, and education (figure 2.4).[62] Smith sacrificed tremendously to fulfill his role; in addition to holding amended hours at his private practice, he traveled six to seven miles almost daily to the institution, sometimes by foot when he was not permitted to use public street cars.[63]

Even before becoming the medical director, Smith had challenged the racialized medical discourses about Black inferior mental and physical anatomical differences that the orphanage physicians, phrenologists, southern medical physicians, and psychiatrists all propagated in their medical writings. In the first years of its opening, the physicians that tended to the health needs of Black children were two well-meaning white men, Drs. James McDonald and James Proudfit. Smith, like other middle-class Black leaders of white-run charities, recognized the doctors' efforts to tend to youth who would have otherwise languished on the streets, in poor houses, or within damp and poorly ventilated city cellars. Despite their laudable work for Black children, however, Smith challenged the racist medical conclusions that McDonald and Proudfit published in white and Black newspapers, including a "Physician's Report," which was republished in the *Colored American* in 1839. The "Physician's Report" included brief case

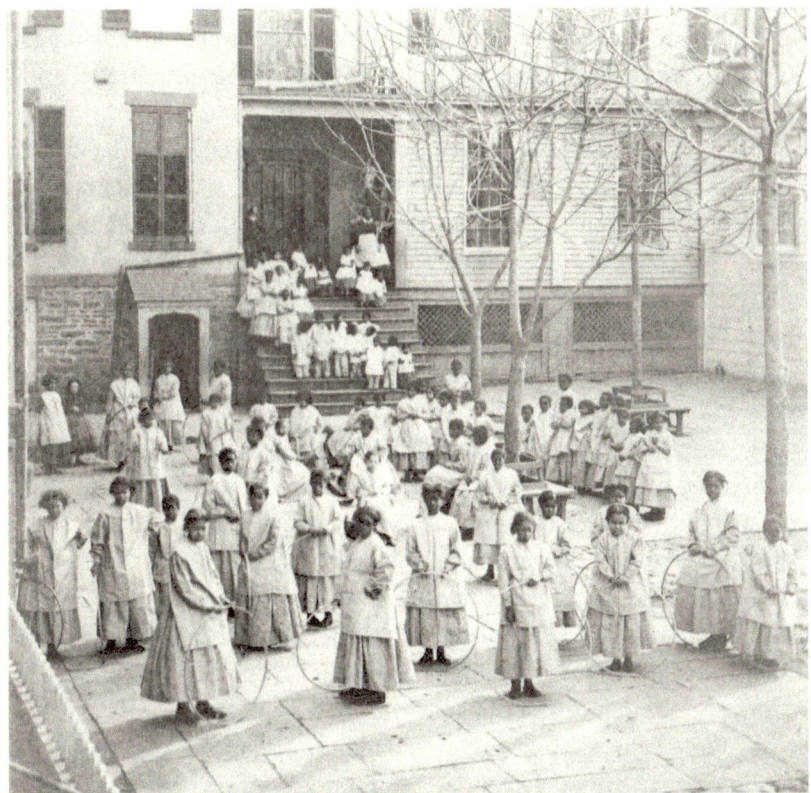

FIGURE 2.4 Children in the courtyard of the Colored Orphan Asylum. New York Historical Society.

studies of nine Black children (out of sixty-four total in house at the time) who had died. The descriptions, only a few sentences each, explained their ailments and symptoms and provided further context for their conditions. Four of the nine children suffered from mental health conditions, which the physicians described with phrases such as "mental imbecility," "disease of the brain," "convulsions," "brain tumor," "inflammation of the brain," and "excitement." Smith contested McDonald and Proudfit's declaration that the children's mental and physical health conditions were caused by factors including their "sickly and feeble" health at admission; poor nutrition, air, and clothing; and epidemic outbreaks in the hospital. In addition to these environmental factors, the physicians included two causes that were innate to the Black children's bodyminds: they were the "offspring of unhealthy parents," and their ailments were due to the "peculiar constitution and condition of the colored race."[64]

In a reply, Smith cross-examines the "Physician's Report" with both scientific precision and argumentative sarcasm. He expresses the hope that his medical research will administer to the doctors "a rebuke more stern than [he could] pen." As a medical doctor, Smith believed whole-heartedly that medicine should not minister "to public prejudices" as the report did. In the midst of presenting alternative figures, mostly from city inspector mortality reports on childhood mortality, and citing medical research on climate and chest anatomy, he reminds readers several times that he is searching for the supposed "peculiarity in the constitution of the colored people."[65] Smith points out the absurdity of the doctors' references to parental health in the case of a child named Sidney. This child, Smith insists, died of natural causes, not the "imaginary diseases" the doctors, without evidence, assigned to her parents.

Smith argues that, when it comes to mental health conditions, white children suffer in greater numbers than Black children. In conditions involving the brain, evidenced by symptoms such as "convulsions," he writes, "one colored to 21.36 white children die of convulsions, which leave the balance of 20 percent of 'peculiarity' on the side of the whites." Likewise, in the case of mental disabilities arising from a "tumor on the brain," Smith declares that the inspector report statistics show that "1 colored to 26 white persons died of [the] complaint." He sarcastically notes that the condition plagues whites more by far, so "'peculiarity' is "on the side of the whites." He also includes statistical data that mental health conditions such as "dropsy of the brain" occur more often among whites, listing that the position was "22" Blacks to "343" whites in 1837.[66]

Smith not only directly challenged the doctors' claims about Black constitutions but also attacked other ways in which medical logic supported slavery, such as the debate that A. P. Merrill put forth in his article about harmful impacts of the northern climate on free Blacks' bodyminds.[67] Smith takes an antiessentialist stance on race by noting that Black people in the United States are not purely of Black or European ancestry, but rather preeminent examples of the national motto "E pluribus unum" (Latin for "out of many one") and that their mixed-race heritage makes them "best fitted" for every climate, including northern ones, which fluctuate between warm and cold temperatures across seasons. He cites a climate medical researcher to support his claim that Blacks born in the United States have a chance to adapt to the climate slowly and therefore are not prone to diseases associated with migration from different climates: "Those who change the climate progressively, or who are born in countries of an intermediate temperature, suffer much less than those who migrate in a more direct manner."[68]

Smith also went on the offensive about the cultural context of Black people's health. He declared that innate differences in Black bodyminds did not determine the frequency of disease among Black people, stressing instead the paramount importance of social and cultural factors. Taking consumption (tuberculosis) as an example, he argued that the avenues for treating the disease were unavailable to Blacks for social reasons. White people, he noted, are able to stave off death from consumption by relocating to the West, South, the Caribbean, or even Europe, where their mortality rates diminished drastically. But the "colored" consumptive, he declared, had many fewer treatment options. Free Black people in the North could not enjoy the "genial clime of the South" for financial reasons. Discussing the consequences of such constraints, he writes, "all the colored persons in [New York] who are seized with consumption, die in the city of consumption; whilst the whites fly and obtain a reprieve, or die elsewhere." He believed such constraints skewed the consumption death rate numbers, which presumably would be equal to those of whites if Blacks had easier access to favorable health environments. Smith directly names American social systems as the culprits for bad health, which differ in kind but not degree in the South and North: "To him the avenues to wealth and the genial clime of the South, are barred by the same relentless spirit of aristocracy, which is prejudice in the North, and slavery in the South."[69]

Smith further included a discussion of social predictors of adverse health consequences across the Black lifespan. He acknowledged that Black children's favorable statistical health figures could be reversed in adulthood. This reversal, he insists, is not based on innate Black characteristics: "And even if, as these children advance in life, the proportions in mortality be reversed, it cannot be the result of any 'peculiarity of constitution.'" Rather than Black bodyminds themselves, Smith argues that increased Black mortality results from a "suicidal" social structure that causes Black mental destruction and intellectual exclusion.[70] At the end of his medical analysis of the children in the orphanage, Smith departs from attacking medical discourses to make a more philosophical assertion about the limited possibilities for Black excellence: "[Black mortality arose from] that legalized curse which drives colored mind to prey upon itself—that hell-born prejudice which shuts out from its proper sphere the patriotic intellect of colored men, in crushing whom the state suicidally destroys the hardiest frames with which she is blessed."[71]

To Smith, the racist state destroyed the health of Black people and, in turn, damaged the health of the nation as a whole. In Smith's paradigm of health, Black people were not only integral to society but also a blessing to the nation. Smith did not elaborate on what made Black people a "blessing" in his report or on the characteristics of the cultural context of their experiences of health. He saved such descriptive detail and insights for his literary writings, through which he offered readers access to the interiority of everyday Black people. Through Smith's portraits of ordinary Black people, we observe how mental disability takes shape in response to normal social conditions. Smith grants his readers access to the social contexts and life circumstances in which working-class Blacks battled for their sanity daily.

"HEADS OF THE COLORED PEOPLE"

Smith's most singular cultural productions on race were not his medical writings but those in which he wrote creatively about Black life in the big city. Although they are separate modes of production, Smith's medical and scientific writings provide context for the literary ones and shape their themes and points of emphasis. Writing under the pen name "Communipaw," Smith announced that his stories would be a contribution to the "Republic of Letters."[72] He published a series of nine fictional sketches of individual Black working-class people in *Frederick Douglass' Paper* from 1842 to 1854. The title of the sketches, "Heads of the Colored People," was a direct response to the field of phrenology, which (as previously discussed) proposed that Black people's skulls disclosed everything from their mental capacity and morality to their fecundity.[73] Smith's "word paintings" reveal that phrenology's trite racist assessments of Black people belied the richness of character, personality, and emotional depth that emerged from a true examination of their lives.[74] Through sketches that are stylistically a mixture of reportage, biography, and witty commentary, he renders textured and multidimensional treatments of various skilled trades people, including a news vender, bootblack, washerwoman, sexton, steward, editor, inventor, whitewasher, and schoolmaster. My analysis focuses primarily on "The Black News-Vender"; however, I include a survey of the ways mental disability arises throughout the collection. The other stories offer slightly different vantage points on issues of mental disability in the lives of the Black city dwellers. They collectively provide portraits of mental fortitude and genius; mental coping and avenues of improving mental and physical health; and challenges to "crazy" (irrational) social systems and perverse exploitation of Black communities.

Smith wrote the stories at a particularly trying time socially, economically, and politically for Black people in New York City. Black skilled workers were under strain from competition with white immigrant laborers and sometimes faced violent assaults from them. Contending with low wages and high rents, Blacks faced what William Fogel calls a "hidden depression" as they "suffered one of the most severe and protracted economic and social catastrophes of American history."[75] Smith was keenly aware of these economic challenges. A year before publishing "Heads of the Colored People," Smith discusses in an article how both working-class and middle-class Blacks struggle to find work and secure livable wages amid the rising costs of living, conditions deleterious to their human dignity:

> From the necessity of seeking employment in the city, as servants, porters, &c., our manhood is, in a measure, demeaned, lowered, kept down; and I doubt much whether manhood flourishes very much among citizens of any class. . . . The enormous combination of capital which is slowly invading every calling in the city, from washing and ironing to palace steamers, must tend more and more to grind the face of the poor in the cities, and render them more and more the slaves of lower wages and higher rents.[76]

To alleviate the economic pressures Smith outlines above, he urges Black people to look for practical ways to improve their conditions, including self-help initiatives such as consolidating financial resources. In the article, Smith calls for the creation of Black-owned banks, real estate vendors (to earn income from renting out properties), and communal purchasing projects that would buy fuel, food, and household goods wholesale on behalf of the entire community. Smith also cautions Black readers against wasteful spending, most notably gambling. Above all, Smith advocates for Blacks to abandon city life for more affordable rural communities in which they could farm or start businesses. This is a rational and "sane" path forward: "No sane man can doubt, from this or any comparison of the kind that country life is the better choice for our people; not consolidated, isolated country-life, but a well mixed country and village life." He notes further that city life expectancy is shorter than that in the country and that there are a preponderance of "seductions of the city." True to medical beliefs connecting social behavior to physical health, he maintains that supposedly harmful social vices, like gambling, sex work, unrestrained expressions of sexuality, and idle hanging out on street corners, cause rampant sickness and can lead to the formation of a "gang of lazaroni of both sexes."[77]

In addition to severe economic strain, the passage of the draconian Fugitive Slave Law sent shock waves through the free and fugitive slave community; it created widespread anxiety that led many Black people to flee to Canada and Europe. Smith understood the difficulty of existing under these circumstances and acknowledged that Blacks sought to improve their lives while "in the teeth of the most tremendous opposition ever encountered by men."[78] Nonetheless, in the midst of it, they led meaningful lives that he put on vibrant display in each life portrait. The social context of Black life in New York deeply informed how Smith represented health, including mental health and mental disability, in the sketches. As a whole, the vignettes are counternarratives to medical and scientific thought about Black people's inherently inferior mental capacities, ideas that began with Thomas Jefferson at the end of the eighteenth century and continued through to the 1850s; and as later chapters will show, such ideas lingered well into the late nineteenth century. Smith engaged the racialized medical discourses only to topple them in his descriptions of what the heads of Black people *actually* revealed, as details of Black actions contradicted any notion of innate inferiority. The sketches challenged the medical and psychiatric ideas that Black bodyminds were less intelligent, lacked emotional depth, and were prone to disease. Smith's "Heads of the Colored People" was equally significant for unveiling the meaning of mental disability on Black people's own terms as it was intertwined with their conceptions of self-reliance, social progress, exploitation, and psychological coping strategies. The social value, and sometimes superiority, of the Black people Smith profiled were indexed not in their acquisition of elite education but rather in the ordinary work they performed within their communities. In this section, I discuss several instances in which mental disability or mental health figures as a theme across the sketches.

First, though, it's important to mention that Smith's vision of Black people's path forward clashed with the stance of Frederick Douglass, who saw the sketches as demeaning. He felt that portraits of Black people should be performing a particular cultural work to unequivocally dismantle notions of Black innate inferiority: "If those who are everlastingly harping upon the natural inferiority of our race would look in occasionally upon these churches and witness the evidence of the good character and intelligence of their colored congregations, they would see that they have formed their opinions before learning the facts."[79] Although Douglass and Smith both opposed phrenology, they had different ideas about how best to respond to its racist discourses. Douglass believed that Black thinkers needed to generate representations of Black people as intelligent, virtuous, and moral. For Douglass, these traits were most evident in members of the Black middle class. Douglass published a response, "Letter from the Editor," to Smith's sketches in which he included his own portraits of respectable, refined, and educated Black men in their churches, literary societies, and businesses, all being "productive" citizens. Smith's vision did not require the attainment of middle-class status. Smith's portraits showed Black people embracing the world that countless working-class people had already built.

Middle-class respectability politics of Black social success were not the only grounds on which Douglass objected to "Heads." Douglass was a part of a larger trend within Black middle-class circles in which members adopted and reformulated ableist discourses that deemed disabled Blacks as ill-equipped to contribute to society.[80] Jacob Crane contends that Douglass was invested in the figure of the able-bodied hero, epitomized in his only fictional work *The Heroic Slave*, and was uneasy with Smith's representation of disability, particularly in "The Black News-Vender," stating that Douglass's letter "contests and even erases representations of black disability."[81] Indeed, disability figures importantly in the sketch; Smith's only physically disabled subject in "Heads" is mentally, emotionally, and economically striving—a premier illustration of self-making. Tobin Siebers contends that oppressive systems like ableism function "by reducing human variation to deviancy and inferiority defined on the mental and physical plane."[82] In many respects, "The Black News-Vender" disrupted ableist narratives of the Black body that diminished his contributions to his family and society. A fugitive slave, the news vender becomes disabled while working on a ship traveling from Liverpool to New York. During the voyage, the ship, the *Tuscarora*, wrecks, and the man washes up in New Jersey, where his frozen legs are determined to require amputation. Despite the fact that sometimes the cold weather "troubles" his "stump," he sells his newspapers faithfully "fastened near the ground." With the same devotion to craft as Smith's other subjects, his power is tied to his labor. More than the other portraits, his actual body blends with his products; with his proximity to the ground and the newspapers, his figure is "almost part of [the papers]."[83] "A black man razed to the knees," for Smith, he symbolizes the Black community's strivings despite enduring legal, political, and cultural hindrances, all of which (like the news vender's accident) are outside their control. At the same time, the story reveals the ways race and disability function as mutually constitutive social categories. It is impossible to disentangle the news vender's experience as a disabled person from his status as a fugitive slave. Dea Boster reminds us of the nature of this entanglement: "[The] stigmatized social constructions of race and impairment often coexisted in complicated and dynamic relationships in antebellum social and cultural discourse."[84] Before he became physically disabled, the news vender escaped the potentially disabling system of slavery, having "made [him]self free," only for his physical body and movement throughout the North to be restricted. When slave catchers came into town, he went "straight to the dock, [took] ship, and [was] away two or three months."[85] This physical restraint led to the dangerous conditions and the outcome of physical disability that circumscribes his life in freedom.

Smith clarifies for the reader how the news vender's life is shaped by dual systems of racial exclusion: economic exploitation and ableism.

Slavery was steeped in an ableist rubric that was profit driven, as Jennifer Barclay outlines: "Under slavery, bondpeople were valuable 'property' as laborers and potential reproducers of future generations of slaves, so the condition of their bodies and minds were central to slaveholders' pursuit of economic gain."[86] The news vender directly acknowledges chattel slavery's profit rubric in which able Black bodies were accessed as more valuable than disabled ones.[87] The narrator-turned-direct reporter asks the news vender whether he fears recapture given his inability to escape on ships. Speaking of the slave catchers, the news vender asks, "But now— what would they want with me?" Despite his acknowledgement of its organizing force, the news vender neither subscribes to this value system nor becomes resigned to remaining hidden because of his disability. He is able to sustain his livelihood with the help of his wife, who physically brings him the papers each morning, and as a result of his own mental prowess, demonstrated by his ability to "judge very nearly . . . the quantity that will sell" each day.[88]

In "The Black News-Vender," Smith participates in the Black literary tradition of "bearing witness," which entails giving voice to the experiences, passions, and inner motivations of Black people.[89] This tradition occurred most notably in the slave narrative genre, none more iconically than in his friend Frederick Douglass's narrative. Unlike the most popular slave narratives that usually conclude with the fugitive's escape to freedom, the Black news vender's story begins with the life of a fugitive after attaining freedom. The memory of slavery appears primarily on the body of the enslaved man.

Pushing back on the phrenological impetus to read the heads of Black people, Smith makes a parody of the fact that the news vender's head tells a story not of his individual personality traits but rather of the unspoken cultural narratives of racial mixing and the falsehood of scientific racism.[90] The news vender's bodymind is depicted in observable terms; he has "black transparent skin" and "prominent perceptive faculties," and he has a "fine long hooked nose, evidently from the first families," which the narrator presumes was a product of Thomas Jefferson and Sally Hemming's lineage.[91] By acknowledging the biracial realities of Black people, Smith disrupted the racial purity narratives of scientific racism. He questioned the validity of making race-based claims about Black inferiority when the history of Black people was a history of white people's capacities as much as Blacks. Smith explicitly called into question the "anti-negroisms" of Jefferson's *Notes on the State of Virginia*. In *Notes*, Jefferson presents Black men as sexuality driven in an animalistic way and more given to lust than love: "They are more ardent after their female: but love seems with them to be more an eager desire, than a tender delicate mixture of sentiment and sensation."[92] Yet, as Smith declares, this statement more accurately represented Jefferson's sexual desires for Black women: "[I]t is well known that Jefferson contradicted his philosophy of negro hate, by seeking the dalliance of black women as often as he could, and by leaving so many descendants of mixed blood, that they are to be found as widely scattered as his own writings throughout the world."[93]

In addition to vociferous sexual appetites, Jefferson wrote that Black people lacked the psychological and emotional capacity for deep feeling. In *Notes*, Jefferson explains that Black people's "griefs are transient" and major life calamities such as death and separation from kin are "less felt, and sooner forgotten."[94] Smith, however, was well aware that psychiatrists and physicians located the cause of many cases of mental instability in major life events such as the death of a close loved one. Smith's insistence that Black people had the capacity to suffer emotionally was an assertion that Blacks were equally vulnerable to experiencing mental breakdown as their white peers. Smith, as the narrator, performs the emotional capacity for deep feeling in response to both the news vender's story and the death of the narrator's own young child. The narrator is also inspired by the news vender's tenacity in the face of past and ongoing barriers. The news vender shares how he tried to save money, but his savings were often depleted because of sickness. Still, he continuously resumes his saving efforts in hopes of buying a better venue: "Last summer, a year ago, and winter, I saved up fifteen dollars; but was taken sick and most of it went; but now I am coming up again. I wish to get a place, a stand or shop in doors to sell papers and stationery; when the weather is cold and frosty, my stump troubles me and may lay me up."[95] As Smith's editorial writings demonstrate, he was aware that health struggles, what he called "calamities of mere sickness," limited Black prospects for uplift.[96] The narrator is moved by the news vender's story of loss and aspiration against impossible odds. Learning that the news vender lost his legs on the same day as his own child's death, the narrator resolves to give the news vender money from a life insurance policy to help him attain a shop. Smith wrote partially from personal experience—he was openly distraught after losing three of his children, who had died by 1854.[97] The narrator's deep emotions are articulated in language he uses to describe his emotional state during his child's sickness. He experienced a range of mental states, a mixture of "hopes and fear," "deep agony," and "distress."[98]

To drive home the extent of the narrator's psychological suffering, Smith quotes lines from Alfred Tennyson's poem *In Memoriam* (1850), which is part of a collection of verses written for the poet's friend Arthur Henry Hallam, who died in 1833. Smith's choice of Tennyson is evocative for conveying the narrator's psychological distress. In 1850, two years before Smith's sketch of the Black news vender, Lord Tennyson was appointed Queen Victoria's poet laureate after the death of William Wordsworth. Tennyson was a perfectionist, continuously editing his work, a practice that led his contemporary Robert Browning to call him "insane" and his habit of pouring over his writing a symptom of "mental infirmity."[99] Tennyson also suffered from lifelong and debilitating depression, which helped shape his poetry. He was known for his technical mastery of verse and capturing the language of sorrow. He was called "the saddest of all English poets" by T. S. Eliot.[100] Even writers who were not laudatory of his literary talent affirmed his gift for capturing emotional agony in words: W. H. Auden wrote, "There was little about melancholia that [Tennyson] didn't know; there was little else that he did."[101] True to his talents, *In Memoriam* explores themes of faith, grief, and love in the face of loss. The poem is a sustained meditation on the mysterious question to which neither religion nor science had satisfactory answers: Why was man created to die? In stanza twenty-two, Tennyson's speaker explores how humans cope with the loss of loved ones:

> There sat the Shadow fear'd of man;
> . . . .
>   And spread his mantle, dark and cold,
>   And wrapped thee formless in the fold,
> And dull'd the murmur on thy lip.[102]

Smith taps into Tennyson's expressions of the bewildering fact of life through the personification of death as a fearful "shadow." In the context of the Black newspaper vender's story, Smith stresses the speaker's lack of control over a loved one's life. Death is also personified as a neutral yet compassionate agent with the ability to ease suffering. Although his mantle is "dark and cold," death is not a grim force in the poem. It is a benevolent force because it "dulled" the woman's expressions of pain; it is not to be feared but rather is a partner for the living, picking up where humans leave off. Through his use of literary intertextuality, Smith performs intellectual acuity and psychological depth, defying racist scientific and medical claims that asserted that Black people were incapable of either. Smith the writer, like the narrator, turned to poetry during the hardest times of his life. Having worked through the pain and incomprehensible nature of death, the narrator ends the story with the lesson the reader should take from the Black news vender's story: "There is hope in it for all who, like him, are battling against slavery and caste."[103] As the moral signifies, the Black news vender's story is ultimately one of hope. From the narrator's personal loss, he gives birth to the Black news vender's dream of self-reliance and economic security.

Of the nine sketches in "Heads of the Colored People," the "The Washerwoman" is the most vibrant. In it, we see the ways labor mediates mental suffering and reinforces mental strength. It opens with the deep contextualization of the washerwoman's life, work, and space. Smith describes her signature repetitive action of plunging clothes in water to clean them, her necessary instruments, and the products of her labor: "Saturday night! Dunk! goes the smoothing-iron, then a swift gliding sound as it passes smoothly over starched bosom and collar, and wrists-bands of one of the many dozen shirts that hang around the room on horses, chairs, lines and every other thing capable of being hanged on."[104] In the backdrop of her arduous workspace are photos of men who symbolically overlook her performance of paid rather than slave labor: the British abolitionist George Thompson, the wealthy Black ship captain Paul Cuffe, and the coeditor of *Freedom's Journal*, the first Black newspaper, Samuel Cornish. The white abolitionist reflects her gratitude for white allyship in the fight for her freedom, Paul Cuffe is an example of Black wealth obtained through hard work, and Samuel Cornish represents how Blacks could pursue communal rather than solely individual prosperity.

She is also shown to be a deeply religious person with books representing popular religious reading of the time: "Bunyan's Pilgrim's Progress, Watt's Hymns, the Life of Christ." Part of the rigor of her tasks is the pace at which she works; signaling the rapidness and intensity, Smith uses a repeated word with multiple exclamation points: "Dunk! dunk!!" Smith details that she is on a mission to complete her work before the Sabbath, which is for her "the Day of Rest." Although Sunday is presented as a resting time for the washerwoman's body, her hard work provides mental respite; it takes her mind back to the warm climate of the South, where she is reminded of the comfort that comes from family bonds: "The frame of the washerwoman bends again to her task, her mind is 'far away' in the sunny South, with her sisters and their children." Smith reminds the reader that even in the comfort of her daydream, however, slavery is not romanticized, as her family members "toil as hard [as her] but without any pay!" She takes pleasure in the fact that her labor had uplifted their emotional states in the crucible of slavery, a sentiment that motivates her to work even faster and harder: "And she fancies the smiles which will gladden their faces, when receiving the things she sent them in a box by the last Georgetown packet. *Dunk! dunk!! dunk!!!*"[105]

The most mentally liberating sentiment for the washerwoman is not religion but the possibility that she and her kin could relish "sweet" freedom, unconstrained by legal or political mandates. In the sketch, the washerwoman's concept of freedom takes on a more timeless, universal, and existential character as her only prayer is that it be extended to her kin:

> Oh Freedom! No *Prie Dieu* in reverential corner, no crucifix and lugubrious beads pendent from the sidewall, no outward and visible sign, but the great impulse of progressive humanity has touched her heart as with flame, and her tried muscles forget all weariness, the iron flies as a weaver's shuttle, shirts appear and disappear with rapidity from the heated blanket and at a quarter to twelve, the groaning table is cleared, and the poor washerwoman sinks upon her knees in prayer for them, that they also may soon partake of the freedom which, however toilsome, is yet so sweet.[106]

Smith demonstrates that the washerwoman's belief in freedom is not just philosophical but also borne of her own mental fortitude to stand up to her northern master, who one day threatened to whip her. Disobeying this man in the same fashion as Douglass famously did to Covey, a pivotal moment in his quest for manhood, she tells him that if he "touch[es]

[her] with [the] lash," then she will "tear [him] to pieces." Her master backs down; "the whipper" is "whipped." As John Stauffer contends, her work becomes a place where she can exercise her power and enter a realm of consciousness in which she rises above her condition as wage laborer: "In McCune Smith's view, 'hard work' combined mental and physical powers, and it enabled workers to achieve an alternative consciousness that was immune to racism."[107] The washerwoman's work itself is a reservoir for her spirit of freedom, physical and mental mastery, and a resting place in the midst of the racial challenges with which Blacks in New York City contended.

In his sketch "The Whitewasher," Smith not only locates mental genius in ordinary work but also demonstrates that "craziness" is a rational response to the irrational system of human bondage. He remarks that the whitewasher, although doing particularly arduous and dirty work, is also "a chemist" who is attuned to the mixing of actual colors—and to the racial mixing that defines American culture. His access to "secrets about lime and lamp black," whites and Blacks in America, respectively, enables him to charge high rates for his services.[108] Smith tells the story of an enslaved whitewasher named Surrah Carrtarr, an Arabic-speaking African-born man, who became privy to the knowledge of his right for freedom on a visit to New York with his master.

Surrah's story is one in which the subject either is genuinely driven "crazy" or intentionally embraces mental disability; the sketch does not clarify which is the case. Boster argues that for enslaved people, mental disability could take on different valences and offered alternative avenues for agency: "In many cases, slaves shared assumptions about impairment and weakness, but slave perceptions of disability could be influenced by the possibility of self-control or resistance, and bondspeople actively negotiated meanings of disability with each other and with their masters."[109] Surrah demands wages from his master but is "rebuffed." A few days later, he starts throwing apples at his master in an orchard while speaking Arabic; "thought to be crazed," he is "seized and secured in an upper room until officers could be sent for." He escapes from his confinement by running "head foremost" into the thick oak door of his cell. Although a man of a "well developed head," thus by phrenological standards intelligent, Surrah lives in the city for twenty-five years muttering "apt proverbs" in broken English that are "often ludicrous, always hot and pithy." Smith plays with the irony of an enslaved man who is seen as crazy for wanting his freedom, and the whitewasher's seemingly crazed sayings are of the same tenor as the most "rational" minds of the time: "And as to his sayings, is not Wall Street full of them?"[110]

In the sketch "The Boot-Black," Smith challenges the notion that Black bodyminds are inherently prone to disease by connecting the choice of hard work with the attainment of good mental and physical health. The bootblack is described as a man who rises from poverty through the work of his bare hands and is finally rewarded with great wealth. He is able to purchase a home with a view of the wealthy Livingston Manor, the plantation on which he was once enslaved. The narrator finds the bootblack admirable because he seized the opportunity for self-determination on the 1827 Emancipation Day in New York; when he "found himself in possession of himself," he took a seemingly lowly job and made the best use of it. Smith depicts him as an industrious man. The bootblack's work, he writes, led him to "*stoop to conquer, and he has conquered.*"[111] Further, Smith presents the bootblack as a man who maximizes his mental faculties; in opposition to phrenological stances on Black people, the bootblack's faculties are not predetermined or fixed by his race: "He knew, years ago, that his calling was looked down upon. But wiser than dandy opinion, he found it and has proved it . . . well fitted for him to exercise by means of it all the faculties which make a man useful to his family and a credit to the State." More than being useful to his family prosperity and contributing economic benefits to the nation-state, the hard-working bootblack attained the optimal mental and physical health. At the end of the sketch, Smith switches the narrative perspective from that of the narrator to the subject himself, thereby casting the bootblack's voice and logic on the reader. Any reader who would be dissuaded from following his example on account of the seemingly low-level work is scorned: "[He] laughs to scorn the vaporing *principled martyrs* who would rather starve for good physical or mental [sic], than handle a shoe-brush."[112]

Although Smith often describes the physical heads of the characters to contradict the logics of racialized science, in "The Sexton," he plays into them to make a point about exploitative behavior within the Black community. The sexton, suspected of making an exorbitant amount of money by burying an unusually high number of Black people, is rumored without proof to have eaten them. This shady figure, whom Smith sarcastically calls a "hero," and his associated dealings are adjoined to bodily disfigurement:

> Our hero was of gigantic height, with broad double-jointed shoulders, bowed legs and a head to match.... His mother must have brooded in charnel houses, fascinated with vampire fancies, or he never would have come into the world with that huge, misshapen head! His eyes were large, prominent and staring, with the whites visible all round, and seemed to have been placed at different times and unsymmetrical places in his head; they were no more than a pair than if they had belonged to different persons.[113]

The sketch ends with a cliff-hanger. The day the city inspector arrives to inquire about whether the sexton is guilty of wrongdoing, he has disappeared, never to be heard from again. Sexton does not merely lack traits highlighted by phrenologists such as benevolence and compassion; Smith points to a more complex behavior—capitalistic exploitation—that was associated with systematic actions that were beyond the scope of personality traits for which race scientists accounted.

In "The Editor," Smith portrays a professional whose mental capacity is deemed inferior by white standards but is highly esteemed within the Black community. Despite the lack of an elite education or even literacy, the editor is respected in the community: "Next to the pulpit, and behind the chairs, no place has greater charms for colored Americans than a seat *in* the chair editorial." When describing the newspaper editor, Smith mirrors the language of his medical writings and comments on his physical characteristics and his temperament: "hair, crisp; complexion, sambo; temperament, sanguine." Yet, he breaks with this static description by offering more context regarding how he is viewed by his own community. The editor's mental state is described in terms that by the standards of racist scientific discourses could be associated with mental disease, particularly emotional excess: "His mental structure is elastic, wiry, with that peculiar disposition to excess, which takes the complexion of the hour and wears it like a well-fitting garment."[114] Here, his flexible yet strong mental state does not overwhelm the editor or lead to mental instability, as medical professionals postulated; the editor has full control over his mind and is able to use it to his advantage. The imagery of the well-fitted garment suggests his "elastic and wiry" mind can be used as an adornment or a means of extending appeal and even supporting his body rather than diminishing it.

Smith undercuts the notion of white innate superiority through an affirmation that Blacks would exceed whites given ample opportunity for betterment in "The Inventor." The sketch focuses on the work of "handicraftsmen," work that he sees as requiring the same intelligence as that of a scientist or any other middle-class professional. By virtue of their struggle to survive stiff competition, Smith affirms that Black workers "must not only *equal* but *excel* their white competitors." This demonstration of excellence is only possible because of the untapped and inherent existence of the "untutored intellect of the negro against the accumulated experience and hereditary skill of the whites." But rather than present white success in terms of their passed down intelligence or skill, he discusses it in terms of the fabrication of artificial power and historical violence, writing that whites were "born to excel" in "contrivance" and "blood shedding." He reveals that white opposition to Black skilled tradespeople is an implicit acknowledgement that Blacks are fully capable of excelling and that Blacks should prove them right: "Their opposition therefore betrays their consciousness that we may compete and win. It is our business to confirm their fears." He uses a southern enslaved mechanic, who is both the "ablest mechanic" in the state and a "mechanical genius," as an example of what Blacks could achieve if given ample opportunity.[115]

In his final sketch, "The Schoolmaster (continued)," Smith returns to his signature style of marshalling statistics to make points about racial equality. Before portraying his subject, Smith addresses readers as if they are students in a classroom where the primary lesson is the refutation of the work of a scientist named David Ansted, who used faulty statistics to say that free Blacks are "idle, useless and unimproving." Smith condemns the conclusions as "the most cruel abuse and misrepresentation of the free colored people of our free States!" Smith accuses Ansted of carrying out a "suppression of the truth" when he presents statistics that suggest the Black population in New England grew only by 6 percent (between 1820 and 1850). Smith writes that the sample size "is too small a number of human beings to afford reliable data in vital statistics." He shows that the statistics actually are more in line with the population of England "who are admitted to be the most normal population on the face of the earth!"

Smith adds that Blacks live longer and that higher proportions of their people in every age group are "physically and intellectually, the superior class" in America. In a final mocking of phrenology, he writes that the schoolmaster has an "average forehead" and is "frank and child-like" but still is fully capable of fostering the promise of these superior Blacks.[116] The end of the sketches is thus forward looking and hopeful that Blacks will be able to break down the challenges of racism through their physical and mental grit and aptitude and to participate as peers in a world more equal and unified irrespective of race.

The sketches served as different weapons on which Smith drew to counter racist medical, scientific, and psychiatric claims. Although at times he engaged in direct refutation of racist medical and scientific claims, with the title "Heads of the Colored People" being a reference to phrenology, for example, there are many more instances in which Smith conceptualized race outside the logics of medicine and science entirely. The "Heads" sketches offered Smith a different avenue for knowing and imagining Black people and Black life. Through them, he created visions of Black futures that were unavailable in the constraining medical and scientific genres in which he frequently wrote. "Heads" had a broader audience that actually included the Black people whom the enterprises of science, medicine, and psychiatry purported to know so well. The short sketches were rooted in Black vernacular and oral traditions in which speakers could impart lessons as a part of parables. Smith's lessons were not for individuals, but for the entire Black community. He proclaimed that the Black bodymind was healthy, capable, and fully poised to create lives outside the choke hold of slavery and racial prejudice.

Together Smith's scientific, medical, and literary writings constitute a powerful Black intellectual counternarrative to proslavery medical and psychiatric discourses and provide a vibrant representation of a thriving Black bodymind in the nineteenth century. He was invested in presenting himself as an intellectual equal to his white learned peers. Fighting fire with fire, he showed himself to be fully capable of making arguments using the modes of analysis that were most respected during his time. Besides proving his points, his mastery of formal medical language, statistical tabulations, and official reportage made him an embodied contradiction to arguments about Black mental debasement. Still, the very characteristics that made him a formidable opponent of proslavery discourses also often trapped him within the frameworks he hoped to critique. His literary sketches are a partial answer to this conundrum, but their reach and appeal were not as broad as other popular forms of Black writing.

Some of the most powerful critiques of the foundational arguments of proslavery psychiatry and racist medical discourses came from nonmedicalized sources and laypeople. The medical and psychiatric claim that slavery was beneficial to Black bodyminds was taken on indirectly by Black writers who furnished electrifying indictments of slavery in one of the most popular literary genres of the nineteenth century—the slave narrative. Writing from the inside looking out and as a fugitive slave, Harriet Jacobs made a convincing case for the various ways that slavery harmed Black bodyminds. As the next chapter shows, her sustained discussion of Black women, whose race and gender informed their embodied experiences of mental disability, challenged the idea that freedom was the source of mental distress. She made a clear argument for the cultural contextualization of slavery as the root cause of not only Black mental disability but also Black mental suffering.

3

PSYCHOLOGICAL COSTS OF BLACK WOMEN'S ENSLAVEMENT IN HARRIET JACOBS'S *INCIDENTS IN THE LIFE OF A SLAVE GIRL* (1861)

> We looked at each other, and the eyes of both were moistened with tears. We had escaped from slavery, and we supposed ourselves to be safe from the hunters. But we were alone in the world, and we had left dear ties behind us; ties cruelly sundered by the demon Slavery.
>
> —HARRIET JACOBS, *INCIDENTS IN THE LIFE OF A SLAVE GIRL*

In June of 1842, after nearly three decades of being enslaved in the home of a sinister white physician by the name of Dr. James Norcom in Eaton, North Carolina, Harriet Jacobs was finally free, at least in one way. Freedom for enslaved women like Jacobs could be formal, in terms of legalized emancipation, but more often it was not state sanctioned. Instead, it meant being free of the physical and emotional brutality of life in slavery. In the first self-authored slave narrative written by a Black woman, *Incidents in the Life of a Slave Girl, Written by Herself* (henceforth *Incidents*), Jacobs writes about her life in slavery and journey to freedom. With the help of well-known abolitionist and suffragist Lydia Maria Child, Jacobs was able to tell her story in her own words. Although the book enjoyed a wide readership during the nineteenth century, it was only in the 1980s that *Incidents* was rediscovered and recognized as a foundational text in the Black literary canon. Audiences then and now have been riveted by Jacobs's account of executing a masterful plan to hide in her grandmother's tiny garret for seven years in an effort to push Norcom to sell her two children.[1] Once certain that they were out of her master's grip, she fled to the North. There, she realized that one of the vilest aspects of slavery—the mental suffering it created—was not peculiar to the South. She was free from some forms of emotional distress but vulnerable to new ones. Even on the ship that took her and her friend Fanny to the "free soil" of Philadelphia, the two grief-stricken mothers did not cry tears of joy for their liberation but somberly meditated on the emotional costs of freedom. The "demon Slavery" had made them alone in a world of strangers, alienated from their children and the family ties that had once sustained them.[2] Even in the land of freedom, they had to be constantly on guard. Legal mandates like the 1850 Fugitive Slave Law made freedom fragile, fleeting, and easily reversible, perversely turning freedom into a new form of mental torture. In her narrative, Jacobs recounts how the law dismantled families in ways similar to southern auction blocks: instead of being forcefully broken up by a slave master on a plantation sustained by southern laws, families in the North were under the constant threat of being fractured by federal laws doing the bidding of a distant master.

Continuing the previous chapter's turn to voices outside the mainstream psychiatric and medical establishments concerning Black mental disability, this chapter focuses in depth on slavery, the most consequential institution of confinement and psychic wounding in the Black experience, from the vantage point of the enslaved. Focusing on practices like the severing of family ties, this chapter uncovers the multidimensional forms of harm slavery created. Although slave narratives did not always include extended discussions about the linkages between these practices and mental disability, it was nonetheless a significant theme. The historian Tyler Parry asserts that even brief reflections in slave narratives "reveal how systemic brutalities damaged the victims' psychological and emotional health." This chapter contributes to scholarship that considers psychic wounding among enslaved and formerly enslaved people.[3] It enhances this literature by accounting for the various ways the violence of slavery specifically affected Black women's and girls' mental health. However, the significance of *Incidents* extends beyond the documentation of instances of mental disability among enslaved people. In the same vein as previous Black feminist scholarship, I view Jacobs as an early Black feminist interlocutor and producer of knowledge.[4] Theri Pickens reminds us that literary writers "speak back to critics." We as scholars can consider the ways that, rather than merely bringing attention to topics that their societies find consequential, writers are "drivers of [such] conversations."[5]

Jacobs presented alternative conceptualizations of Black mental health and sickness that circulated alongside the theoretical assumptions and claims of white, mostly male, nineteenth-century physicians. In other words, Jacobs offered not only historical *facts* about the occurrence of mental disability but also alternative *ideas* about Black mental health that constituted a counter-discourse. Accessing such counter-discourses has been challenging for scholars. Extant work in the history of medicine, asylum studies, and studies on insanity have mostly centered around the perspectives of medical authorities. In part, this omission is a by-product of the sources available. Medical records, physicians' papers, and medical textbooks discussed Black people, but such forms of writing aimed to convey the administrative practices and perspectives of those in positions of authority.[6] With the exception of articles by the prominent Black intellectual and physician James McCune Smith, the subject of the previous chapter, Black discursive conceptualizations of mental health were not formally documented. This dearth of archival materials would suggest, falsely, that Black thinkers and writers were silent on the topic. This chapter follows a Black feminist methodological imperative to turn to Black literary productions to access that which is often silenced in archival sources—the interiority of Black life and thought. In response to the lingering notions of Thomas Jefferson, who questioned Black people's capacity for feeling, Jacobs demonstrates that Black people felt deeply.[7] During the antebellum period, Black voices were most lucid in the abolitionist movement. Black writers produced hundreds of narratives to bring attention to the horrors of enslavement. This chapter aims to bring into view Black people's experiences of mental disability during slavery and uncover sophisticated Black conceptualizations about those experiences in contrast to the discourses of predominantly white medical authorities.[8] To depict the horrors of enslavement, Jacobs drew upon the language at her disposal, which included the vocabulary of the rapidly expanding field of psychiatry. Although she made use of this language, her evidentiary pathway was based in an alternative arena of power often occupied by enslaved healers. As the historian of medicine Sharla Fett argues, in these arenas, enslaved doctoring men and women "asserted the primacy of their experiences and sensibilities."[9] Like enslaved healers, Jacobs's intellectual authority on matters of mental health derived from her empirical experience and existed outside the confines of the medical training undertaken by physicians such as her slave master and antagonist, who was an apprentice of Benjamin Rush, the father of modern psychiatry.

Although today we might easily recognize the causal relationship between the institution of slavery and the psychological strain mothers like Jacobs endured, nineteenth-century mental health authorities, slave masters, and physicians like Dr. Norcom had a different view.[10] Unlike Jacobs, they did not see a major social system of the time—slavery—as a cause. As extant medical records show, physicians relied on slaveholders' descriptions to diagnose mental disability among enslaved people.[11] These included references to psychological and physiological causes but did not mention social order, let alone the views of the so-called "colored insane." Because members of the psychiatric establishment did not see slavery as an incubator for mental disability, they could not imagine the curative methods that surface in Jacobs's narrative. For example, as I discuss later, Jacobs identified the maintenance of kinship networks as a coping mechanism for mental distress stemming from familial severance.

Furthermore, unlike whites with mental disabilities during the nineteenth century, Black people did not write madness narratives.[12] Nevertheless, their ideas about mental disability can be found in hundreds of nineteenth-century songs, plays, poems, folktales, and especially slave narratives, the most popular genre of the period. As the late Black feminist literary critic Barbara Christian contended, Blacks theorize about American culture, society, and life in their cultural productions.[13] Jacobs's "true tale of slavery" provides a window into the conditions under which the "colored insane" labored and a sustained meditation on mental disability during slavery. In contrast to the writings of the white men of psychiatric medicine, Jacobs's narrative reveals that slavery itself was the root cause of mental instability among the enslaved. To pinpoint this theory in *Incidents*, this chapter provides a literary analysis of how language and literary form, historical and cultural context, and authorial perspectives work together to shape meaning about mental disability in the narrative.

The narrative is also an important source of insight into Black women's experiences of mental suffering. Many male-authored slave narratives illuminated the psychological repercussions of slavery for Black women to some degree. However, Jacobs was especially attentive to the distinct experiences of Black women; this is best captured in her oft-quoted proclamation, "Slavery is terrible for men; but it is far more terrible for women. Superadded to the burden common to all, *they* have wrongs, and sufferings, and mortifications peculiarly their own."[14] *Incidents* stands as the most well-developed piece of writing on the intersecting effects of race and gender during slavery.[15] Literary scholars have given apt attention to this aspect of the narrative. Yet to be sufficiently examined, however, are the implications of enslaved women's distinct raced and gendered subjectivity for mental health. Through literary depictions of the stifling that she and "two millions [*sic*] of women at the [South]"[16] faced under slavery, Jacobs articulates various ways the institution psychologically wounded Black women, illustrating the devastating mental harm caused by forms of violence that were integral to the practice of slavery vis-à-vis Black women—sexualized violence, forced and controlled reproduction, separation from children between and within plantations, runaway attempts, exposure to violence, and hazardous labor conditions. To show how these practices hindered mental health, Jacobs chronicles enslaved peoples' experiences of aloneness, anguish, sorrow, sadness, desolation, fear, and anxiety. Her descriptions of these psychological aspects of enslavement rival images of whips, chains, and physical abuse that saturate histories of slavery and contemporary popular culture imaginings. Jacobs's descriptions of psychological forms of pain and illness offer a more textured understanding of the mental health conditions of Black women as part of her abolitionist project.

Approaching *Incidents* as a work of literature, I render an analysis of various themes, narrative sketches, and intertextualities in the narrative that demonstrate Jacobs's conceptions of the "psychological costs" of enslavement.[17] What becomes clear is that Jacobs's narrative troubled visions of resiliency and resistance during slavery.[18] In *Incidents*, enslaved women's embodied experiences of mental suffering were vexed, multilayered, and ongoing. Analysis reveals that Jacobs's outlook aligned with an African-derived healing ontology that drew attention to the holistic, interconnected, and multifactorial nature of mental health. In her literary landscape, mental trauma was not separable from physical trauma and vice versa.[19] For her, health depended jointly on biological and physiological processes, environmental context, and significantly, social position. In this formulation, health status cannot be detached from the cultural and social world in which it is experienced.[20] Jacobs's narrative brought into focus the ways in which early American psychiatry and its handling of Black mental health were inextricably tied to and shaped by the US history of slavery and capitalist enterprise.

"CRIES REPLY TO CURSES, SHRIEKS TO BLOWS": THE MENTAL ASYLUM AS A METAPHOR FOR SLAVERY

One feature of slave narratives is their intertextuality. Slave narrators drew on literary texts to convey new meaning. Jacobs had opportunities to become familiar with popular literary texts after she escaped from slavery. In 1849, Jacobs spent eighteen months in Rochester, New York, where she worked in an antislavery reading room and bookstore above Frederick Douglass's *The North Star* office. She also had access to the library of her New York employers Nathaniel Parker Willis and Cordelia Grinnell Willis. Jacobs's audience was mainly white women in the North, whom she hoped to inspire to act against slavery. That audience would have been familiar with the work of British romantic writers, and Jacobs capitalized on this familiarity through her use of Lord Byron's poem "The Lament of Tasso" to theorize about life under slavery.[21] In "The Lover," a chapter that appears early in the narrative, she meditates on how seemingly universal human desires, such as the pursuit of romantic love, were fraught for slaves. To illuminate the distress, she makes a striking comparison between slavery and asylums. The included Byron stanza suggests that the southern slave system assaulted the enslaved such that its confinement was akin to living in a mental asylum.

The circumstances around the production of the Byron poem are significant for understanding how it aids Jacobs's arguments about mental suffering and slavery. Byron is said to have been inspired to write it after visiting the cell of Torquato Tasso, a prominent sixteenth-century Italian poet confined to the Asylum of St. Anna's in Ferrara, Italy, from 1579 to 1586. That Jacobs, to write about slavery, samples a poem by an allegedly mentally disabled poet, writing about a poet who had been confined to a mental asylum, is more than just evidence of literary sophistication. Jacobs's use of Byron was significant in both its analogical implications and its limitations. In other words, we must consider how she engaged British Romantic poetry as well as how she broke with it to emphasize the particularity of the correlation between confinement and mental suffering for the enslaved in mid-nineteenth-century America. The Byron poem captures the essence of Tasso's lived experiences of mental torment during confinement.

Below the introductory phrase, "A land," Jacobs quotes four lines of Byron's fourth stanza:

> Where laughter is not mirth; nor thought the mind;
> Nor words a language; nor e'en men mankind.
> Where cries reply to curses, shrieks to blows,
> And each is tortured in his separate hell.[22]

Jacobs made a crucial rhetorical move when she included an introductory fragment consisting of only two words—"A land." The fragment prompts the reader to pause and focus on what will be a striking comparison between the southern slave system and the "madhouse." Jacobs's use of metaphor fit within a larger context of Black autobiographical writing that drew on metaphor to convey meaning indirectly. Jacobs exemplified how metaphor made possible new ways of conceptualizing the world of mid-nineteenth-century America. Drawing on Monroe Beardsley's theory of metaphor, William Andrews emphasizes the function of metaphor in slave narratives: "True metaphors reveal new and infinitely paraphraseable [sic] meanings of words in unexpected contexts, by introducing a tension, a 'logical absurdity'... metaphors do not simply adorn arguments for persuasive purposes. *Metaphors are arguments* [emphasis mine]."[23]

Jacobs's narrative used metaphor to make an argument about how best to understand the "land of her birth." Her metaphor did not oppose but diverged from dominant understandings of slavery as gruesome, repulsive, and brutal, primarily because these descriptors are measured by harm to the body. She suggested that slavery is also by definition "mad," in relation to its composition and effect on subjects. In composition, slavery was in equal parts irrational, disordered, and utterly absurd.

Experientially, it was psychologically isolating, torturous, destructive, and ultimately illness-producing. Thus, for Jacobs, the first half of the Byron poem accurately described the character of slavery as an institution of confinement in which there was a disjuncture in the expected correlations between affect and state of mind. In her discussions about madness in the North, Jacobs, like Byron, showed that "laughter" did not indicate happiness, "thoughts" were not linked to a rational state of mind, words did not lend themselves to meaning via language, and men did not embody the ideals of human existence.

Jacobs's metaphorical alignment of medicalized spaces like asylums with slavery allowed her to name social disorder in relationship to "real" health outcomes, which makes *Incidents* simultaneously a slave narrative and an "illness narrative."[24] Bringing mental disability to the fore, Jacobs offered an alternative perspective on Black mental disability during slavery. In contrast to the renowned nineteenth-century asylum reformer Dorothea Dix's claim that there were "comparatively very few" cases of mental disability among the "negro" in the South, Jacobs suggested that southern slavery created psychological illness through confinement, sheer terror, and ongoing abuse.[25] The Byron stanza helped her articulate her experiences within a system that was maddening. It depicts slavery as a torturous form of confinement that entraps each individual, a hellish existence, and an institution in which violence or "curses" beget "cries," expressing emotional distress, and "shrieks," expressing mental torment.

Jacobs's conceptions about how slavery creates mental suffering for enslaved women specifically appear in the chapter titled "The Trials of Girlhood." As Jacobs makes clear, psychological torment caused by sexualized violence and the threat of such violence began early in enslaved women's lives. With this chapter, she planted her narrative squarely within the bildungsroman genre, only to reveal how her own coming-of-age story was perverted by a psychologically assaultive institution. She declares: "But I now entered on my fifteenth year—a sad epoch in the life of a slave girl. My master began to whisper foul words in my ear."[26] Certainly, Jacobs is appealing to her northern audience's sensitivity to gothic fiction's paradigm of "moral insanity." Mid-nineteenth-century writers believed that a woman's purity could be corrupted by captivity in the underworld. Exposure of a woman to illicit sex would serve as "mental rape" or "corrupt her mind" and eventually lead to actual "sexual transgression."[27] Jacobs conveys the mental suffering caused by the physical terror she experienced as she was subjected to moral corruption: "Sometimes he had stormy, terrific ways, that made his victims tremble." She used a semicolon to adjoin the phrase, "sometimes he assumed a gentleness that he thought must surely subdue," which suggests that the threat of violence is exacerbated by the unpredictability of its occurrence. Jacobs informs the reader that such uncertainty produces severe anxiety for a slave girl: "Soon she will learn to tremble when she hears her master's footfall."[28] Dr. Norcom's repeated use of intimidation to pursue his aims is an example of what Saidiya Hartman referred to as "reasoned and routinized terror."[29] Jacobs's experience of fear in and of itself was not a sign of mental disability, but the resulting sorrow and anxiety indicated how slavery was predicated on unremitting mental suffering.

An emblematic, chilling example of this indirect connection between psychic wounding, sexualized violence, and everyday practices of slavery appears in a vignette about a family torn apart by a cruel slave master that Jacobs incorporated into *Incidents*. The family's story, featuring the familiar trope of the "good master turned bad by slavery," includes a portrait of a girl who went "mad." The family, Jacobs explains, lived in a cottage on a plantation owned by a woman who inherited the land and its slaves. The mistress, a "humane slaveholder," allowed the mother, father, and six children to live freely, which meant that they, as Jacobs puts it, "had never felt slavery." But after the mistress took a cruel planter for a husband, the family was "convinced of [slavery's] reality." The new husband insisted on the property relations of enslavement, effectively dismantling the family structure. Jacobs casually chronicles the six children's fates: two male children were sold to Georgia, one girl was too young for work, the oldest girl bore children by the master and was sold with her offspring to his brother, another girl bore five daughters, and the middle girl "went crazy." "The life she was compelled to lead," writes Jacobs, "drove her mad."[30] Jacobs's assessment conveys that the psychological strain of witnessing family dismantlement and sexual exploitation while knowing that the same fate awaits oneself contributes to madness. Some might see the fact that the girl does not become an object of physical and/or sexual exploitation as a subversive use of madness. Indeed, some enslaved people used madness to resist.[31] But more often than not, as *Incidents* repeatedly showcases, the unrelenting forms of violence in slavery psychologically wounded, sometimes chronically, Black female slaves.³² As Byron notes, each was "tortured" in a "separate hell."

Jacobs's appropriation of the Byron poem linked confinement in slavery to confinement in asylums and mental disease, but perhaps most significant is what Jacobs did not use. The remainder of stanza four of Byron's "Lament" features the speaker's decision to abstain from vindictiveness against his oppressors, lines that Jacobs did not include:

> Would I not pay them back these pangs again,
> And teach them inward sorrow's stifled groan?
> The struggle to be calm, and cold distress,
> Which undermines our Stoical success?
> No!—still too proud to be vindictive—I
> Have pardoned princes' insults, and would die.
> Yes, Sister of my Sovereign! for thy sake
> I weed all bitterness from out my breast,
> It hath no business where *thou* art a guest;
> Thy brother hates—but I can not detest;
> Thou pitiest not—but I can not forsake.³³

Jacobs chose to appropriate the description of the conditions of the asylum but not the speaker's *response* to the experience. Because Jacobs was writing a slave narrative, a genre for which the central goal was abolition, there was neither place for such pacifying nor narrative space for an exposition of the irony that would make it suitable for a slave narrative. Thus, in subsequent passages, Jacobs's stance is as clear as it is stringent. Coupled with her summarization of the system—"the degradation, the wrongs, the vices, that grow out of slavery, are more than I can describe"— is a statement that directly opposes Byron's speaker: "My soul revolted against the mean tyranny."³⁴ In the place of restraint is rebellion. Jacobs's project depicted the plight of the enslaved and explicated active *responses* to psychological assault. Her proclamation suggests that, in contrast to Byron's speaker, the appropriate response for the slave was resistance. Jacobs offered a wide range of forms that active resistance might take. Her own grand form of resistance was voluntary confinement, when she concealed herself in her grandmother's attic as part of her plan to free her children and herself.

"THE MAD BLACK WOMAN IN THE ATTIC": MENTAL DISABILITY WITHIN CONFINEMENT

Although Jacobs's use of the Byron poem makes slavery metaphorically confining, an analysis of Jacobs's experiences in actual spaces of confinement draws attention to the multilayered forms of psychological torment enslaved people endured even when resisting. Considering the infamous attic as a space of resistance recalls the tradition of white women writers who showcased the image of the "madwoman in the attic." For feminist literary scholars, the madwoman has signified resistance—either as a reflection of rebellion against nineteenth-century patriarchal authorial authority or as an example of subversive mad female characters. The first generation of Black literary scholars cautioned against faithful comparisons between Jacobs and white heroines. Jean Fagan Yellin does not see Jacobs's garret experience as reflective of the nineteenth-century trope because "she [was] completely sane."[35] Certainly, Jacobs's garret scenes were about a literal experience of confinement. By her own account, however, Jacobs was *not* completely sane throughout her time in the attic. The question, then, is not whether depictions of mental disability appear in *Incidents* but how and for what purposes.

This line of questioning forces us to consider the ways mental suffering became a consequence of Jacobs's attainment of freedom. Although Jacobs's aims differ from those of white women writers of the period, a more historically contextualized reading of Victorian representations of madwomen reveals important insights about the relationship between psychiatric beliefs and literary representation. Consider how Charlotte Bronte's character Bertha Mason echoed the psychiatric thought of the day. Bronte's depiction of the origin of Mason's "insanity"—diseased maternal heredity and the periodicity of her menstrual cycle—aligned with the nineteenth-century belief that "the reproductive system was the source of mental illness in women."[36] Thus, in at least one way—engaging the pathologizing psychiatric thought of the day concerning insanity among women—Jacobs did join such heroines.

Psychiatrists would have read Jacobs more harshly, using different terms than Bronte's readers. For one, Jacobs's engagement with psychiatric thought is embedded in her opposition to slavery and is thus more adversarial than Bronte's. The unique conditions of Black women's mental health were erased in nineteenth-century discourses about the "female insane" in which female inevitably meant *white*. Further, Black women's particular experiences of mental disability were conflated with those of Black men, which is most evident in ubiquitous references to the "colored insane" in medical records and popular culture. This double negation reflects the ways in which Black women are often marginalized in discourses about race and gender when it comes to experiences of mental disability.[37] Jacobs's narrative carved out space for enslaved Black women's particular experiences by insisting on the role of sexual predation in mental suffering. At the same time, she rejected pathologizing narratives around the origins of mental disability, locating the origins instead in the institution of slavery by showing how it created raced and gendered psychological harm. This harm occurred even when she, like other enslaved mothers, resisted ongoing sexualized violence and denials of reproductive autonomy.

Jacobs's description of her seven-year confinement in her grandmother's tiny attic illuminates the correlation between mindful resistance and inadvertent madness. For refusing to be her master's concubine, Jacobs was sent several miles away to his Auburn plantation. When she learned that her children would soon be joining her there in order to "break" them, she decided to execute her plan to hide in her grandmother's attic. Although she could see and hear her children from the attic, only her grandmother and brother knew she was in the nine-foot by seven-foot by three-foot hiding place. Precisely because the attic experience was unfathomable to her audience, Jacobs had the twofold task of authenticating its occurrence and depicting its horror. With respect to the former, today's reader has the benefit of extensive corroboratory archival research.[38] In *Incidents*, Jacobs powerfully depicts the terror of her imprisonment. For example, she suffered from lifelong rheumatism resulting from her long confinement in the tiny space. Jacobs writes about this lasting effect: "But it is a fact; and to me a sad one, even now; for my body still suffers from the effects of that long imprisonment, to say nothing of my soul."[39] Her emphasis on multilayered harm did not reflect seventeenth-century Western philosophical conceptions about the dualism of the mind and body in constructions of the self. Rather, Jacobs's discussion of her long-term emotional scarring reflected what the historian Nell Irvin Painter calls *soul murder*, which "may be summed up as depression, lowered self-esteem, and anger" resulting from physical, mental, and sexualized violence in slavery.[40] Jacobs's discussion of the mental and physical suffering she endured offers a more holistic account of slavery's injuries.

Jacobs begins her portrayal of her psychological deterioration in the attic by highlighting how her long confinement created an array of physical disabilities. During her second of seven winters there, she lost the ability to speak because her face and tongue were stiffened by the brutally cold weather. Under these same conditions, Jacobs lost consciousness for sixteen hours. After regaining consciousness, her speech was disabled again, and this time the manifestation included psychological dimensions: she became "delirious, and was in great danger of betraying [herself] and [her] friends." Whereas the first form of speech impairment was a threat to her health, the second jeopardized her freedom and endangered the entire family. Their initial solution was to "stupef[y] [her] with drugs." The language here is revealing: to stupefy is to make one unable to think or feel properly. In essence, her grandmother and brother chose to fight fire with fire because they recognized that her illness was of a psychological nature. Even after attempts to treat her with drugs, for six weeks Jacobs was "weary in body" and "sick at heart," which suggested that she saw the physical and psychological effects of confinement as separate yet related and equally powerful.[41]

In response to Jacobs's manifestation of mental disability, her brother John brought her drugs from a Thompsonian, a doctor who practiced an early form of homeopathy. Naming the doctor as a "Thompsonian" signaled Jacobs's participation in the nineteenth-century women's health reform movement that opposed mainstream medicine.[42] Jacobs literally opposed her physician enslaver, who knew full well that she had endured psychological illness. In an earlier scene where Jacobs was pregnant with her second child, bedridden, and "ill in mind and body," Dr. Norcom was called. When he entered the room, she became "weak and nervous" and responded by "screaming" as if his very presence was a trigger.[43] Following her family's advice, Norcom retreated so her condition would not worsen. He, like other nineteenth-century physicians, would have recognized this behavior as indicative of insanity. As a former private pupil of Benjamin Rush, Norcom would have likely agreed with his mentor that derangement was characterized by "every departure of the mind in its perceptions, judgments, and reasonings, from its natural and habitual order, accompanied with corresponding actions."[44] He would have not only seen Jacobs's behavior as a form of mental derangement but also agreed that, if it escalated, it could result in death.[45] The ejection of Norcom in the sickbed scene was metaphorical for the rejection of mainstream nineteenth-century approaches to psychiatry. Psychiatric therapeutic practices heralded by Rush included strong drugs, tonics, bleeding, laxatives, warm or cold baths, sedatives, and sometimes physical restraint. Affirming alternative treatments, Jacobs noted that "herbs, roots, and ointments" from the Thompsonian doctor helped her. She explained that her physical scars slowly healed but her "sickness at heart" continued. She was so distraught that she nearly admits to suicidal thoughts: "Dark thoughts passed through my mind as I lay there day after day."[46] Jacobs was not alone in this respect; descriptions of suicidal ideation appear in many slave narratives, including those written by Olaudah Equiano, Frederick Douglass, and Mattie Johnson.[47] Highlighting his own wish to die while enslaved, Frederick Douglass wrote, "I often found myself regretting my own existence, and wishing myself dead; and but for the hope of being free, I have no doubt but that I should have killed myself, or done something for which I should have been killed." Looking out to the Chesapeake Bay, Douglass contemplated both the possibility of escape and the harsh realities of bondage. Rampant thoughts and open dialogues with God, Douglass declared, "goaded [him] almost to madness."[48] Until Jacobs's escape, we find evidence of similar forms of psychological deterioration. In the chapter titled "Preparations for Escape," Jacobs writes, "At times, I was stupefied and listless; at other times I became very impatient to know when these dark years would end."[49] Again she uses the word "stupefy," but in this case confinement, rather than drugs, caused it. Her comments suggest that during her confinement Jacobs oscillated between moments of mental stability and prolonged phases of distress and anxiety.

Beyond its function as a means of achieving freedom, then, the garret *experience* was primarily a place of bodily suffering that combined mental and physical torments. At times, Jacobs claims her mental distress trumped her physical pain. She makes a striking statement when she describes her initial escape from her master's Auburn plantation, during which she was forced to hide in the bushes. Describing a poisonous reptile bite, she comments, "The dread of being disabled was greater than the physical pain I endured." The opposition she sets up between "dread" and "physical pain" reflects her belief that the latter was neither her sole form of suffering nor the dominant one. This hierarchy also appears in depictions of another stop on the journey to the attic, a temporary hiding place at her friend Betty's home. She begins with vivid descriptions of her physical affliction: "The pain in my leg was so intense that it seemed as if I should drop," but after noting that Betty offered "some nice hot supper," Jacobs writes, "Betty's vocation led her to think eating the most important thing in life. She did not realize that my heart was too full for me to care much about supper." Jacobs not only indicates a distinction but also places more weight on the emotional challenges she faced. It was with this state of mind, the belief that physical pain was often secondary to mental suffering, that Jacobs spent seven years in the attic. This continued even as she fled to the ship that would carry her to freedom: "My brain was all of a whirl, and my limbs tottered under me."[50] Jacobs presents the struggle for freedom as affecting her body in both mental and physical ways. Her depiction, however, stands in opposition to the perspectives of physicians like Samuel Cartwright, who pathologized "absconding from service" as indicative of the so-called mental disorder drapetomania.[51] Jacobs's emphasis on the mental suffering that accompanied running away suggests that slavery created the conditions for ill health but escaping it posed another set of health risks.

Jacobs not only articulated a theory about the origin of mental disability among Black Americans in slavery but also suggested preventative measures and coping mechanisms. The choice not to remain in bondage in narratives of slavery, the "goal of freedom," was not limited to an absence of physical bondage or the acquisition of legal rights but included maintaining intradependence.[52] Escapees underwent tremendous psychological turmoil, but those they left behind were equally distressed. When Jacobs's grandmother learned that her grandson and Jacobs's brother William had gone to the North, she was overcome by despair. Jacobs illustrates the complicated feelings that accompanied the pursuit of freedom: "If you had seen the tears, and heard the sobs, you would have thought the messenger had brought tidings of death instead of freedom."[53] Other slave narratives include stories of women who endured tremendous distress from the threat of being separated from their loved ones. John Brown told the story of a woman named Critty who was married to a man of her choosing before being forced to marry a man her master chose for her. From that union she had no children, which dissatisfied her master so much so that he sold her away to another plantation. She did not recover emotionally from being separated from her husband and kin; within four days, "she died of grief."[54] These examples bear out how being separated from one's family created the circumstances from which mental distress arose for many enslaved women.

These conceptualizations of the roots of mental disability contrasted sharply with the psychiatric thought of the day, which was more interested in the mental suffering of white enslavers. Psychiatrists saw the loss of property, including human property, as a causative condition for the onset of insanity. It followed that because slaves owned no property, their circumstances protected them from insanity. John Minson Galt claimed that "insane slaves" had less severe cases of insanity because they were free of the stress of holding property.[55] Intertwining causation and therapeutics, on the supposedly rare occasion when they did become mentally ill, Galt believed slaves were "more readily yielding to remedial means."[56] Limiting family connections figured importantly in mainstream psychiatric "remedial means," for these practitioners believed that mental healing depended on removing people from their homes and restricting contact with families.[57] In stark contrast, Jacobs's text is concerned with the perils of *being* property rather than losing it. Other slave narratives also point to family bonds as sources of coping and recovery from the psychologically damaging effects of slavery. Charles Ball conveyed that his fraternal connections to his father and son functioned as a source of solace and knowledge about religion-based mental restoration. After a bout of suicidal ideation, Mattie Jackson's grandfather was restored mentally through his connection with his wife.[58] In Jacobs's narrative, preserving family ties was less of an expression of individual liberty and more of a means of maintaining individual and communal sanity.

"SORROWFUL MOTHERS": THE LINKAGES BETWEEN MOTHERHOOD AND MENTAL DISABILITY

Slave narratives as a genre included the theme of motherhood and severed family ties to demonstrate the ruthlessness of slavery. Considering the cultural factors that informed Jacobs's desire to preserve her family in the first place offers a fuller grasp of mental suffering particular to enslaved women. Jacobs suffered in the attic to carry out her obligations as a mother. Enslaved women asserted their womanhood through a variety of gendered subjectivities, including appealing to narratives of collective responsibility, spirituality, and significantly, motherhood.[59] Jacobs's narrative detailed how strained experiences of motherhood led to mental suffering, chiefly as a result of being severed from children. Separation from kinship networks, or "natal alienation," was a defining feature of slavery; as Orlando Patterson asserts, "nothing comes across more dramatically from the hundreds of interviews with American ex-slaves than the fear of separation."[60] Some mothers "went crazy" on account of being separated from their children.[61]

One of the most complete portraits of a sorrowful mother's life appears in Solomon Northup's *Twelve Years a Slave*, which tells the story of a woman named Eliza. Tricked into thinking she would be granted her freedom, Eliza found herself and her children in a slave pen in Washington, DC. At the realization that she was actually to be sold and likely away from her children, she "filled the pen with wailings and expressions of heart-rending woe." When she, her children, and other slaves arrived at a New Orleans slave market, her worst fears were realized. As her son Randall was instructed to run and jump across the floor, Eliza watched, "crying aloud, and wringing her hands." She begged his purchaser to buy the entire family, pleading with him that she would be faithful and obedient. When the man said he could not afford to meet her request, Eliza "burst into a paroxysm of grief." In her final moments with her son, she kissed him profusely and admonished him to remember her. Randall, too young to fully understand, promised his mother that he'd be "a good boy."[62] Only a few weeks later, Eliza's sorrows deepened when she was separated from her daughter, a frightful scene (figure 3.1). Northup imparts that his words were insufficient to capture Eliza's emotions during the ordeal. Her sorrow dwarfed even the natural grief that a mother would have for a dead child:

> It would be a relief if I could consistently pass over in silence the scene that now ensued. It recalls memories more mournful and affecting than any language can portray. I have seen mothers kissing for the last time the faces of their dead offspring; I have seen them looking down into the grave, as the earth fell with a dull sound upon their coffins, hiding

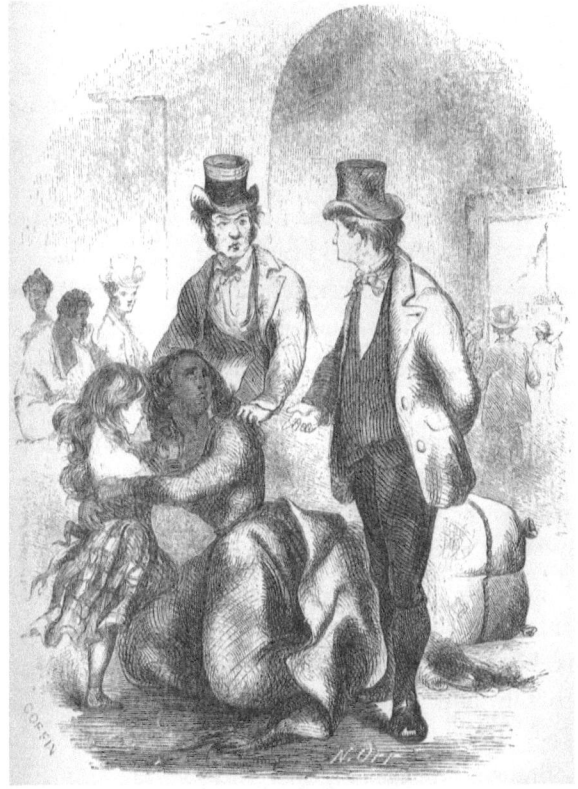

FIGURE 3.1 *Separation of Eliza from Her Last Child.* New York Public Library.

them from their eyes forever; but never have I seen such an exhibition of *intense, unmeasured, and unbounded grief,* as when Eliza was parted from her child [emphasis mine].[63]

Eliza had the heart-wrenching experience of being pulled away from her child as they embraced one another tightly. The weak mother, who before the ordeal was already "haggard and hollow-eyed with sickness and with sorrow," pleaded to be sold along with her daughter to no avail. That day, Eliza felt the deep agony and helplessness that came from having to hear the screams of her child; Emily wailed, "Come back—don't leave me—come back, mama," as she was hauled away.[64]

Northup writes that Eliza broke under the "burden of maternal sorrow," and she never recovered. Her body became physically weak and her approach to life apathetic. Her master was displeased with her work both in the house and in the field; in response, he "lashed and abused her most unmercifully." After all the beatings, her master finally left her alone but with no provisions. For several weeks, she lay motionless on the floor of a ramshackle cabin, left to "linger through a life of pain and wretchedness" until she was found dead by field hands.[65] Eliza's story reveals why enslaved women had such anxiety about being separated from their children, a practice that was inherent to the system of slavery. The law prescribed Black women's relationships with their children even before conception; children belonged to their slave masters even before they were conceived. After children were born, enslaved mothers' workloads made it difficult to attend to their children's needs, causing a substantial amount of sorrow to these mothers.

In *Incidents*, an example of this kind of sorrow appears in Jacobs's description of her daughter Ellen's reaction when they were sent to the Auburn plantation. Much like Jacobs, who did not know she was a slave until age six, Ellen had not felt the sting of slavery growing up. According to Jacobs, Ellen, unaccustomed to abandonment, "broke down under the trials of her new life." Jacobs's ability to protect her child through such turmoil was limited. Immediately upon their arrival, she was sent to work while "[her] little Ellen was left below in the kitchen." The distraught child "wandered about" until she "cried herself sick." Jacobs indicates that witnessing her daughter in such a terrible condition was distressing: "One day, [Ellen] sat under the window where I was at work, crying that weary cry which makes a mother's heart bleed. I was obliged to steel myself to bear it."[66] Jacobs's description, particularly her emphasis on the "cry" that made a mother feel distress, alerts the reader to both her pain as a mother and a strategy she was forced to adopt to cope. Many enslaved mothers had to endure violence toward their children, making it a common source of mental breakdown.[67] Although some mothers, like Jacobs, were able to "steel" themselves, others were unable to handle the grief that came from strained experiences of motherhood and "descend[ed] into madness."[68] Because separation occurred whether or not children were sold, unfortunately this kind of incessant suffering rivaled forms of brutality such as whippings or beatings in scope and prevalence.

Dread over the possibility of separation was also a torture enslaved mothers had to confront. Potential separation "[struck] terror in the hearts of all slaves."[69] This general emotional climate took on a special character for mothers, which Jacobs represents through depictions of their constant feelings of uncertainty and anxiety. In his slave narrative, Henry Bibb describes how his wife Malinda found herself "under great distress of mind" when she learned that her deacon slave master planned to have her husband whipped with five hundred lashes for attending a church service without permission. Henry Bibb decided to run away to avoid the harsh punishment. As a result, the deacon threatened not only the lash but also to sell him away from his family. Malinda was mentally devastated by the proposition. As Bibb reflects, "This was truly heart-rending to my poor wife; the thought of our being torn apart in a strange land after having been sold away from all her friends and relations, was more than she could bear."[70] Because of the potential of family separation, the slave mother, Jacobs contends, was "very watchful" and "[knew] there [was] no security for her children." This watchfulness, Jacobs writes, increased as children aged: "After they have entered their teens she lives in daily expectation of trouble. This leads to many questions."[71] Impending violence created anxiety-laden behaviors such as "watchfulness" and "questioning," as ongoing feelings of insecurity weighed heavily on enslaved women's minds.

Jacobs recounts stories of mothers who experienced a great deal of sorrow, agony, and even thoughts of suicide because they were separated from their children. To illustrate these heightened emotions, Jacobs provides a sketch of an auction from the perspective of an enslaved mother: "But to the slave mother New Year's day comes laden with peculiar sorrows. She sits on her cold cabin floor, watching the children who may all be torn from her the next morning; and often does she wish that she and they might die before the day dawns." Jacobs reveals that the practice of selling children, a mainstay of the institution of slavery, inscribed mental suffering into Black mothers' lives. The institution shaped their perspectives on life and death: from a sense of sorrow about the structure of slave life came a death wish. Among many sketches of sorrowful mothers in the narrative, Jacobs includes one that made a lasting imprint on her. Referring to how one anguished mother watched all seven of her children be sold, Jacobs writes: "I met that mother in the street, and her wild, haggard face lives to-day in my mind. She wrung her hands in anguish, and exclaimed, 'Gone! All gone! Why *don't* God kill me?' I had no words wherewith to comfort her. Instances of this kind are of daily, yea, of hourly occurrence."[72] By juxtaposing the woman's misery and despair with her own inability to console her, Jacobs redirects the question to a broader analysis, illuminating her antislavery theorization. According to Jacobs, only the end of slavery could ensure that future mothers would not suffer in this way. This conclusion stood in contrast to psychiatric conceptions about how mental disability could be cured and treated. Whereas nineteenth-century psychiatrists prescribed more control and constraint, Jacobs's narrative pointed to the dismantling of the institution of slavery as the most effective curative model for Black women's mental health.

Not fastened to any specific diagnosis invented by nineteenth-century psychiatrists such as lunacy, idiocy, or epilepsy, *Incidents* shows that mental suffering included both temporary and prolonged psychological breakage in a slave's life that altered her usual functioning and mental state. Considering changes in behavior as evidence of mental suffering showcases the fact that physical and emotional harm done to enslaved people was tied to pain that in turn registered on their bodies even if it was not apparent. Only one formal photograph of Jacobs is extant (figure 3.2). Three years before she died, Jacobs sat in an ornately carved wooden chair.

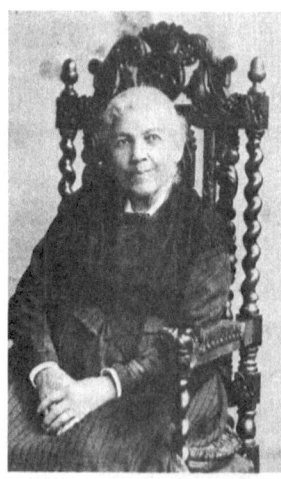

FIGURE 3.2 Harriet Jacobs in 1894. Schomburg Center for Research in Black Culture, Photographs and Prints Division, The New York Public Library.

She sat dignified, with a content expression, a mouth-closed half smile, gentle eyes, and folded hands, the left lightly clasping the right. The chair she sat in upheld her, supporting her chronically ailing body. Even more hidden from view are her mental scars. Invisible are the apparatuses that upheld her mind. Her half smile suggests that in the end, she was happy to some degree. At the time of the picture, Blacks were free, but the racial uplift projects she and her daughter engaged in were curtailed by violent racist backlash in the South.[73] Although she was sadly forced to stop her work educating southern Blacks after the Civil War, she was united with her daughter Louisa. As her narrative suggests, such familial bonds were her source of mental solace.

Incidents' treatment of mental suffering urges us to reassess the fundamental nature of female enslavement and possible responses to domination. We can no longer rely on conclusions about slavery or the health of enslaved people that underemphasize psychological harm. Repeatedly, *Incidents* conveys that the raced and gendered nature of mental suffering in slavery was not trivial; its existence was commonplace. Any assessment of the costs of enslavement for Black women, or enslaved people more generally, must calculate the substantial weight of psychic pain and injury. Further, literary accounts of the enslaved offer insights that nineteenth-century psychiatric accounts completely obscure. Not only did psychiatric thought obfuscate the causes of mental disability, but it also erased enslaved people's strategies for coping and healing. Beyond a more robust understanding of health in slavery, theorizations about mental disability in *Incidents* broaden the conversation about the lasting effect of enslavement and possibilities for redress.

Although her theorizations about Black women's experiences of mental disability are rooted in the Black American experience, Jacobs's ideas are fertile ground for understanding mental disability in other temporal contexts. Her sensitivity toward the ways in which cultural conceptions about Black femininity and routinized practices of terror can create harmful medical conditions makes clearer how trauma is created in communities faced with ongoing practices of police brutality that are inflamed by cultural stereotypes about Black criminality. Her descriptions of the psychological costs of resistance urge us to consider the radical nature of self-care even in the midst of activism and resistance. Above all, *Incidents'* meditations on Black women's psychological wounds during slavery do not make them "crazier" than any other group; in fact, their wounds make them equally human.

Harriet Jacobs, like her younger contemporary Harriet Tubman, was committed to garnering sympathy for Black people for the cause of abolition. But for all her descriptions of mental suffering, Harriet Jacobs never identified as or was labeled "colored insane." Harriet Tubman, as the next chapter will show, not only experienced mental suffering but also lived with a host of symptoms that were seen as evidence of insanity. Through Tubman's life, we see a striking example of how the embodied experiences of mental suffering, to which Jacobs so eloquently alerts us, are always already shaped by culturally informed discourses on mental health.

4

HARRIET TUBMAN AND NINETEENTH-CENTURY CONCEPTIONS OF MENTAL DISABILITY

Harriet Tubman led one of the most remarkable lives of public service in US history. She was born Araminta Ross in 1822 on a plantation in Dorchester County, Maryland. In 1849, she escaped from slavery and arrived in Philadelphia, Pennsylvania. Within a year, she returned to her plantation to help her relatives. Earning the affectionate title "the Moses of her people," Tubman led at least seventy enslaved Black people out of slavery between 1850 and 1860. She also spoke and organized for abolition and women's suffrage. At the start of the Civil War, she enlisted as a spy and nurse in the Union Army. Her last great act of service was opening the Harriet Tubman Home for Aged and Indigent Negroes (1908) in Auburn, New York, which provided a homelike setting where Tubman cared for a few dozen poor, sick, mentally and physically disabled Black people. She lived in Auburn until her death in 1913 at the age of ninety-one. In 2016, the US Treasury Department announced that Harriet Tubman would replace Andrew Jackson on the twenty-dollar bill, a promise unfulfilled at the time of this writing.

Harriet Tubman's life was extraordinary for reasons beyond her exemplary contributions to humanity, however. In this chapter, I argue that in the history of nineteenth-century mental disability, Harriet Tubman is an emblematic figure because of popular discourses on insanity that circulated around her. Nineteenth-century psychiatric discourses misidentified her as a "colored insane" based on her signature religiosity and

African-derived spiritual beliefs and practices. Yet, I contend that Tubman was never constrained by people's efforts to color her "insane." Instead, she successfully integrated nineteenth-century markers of insanity, such as seeing visions, singing, having hallucinations, and hearing voices, into her life and used them as assets across her full and productive career.

Like Harriet Jacobs, whose discussions of mental suffering among enslaved people I examined in the previous chapter, Harriet Tubman openly shared the mental and physical toll of slavery on her bodymind with northern whites and abolitionist allies. As I explore in this chapter, Tubman was a Black woman whose mental suffering during slavery led to subsequent charges about her sanity, and such indictments were entangled with then-dominant psychiatric beliefs about the etiology and treatment of mental illness. By today's medical standards, Harriet Tubman was not mentally ill, but in the nineteenth century, there was no such consensus. Questions about her sanity circulated among her enslaver, abolitionist allies, and loved ones alike. In this chapter, I introduce the physical injury that disabled her as a child and then turn to nineteenth-century speculations about her mental health. I delve into the psychiatric and medical theories pertaining to Tubman's African-derived religious expressions, including those of psychiatrists and physicians. In the second half of the chapter, I discuss how Tubman and her community understood the symptoms psychiatrists categorized as mental disabilities. I show that Tubman saw her unique embodied experiences not as "symptoms" but rather "gifts" not to be wasted. I present the various ways she understood her experiences and instances in which she conceptualized insanity. I conclude the chapter with a discussion of how she used her abilities and African-derived sensibilities in her small-scale healthcare work on the Underground Railroad, during the Civil War, in her home, and in her institution for vulnerable Black people. Ultimately, the chapter uses Tubman's rich story and work as a prism through which we witness the deeply ingrained meanings of mental disability in the lives of nineteenth-century Black Americans.

TUBMAN'S HEAD INJURY

In present-day narratives, as in those from her own time, authors depict Tubman's severe skull fracture as a "head injury." The stories usually describe how an overseer wounded Harriet while she was on an errand

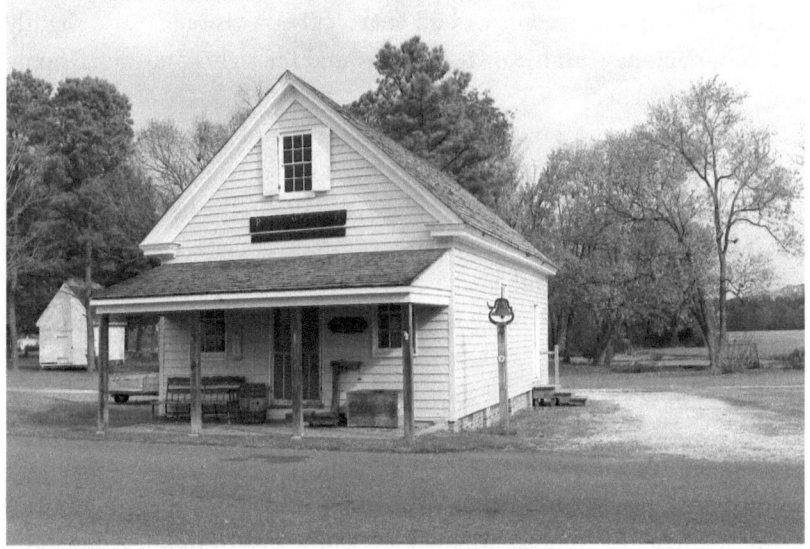

FIGURE 4.1 Bucktown General Store. National Park Service.

to Bucktown General Store (figure 4.1). The overseer chased a field hand because the enslaved man left his post without permission. The overseer hurled a two-pound iron weight at the escaping man but missed, striking Tubman instead. In lieu of medical treatment for her injury, Tubman lay down for two days, during which period she repeatedly went in and out of consciousness. After the incident, Tubman's slave master quickly attempted to sell her, but he was unable to find a buyer. She became a risky investment in the economy of chattel slavery.

After several gruesome weeks, the wound healed, but Tubman's bodymind was forever changed. Along with a physical scar from the childhood incident, Tubman lived with a host of physical and psychological symptoms into adulthood. She suffered decades of headaches and bouts of extreme fatigue. Among her afflictions were sudden sleeping spells, during which she lost consciousness for several minutes. When she awoke from these spells, Tubman was able to pick up a conversation without losing her train of thought.[1] The sleeping spells were often followed by extreme exhaustion.[2] She often experienced hallucinations, including seeing visions and hearing sounds and voices to which others were not privy.[3] In her novelistic portrait of Tubman's life, Beverly Lowry poignantly describes the major changes the head injury brought on: "At thirteen, Minty has become a child apart, either a visionary or a slightly crazed girl, alone with her own certainty and the sights and sounds only she can see and hear."[4]

According to the logics of nineteenth-century psychiatry, Tubman could have suffered the fate of the many "colored insane" in preemancipation asylums. As I discussed in chapter 1, a "blow to the head," such as the one Tubman experienced, was a fairly common somatic cause of "insanity," and she exhibited other characteristic signs of nineteenth-century psychiatric illness, such as hearing voices and experiencing episodic unconsciousness. Instead, when she escaped slavery, she became one of the most famous examples of Cartwright's mental disease, drapetomania, also discussed in chapter 1. Moreover, because she facilitated the escape of so many Black people, Cartwright might have well charged her with spreading drapetomania. Although she neither bore the title nor lived the life of the "colored insane," Tubman was never free from the association. Emma Paddock Telford writes in her biography of Tubman that as a result of the impairment, Tubman was not worth a "sixpence" to her master.[5] Tubman's injuries made her "unsound."

Soundness was a concept used by enslavers within the system of chattel slavery to consider the mental and physical health of enslaved people and to determine the potential value of their labor on the slave market.[6] Yet, members of the medical field were hardly on the sidelines in matters of enslaved people's mental health. In fact, medicine was often marshaled to maintain the economic and social hierarchies that characterized nineteenth-century life. The southern physician Juriah Harriss explained that unsoundness was characterized by "any deformity which materially diminishes the value of the negro, or disables him for the performance of such labor as is usual for him to perform, or prevents the execution of natural functions which are necessary to the preservation of health or life."[7] Harriss was critical of a Georgia Supreme Court ruling that defined medical health only in terms of physical infirmities. In line with the conclusions of psychiatrists, he contended that mental conditions such as insanity should be considered as abnormalities of the brain and thus constitute disease like other diseases of the body. Harriss's commentary on the Supreme Court decision reveals that defining disease was both a medical and legal matter. The grounds for legal protections and defenses that appeared in reference to enslaved people's soundness were written into bills of sale. In the case of a thirty-five-year-old enslaved man named Wade, who was sold in Macon, Georgia, in 1859 for the considerable price of one thousand and twenty dollars, the relatively high price was in part justified by his master's claim that he was "sound and healthy both in body and mind."[8] As Harriss made clear, unsoundness was also characterized by mental or physical "deformity," which could be "congenital or accidental."[9]

Tubman's injury helps to make her a pivotal figure in the history of mental disability, not only because of the ways in which her life was extraordinary but also for the ways it was ordinary. Among the enslaved, she joined hundreds of thousands—whose numbers have not been accurately recorded—who suffered disabling injuries, experiencing acute and enduring impacts on their health in general and mental health in particular. Statistical data about the prevalence of disability during the period have not been systematically or accurately documented, but we know from Tubman's story and others that disability was common.[10]

Enslaved people were often injured or killed, sometimes through the violence of discipline or punishment, sometimes by accident, and sometimes in fights. For example, in 1842, an unnamed enslaved man between the age of thirty and forty years old was struck on the head with the edge of a hoe in a fight.[11] A young enslaved girl named Peggy, who was about Tubman's age when she was injured, was struck on the left side of her head while drawing water from a well.[12] Both the man and Peggy succumbed to their injuries and died within a few years of these incidents. Many others who sustained injuries had to live with them, as Tubman did. After defending himself against an attack by a white young man, William Wells Brown was attacked by the young man's father, seeking revenge: "A few days after, as I was walking along Main street, he seized me by the collar, and struck me over the head five or six times with a large cane, which caused the blood to gush from my nose and ears in such a manner that my clothes were completely saturated with blood."[13] Sometimes such blows to the head left physical scars. John Brown, a former slave from Georgia, compared the blow to the head his enslaver gave him to a gunshot wound. In his narrative, he described not only the brutality of the assault but also its enduring mark: "When I recovered,

I found myself stretched on the ground, my head bleeding fearfully, and my master standing over me, with his foot on my forehead. The scar that blow made, I retain to this day."[14] Tubman, too, carried the mark of the assault on her body, but she was fully aware that the wounds she endured extended beyond physical scarring.[15]

NINETEENTH- TO TWENTY-FIRST-CENTURY SPECULATIONS ON TUBMAN'S SANITY

Some of the most influential assessments of Tubman's sanity came from her biographers. In addition to writing about John Brown and other notable cultural figures, including Ralph Waldo Emerson, Nathaniel Hawthorne, and Henry David Thoreau, Franklin Benjamin Sanborn penned the first biographical sketch of Harriet Tubman entitled, "Harriet Tubman," which was published in *The Commonwealth* in 1863. He also contributed to the first full-length biography of Tubman, put together by Sarah Bradford.[16] Echoing the slave narrative genre's inclusion of white-authored prefatory testimonies as to the veracity of the account and the purity of character of its subject, Bradford's *Scenes in the Life of Harriet Tubman* contained several letters and testimonials from Tubman's friends and fellow activists, including Wendell Phillips, Frederick Douglass, and Gerrit Smith.[17]

Included among the documents in the biography was a letter from Sanborn to Bradford, in which he poetically aggrandized the mystical nature of Tubman: "There is a whole region of the marvelous in her nature, which has manifested itself at times remarkably." Believing that the supernatural aspects of Tubman's life were critical to her story, Sanborn instructed that retellings of her life should include "her dreams and visions, misgivings and forewarnings." Sanborn's familiarity with nineteenth-century discourses on mental disability did not dissuade him from publicly amplifying the "marvelous" aspects of Tubman's story. However, other nineteenth-century allies were more wary about associating Tubman with insanity. Immediately following Sanborn's gesture, Bradford penned lines that defended her editorial choices and hedged against any judgment of Tubman's mental state: "Of the 'dreams and visions' mentioned in this letter, the writer might have given many wonderful instances; but it was thought best not to insert anything which, with any, might bring discredit upon the story."[18] As if to satisfy Sanborn's request, Bradford perfunctorily described the characteristics of the remarkable that she observed in the company of Tubman. She explained how Tubman believed that her spirit left her body during the sleeping episodes, referenced Tubman's psychic powers, and relayed how Tubman sometimes broke out into a scripture-inspired "rhapsody."

Appealing to her audiences' probable knowledge of nineteenth-century anthropological and scientific accounts of mental capacity, especially between races, Bradford repackaged Tubman's supernatural exhibitions as evidence of a superior, rather than inferior, mental aptitude. However, her investment in this argument was precarious. Bradford knew the metrics of insanity by which Tubman's experiences and behavior would be judged. Thus, her final statement on the matter is both a concession and a sidestep: "There was a wild poetry in these descriptions which seemed to border almost on inspiration, but by many they might be characterized as the ravings of insanity. All that can be said is, however, if this woman is insane, there has been a wonderful 'method in her madness.'"[19] Bradford left open the possibility of Tubman's madness. But her proclamation was also subversive in that she, as a lay woman, postulated that there was ground yet undiscovered and unappreciated in the white, male-dominated domain of theorizing about mental disability. Her declaration not only exposed the precarity of the observational and often idiosyncratic means by which mental disability was determined but also rhetorically constructed Tubman as an agent of her own life, in full command of herself and purposes. Bradford's framing of Tubman's expressiveness was just one strategy to shield Tubman from associations with insanity.

More often Bradford and others openly described Tubman as mentally disabled. In Bradford's 1886 version of the narrative, *Harriet, the Moses of Her People*, she describes Tubman from the vantage point of other enslaved children witnessing one of her sleeping episodes: "She seemed a dazed and stupid child, and as her head hung upon her breast, she looked up with dull blood-shot eyes towards her young brothers and sisters, without seeming to see them."[20] Drawing from Tubman's interview with Emma Telford, the narrative describes her as being in a "dazed" and "stupid condition."[21] John Tubman, Harriet's first husband, found her desire for freedom troubling and far-fetched and the prospect of escape from slavery to be a crazy, outrageous, and outlandish pursuit. Turmoil in the marriage resulted from the fact that her husband also dismissed her visions as frivolous folly and thought they reflected mental disturbance. Bradford writes that Tubman's husband "thought her a fool" and perceived her as having cognitive deficiency or delayed comprehension. She imparts that John Tubman said Harriet was "like old Cudjo, who when a joke went round, never laughed till half an hour after everybody else got through, and so just as all danger was past she began to be frightened."[22]

In many retellings of Tubman's story, authors affixed Tubman's head injury to a host of spiritual gifts and supernatural abilities, including hearing the voice of God, forewarnings, dreams, visions, and out-of-body experiences. In her visions, for example, Tubman foresaw the commencement of the Civil War. She also had visions about John Brown and his demise before ever meeting him and had several premonitions of visitations from friends bearing monetary aid before these events occurred. Those who knew her also believed that the injury awakened a vibrant spirituality that was reflected in her Black religious practices, characterized by the wielding of divine power, ecstatic singing, praying, and shouting, and a belief in supernatural signs, symbols, and entities.

Twentieth-century keepers of Tubman's story have attempted to demystify the head injury and its aftermath by placing it within a biomedical framework. Focusing on the sleeping spells, Tubman's mid-twentieth-century biographer, the journalist Earl Conrad, settled on a diagnosis of narcolepsy, after communicating with several psychiatrists and physicians who speculated that her condition might be one of several mental illnesses, such as hysteria, dementia praecox, or schizophrenia. Conrad believed her supernatural experiences were linked to her head injury but refrained from including references to her religious expression in what he claimed was Tubman's "definitive" biography.[23] Conrad, who had a genuine respect and admiration for Tubman, guarded against the potential of Tubman's legacy being sullied by what he saw as the stain of mental illness or religious zealousness.

A self-proclaimed agnostic Jew inspired by Marxist thought, Conrad could neither imagine nor entertain the possibility that the greatest woman in American history could have been an insane zealot, let alone mentally disabled and in possession of spiritual gifts. Even when implored by Tubman's great-niece Alice Brickler to capture the ways "Aunt Harriet" was "in touch" with a "mysterious central originating Force," Conrad was steadfast in his stance: Tubman's psychohistory was irrelevant. In the end, he remained firm in the supposition he expressed in a letter to the medical authorities at Battle Creek Sanitarium in Michigan: "The measurement of the woman must finally rest upon her deeds rather than upon her visions."[24] His references to religion in the biography were relegated to a description of how Tubman prayed that her master would either have a change of heart or die, captured in Tubman's phrase that he be "taken out of the way," which Conrad referred to as a "strange kind of prayer." Reconciling his Marxist view on the distracting nature of religion, he categorized her faith as "applied religion." By this he meant religion in the service of revolution, as seen in the historical examples of the large-scale slave revolts of Nat Turner and Denmark Vesey.[25]

Twenty-first-century Tubman historians have also deciphered her condition by drawing associations between her symptoms and present-day medical diagnoses.[26] Catherine Clinton especially embraced Conrad's identification of narcolepsy because she believed medical knowledge that narcoleptics can "suffer from hypnagogic hallucinations—vivid images that emerge at the onset of sleep." However, Clinton was more skeptical about the linkages between Tubman's head injury and psychic abilities. She writes, "It is impossible to say if there was some physiological or neurological root cause of her visions."[27] Similarly, in a recent book about Tubman, stylized for contemporary popular audiences, *She Came to Slay: The Life and Times of Harriet Tubman*, the historian Erica Armstrong Dunbar speculated that "though in the 1830s there was no fancy term to describe Araminta's condition; her grave head injury likely induced a form of epilepsy that was accompanied by seizures."[28] The historian Kate Clifford Larson identified the condition as temporal lobe epilepsy (TLE) and sought to stress the possible "symbiotic" relationship between Tubman's spirituality and head injury.[29] Larson's claim was based on the overlap between the symptoms Tubman's interlocutors described and present-day medical descriptions of the disease: "seizures," "sleeping spells," and "bright lights, colorful auras, disembodied voices, states of tremendous anxiety and fear alternating with exceptional hyperactivity and fearlessness, and dreamlike trances while appearing to be conscious, followed by the episodes of overwhelming and crippling fatigue."[30] TLE would have satisfied Conrad; the condition is identified first and foremost by its primary symptoms—sleeping and staring spells—and only includes hearing voices and anxiety as secondary symptoms, often associated with psychotic illnesses like schizophrenia. Neither TLE nor schizophrenia were available diagnoses in the nineteenth century. Attempts to medicalize Tubman's disability draw attention away from the implications of her disability in her time period. Like many enslaved people, Tubman's injuries often led to precarious encounters with medical institutions and/or medical practitioners, some of whom specialized in the treatment of mental disabilities. Modern explanations also overlook the circumstances in which Tubman transformed her disability into a strength in a world in which it was seen as a fault, misfortune, or imperfection. Paying attention to her disability as she experienced it in the nineteenth century sheds light on how she might have seen it and how those who knew her, many of whom were devout believers in an age of reform, made sense of her disability and religious expression and, further, how they incorporated it into the mythology of Tubman.

Psychiatric authorities of Tubman's day would have scrutinized the various and curious aspects of her story to judge her sanity—the blow to her head, her animated (or charismatic) religious expression, and her earnest belief in the supernatural. There is no record of Tubman being seen by a psychiatrist, but she had medical encounters on account of her head injury and spiritual expressivity. In her seventies, she sought out brain surgery at Massachusetts General Hospital to alleviate the "fits of insensibility" and headaches that had kept her up at night for decades.[31] There is no record of a surgery, but quite a bit of lore exists around the procedure—she is said to have undergone the surgery without "ether" (anesthesia), while "mumbling prayers" and clenching a bullet between her teeth like so many of the Civil War soldiers that she nursed.[32]

On an earlier occasion, it was others who called a physician in response to Tubman's behavior. In 1884, Tubman was praying at an Auburn jail for Moses Stewart, a relative who had been arrested. She cried, shouted, and sang in hopes that he would be released thanks to her spiritual intercession. In the midst of her expression, she was "seized" by the "power." In response to her supposed overexcitement, Deputy Sheriff Stiles and another officer summoned physician F. M. Hamlin, who "succeeded in quieting her, after a time."[33] There is no record of the doctor's assessment of her mental health, but the very fact that he was called establishes that onlookers found Tubman's spiritual expression concerning. Physicians followed the lead of psychiatrists on the relationship between religiosity and mental disability.

NINETEENTH-CENTURY PSYCHIATRIC PERSPECTIVES ON RELIGION AND MENTAL DISABILITY

To situate Tubman in her own time period, it is necessary to consider the relevant medical and popular understandings of mental disability. Of great import is the fact that Tubman and her peers were products of an electric age of social reform on multiple fronts. She was connected to prominent nineteenth-century social reformers such as Franklin Benjamin Sanborn, Horace Mann, and Samuel Gridley Howe, who are usually associated with abolition but who were also active in mental health reform circles. They were versed in psychiatric doctrines and assessed Tubman's sanity in light of them, particularly as it related to her charismatic religious expressions. The Harvard-educated Sanborn published a memoir of the "Father of Psychiatry," Pliny Earle. He also publicly criticized the efforts of the darling of the asylum movement, Dorothea Dix, arguing that the more than thirty asylums she helped found were failing because she had not attended to the training of asylum superintendents. Dix worked with other reformers who operated behind the scenes in the world of asylum building, including Horace Mann, who hosted Tubman in his home on her trips to Boston. Mann was instrumental in the establishment of the Worcester Lunatic Asylum in Worcester, Massachusetts, in 1833, choosing Samuel Woodward, a founding member of the Association of Medical Superintendents of American Institutions for the Insane (AMSAII), as the superintendent.[34] Mann's writings reveal a keen interest in psychiatric conceptualizations, and he likely applied what he learned about insanity to his educational theories.[35] Mann was close friends with other notable men in the world of psychiatry, including Dr. Samuel Gridley Howe, who was both a trustee of the Worcester Hospital and another host to Tubman. Howe was also involved in the establishment of institutions for the "insane," "deaf," and "blind."

Peers of Tubman's friends, psychiatrists would have likely associated Tubman's sleeping spells, convulsions, and "excitability" with epilepsy. Unlike other nineteenth-century diagnostic terminology such as "idiocy" and "lunacy" that became defunct and derogatory, the term "epilepsy" persisted in the medical field for two centuries. Epilepsy has now largely been excised from categorizations of mental illnesses, but in the nineteenth century, it fit squarely under psychiatry's purview. Still, despite the fact that roughly 10 percent of asylum cases involved epilepsy, there was little in the way of clearly demarcated or shared definitions about the condition or its prognosis.[36] Nevertheless, epilepsy was mostly associated with a range of symptoms such as uncontrollable convulsions, excessive shaking, spasmodic movements, staring spells, and periodic losses of consciousness and awareness.

Psychiatrists believed that, like insanity, epilepsy had physiological manifestations and that its symptoms were the result of abnormalities in or injuries to the brain. In other words, insanity and epilepsy were both seen as diseases of the brain. In keeping with the medical taxonomies of the nineteenth century, which favored somatic causes for mental illness, the New England reformer and suffragist Edna Dow Cheney called Tubman's injury "a disease of the brain" in an 1865 biographical sketch.[37] Psychiatrists applied the same etiological principles and treatment practices to epilepsy as they did to insanity. Often, they resigned themselves to not having good answers. For example, in response to requests by political leaders to define insanity for the purposes of criminal cases, Isaac Ray, who concerned himself with matters of the law more than his peers did, argued that it was too complicated a task, admitting there was no uniform definition of insanity. Instead of defining insanity, historians of psychiatry contend that psychiatrists preferred to spend the bulk of their efforts in describing their treatment practices.[38] Even with this emphasis on treatment, however, and despite the fact that asylum doctors went to great lengths to declare that their facilities were curing people, their cure rates were dismal.

Segregation by diagnosis was seen as vital for effective treatment; thus, mental asylums had separate wards for people with epilepsy, which remained a significant diagnosis for people in asylums throughout the nineteenth century. Some psychiatrists warned that if left untreated, epilepsy could lead to other forms of insanity.[39] They also believed that epilepsy was hereditary, brought on by physical trauma to the brain, or the product of a separate disease such as a tumor.[40]

Like other movement disorders, such as Sydenham's chorea (St. Vitus's dance), psychiatrists often made associations between epilepsy and religious expression. John Minson Galt, who fashioned himself an expert on the care of the "colored insane," claimed there was a significant correlation between religious enthusiasm and epilepsy: "There is not a more common symptom of epileptic insanity than an exaltation of the religious feelings."[41] American psychiatrists' critical views of religion and its negative influence on mental health reflect their complicated relationship to religion in general.

Religion figured importantly in psychiatrists' claims about the etiology of mental disability and, by extension, to other brain diseases, epilepsy included. Psychiatrists all agreed that mental disabilities did not have supernatural origins. In their new medical science, there was no place for divine visitation or demonic possession.[42] They were primarily influenced by the Enlightenment idea that scientific inquiry was the key to uncovering the principles or natural laws that governed the God-designed universe. They believed that the truths produced by flourishing and bourgeoning scientific fields—such as medicine, statistics, and anthropology—aligned with the truths that were found in so-called "rational" religious beliefs and practices. Psychiatrists held that there was a blueprint or formula for perfect mental health and that they were best positioned to discover it and to implement it in the lives of the afflicted. They contended that the universe had an order that came initially from a supernatural being, a monotheistic God, who was manifested in the form of natural laws. Although they believed that God designed the inner workings of the universe, the source of ill health was not in the cosmos. Mental disease was rooted in the material body—not the spiritual realm. As historian of psychiatry Norman Dain explains, mental illness for nineteenth-century psychiatrists was "a pathological brain condition that had psychological symptoms, the origin could be psychological or organic, but the pathology was somatic."[43] However, usurping mental illness from the province of the church did not lead to the total severance of religion from the treatment of mental illness in the United States. American psychiatrists were committed to an understanding of disease that located its origins and treatment in the realm of science and medicine, but they were not willing to completely part with the religious doctrines that shaped the period's cultural and political life.[44]

Most psychiatrists often incorporated religious instruction into their administration of the main therapeutic modality—the moral treatment.[45] Religious observance was built into people's daily activities along with amusements, gardening, and handicrafts like needlework or carpentry. Often asylums had their own chapels and assigned chaplains, even though there were conflicting views about the place of religion in the rubric of the moral treatment. A few Christian psychiatrists saw religion in the asylum as part of their own faith commitments to missionary work; the people in asylums were thus viewed as potential converts or religious adherents.[46] Others had reservations about their medical authority being undermined by clergy or about services worsening peoples' conditions through depressing or terrifying sermons.[47] Still, most asylums maintained the practice of religion. Even though clergy were allowed into asylums, often reluctantly, psychiatrists had definite ideas about what kinds of religious expression were acceptable. They approved of "rational" religion, exemplified by Protestant sects such Methodism, Presbyterianism, Episcopalianism, and Orthodox Quakerism. But they were critical of what they deemed fanatical practices—exemplified by the evangelical tent revivals that animated the Great Awakening. In addition to a general belief in the supernatural and its direct influence on human existence, the glossolalia (speaking in tongues), falling down, loud weeping, prolonged singing, shouting, praying, and "catching the spirit" on display at tent meetings all constituted fanaticism to psychiatrists.[48] Pliny Earle explained that "true religion" aided in mental stability, whereas "fanaticism" overtook its adherents.[49] Still, psychiatrists did not believe that even fanatical religion was the root cause of mental disability. For individuals with a predisposition toward mental disability, it was at most a precipitating factor that could lead to "religious excitement"—a term that was used as both a formal diagnostic category and a descriptor for an individual's behavior.

One of the most well-known psychiatric writings on mental disability and the dangers of "religious excitement," especially evangelical religious expression, was Amariah Brigham's 1835 book *Observations on the Influence of Religion Upon the Health and Physical Welfare of Mankind*. Of the thirteen founding members of the AMSAII, Brigham was one of the most highly respected. He was the first director of the New York State Lunatic Asylum at Utica and the first editor of the *American Journal of Insanity*. In his book, he warned that certain religious services caused increased mental activity, which had dangerous consequences. He wrote that "mental excitement, by increasing the momentum of blood to the brain, causes insanity, epilepsy, [and] convulsions." Brigham was particularly concerned about the content of evangelical pamphlets because they promoted and perpetuated belief in the "marvellous" and "mysterious," including the "fulfilment of dreams of pious people" and "immediate answers to prayers [and many other accounts far more wonderful]." He speculated that the "fits" and "seizures" of participants were clear evidence of the inherent excitability of their religious expression.[50]

Even when it was not tethered to church-based religious practice, an individual's belief in the supernatural was seen as harmful to mental health. Brigham, like his peers, believed that Black people were especially superstitious, but psychiatrists also encountered whites who were supposedly susceptible to superstition as well. White people were influenced by Black religions such as Hoodoo and Conjure, as well as Anglo-American spiritual traditions that existed within Christianity and those that developed alongside it, such as demonology and witchcraft.[51] Belief in superstition was risky, in Brigham's estimation. He warned that believing in bad omens and signs or laying claim to supernatural abilities, such as "hearing voices which do not really sound," made individuals especially susceptible to mental disability.[52]

TUBMAN AND THE TRANS-SENSE

Tubman's sanity is best understood in light of the predominance of her African-derived spirituality in her life and work. Many facets of Tubman's life revealed the strong imprint of African-derived ontologies, manifesting in her embodiment of spiritual power and her belief in the supernatural world. Tubman's contemporaries hence saw her as a person of great spiritual power, authority, and metaphysical abilities. Bradford went to great lengths in her biography to depict Tubman as saintly and self-sacrificing and compared her to Joan of Arc.[53] The Tubman scholar James McGowan argues that what she most shared with Joan of Arc was not piety or a singular devotion to a cause but the fact that she heard voices and had visions.[54] Figures like Tubman are common in African diaspora religious traditions. The historian of religion Diane Stewart argues that people with extraordinary gifts, such as perceiving the realm of the invisible or reading undisclosed phenomena (past, present, and future), are often referred to as "'seers' possessing more than two eyes."[55] One of Tubman's most well-known premonitions was about John Brown. Before meeting Brown, Tubman had a puzzling reoccurring dream about him. Sanborn records her often-recited story of the dreams in his 1869 biographical sketch:

> She thought she was in "a wilderness sort of place, all full of rocks and bushes," when she saw a serpent raise its head among the rocks, and as it did so, it became the head of an old man with a long white beard, gazing at her "wishful-like, jes as ef he war gwine to speak to me," and then two other heads rose up beside him, younger than he, and as she stood looking at them and wondering what they could want with her, a great crowd of men rushed in and struck down the younger heads, and then the head of the old man, still looking at her so "wishful."[56]

When Tubman finally met John Brown in April 1858 in Canada, she recognized him as the "wishful" face she had dreamed about. Her clairvoyance concerning Brown's life did not end with the serpent dream. On the day before Brown's October 1859 raid, Tubman woke up uneasy in New York City. She alerted those who were hosting her that Brown was probably in danger. Her forewarning was fulfilled, as the next day reports of the raid surfaced.[57]

Tubman's gifts are best understood in the context of Black American communal values and family legacies. Although psychiatrists have been skeptical of spiritual gifts, seeing them as signs of mental disturbance that without question have a hereditary basis, Tubman was proud to proclaim that her gifts were inherited from an earlier generation. As Emma Telford noted, "Harriet declare[d] that she inherited [her] power of foresight;

that her father could always predict the weather and that he foretold the Mexican war."⁵⁸ Tubman herself had a prophetic vision of a consequential armed conflict, the Civil War. After Brown's raid, Tubman sensed war on the horizon. She told Sanborn, "They may say 'Peace, Peace!' As much as they like; I know there's going to be war!"⁵⁹ When Tubman visited New York City in early 1860, she stayed with the Black minister and ardent abolitionist Henry Highland Garnet. One morning, Tubman woke up singing in an ecstatic episode, proclaiming, "My people are free! My people are free!" Garnet was startled at her behavior and said, "Do cease this noise!"⁶⁰ He insisted that his grandchildren would see the end of slavery but that he and Tubman would not. Tubman was unwavering in her reliance on the power of her dreams and rejoiced throughout the day. When the war started, there was an incredible sense of joy about the end of slavery. When asked why she was not jubilant, Tubman reminded people that she had already celebrated. Telford relayed her sentiments in her biography: "I had my jubilee three years ago. I 'joiced all I could den; I can't joice no mo.'"⁶¹ On other occasions, Tubman had dreams predicting a maritime accident in the city of Columbus, Ohio, and an earthquake in South America.⁶² Tubman's premonitions were not just of grand historical events; they also pertained to the everyday concerns she had, such as providing for herself and those she cared for. On numerous occasions, she predicted that money would be sent to her and sometimes anticipated the amount. Telford narrated a time when she received a donation for Tubman and Tubman, upon arriving at Telford's house, exclaimed, "I knowed it was comin'."⁶³ When Telford asked what was coming, Tubman replied correctly that it was ten dollars. Tubman explained that she had been praying for the money to pay her taxes and that God had spoken to her and told her it would come.

Tubman's spiritual power was evidenced not only in her third sight and rhythmic trances but also in her understanding that she lived in a world that was animated by seen and unseen forces. Alexis Wells-Oghoghomeh, a historian of religion, explains that enslaved families and communities depended on such women, often maternal figures such as aunts, mothers, and grandmothers, who were respected as spiritual authorities: "Though flesh and blood, they resided alongside hags, witches, and other entities in the sacred imagination—the realm of the spirit powers that animated the sense world and imbued its material elements with spiritual meanings."[64] Tubman's belief in what Wells-Oghoghomeh calls the "trans-sense" world, or "the realm of, beyond, and between the visible and invisible," appears in accounts of the infamous gold swindle incident.[65] In October 1873, Tubman found herself deprived of a government pension and in desperate need of funds to maintain the seven-acre property that had been signed over to her for twelve hundred dollars by Frederick Seward, son of the late senator, governor, and secretary of state William Seward. Tubman learned from her brother, John Stewart, that there was an opportunity to make extra money fast. Two Black conmen from out of town, John and Stevenson, claimed not only that they knew Tubman's nephew who was working in the South but also that they were acquainted with a Black contraband runner from Charleston who had discovered a trunk full of gold worth five thousand dollars. The swindlers said that the South Carolina man was willing to part with the gold for the discounted rate of two thousand dollars in "greenbacks" or paper money. Despite warnings from her well-to-do white friends, Tubman agreed to the deal; her brother acquired the cash from a wealthy Auburn man, Anthony Shimer, for exchange. When the time came to meet with the Charleston man, the fifty-one-year-old Tubman, with the cash on her person, went with Stevenson alone to retrieve the gold. The Charleston man turned out to be Harris, a known confidence man from Seneca Falls. The two men beat and tied up Tubman and stole the cash.[66] Several stories about the robbery appeared in Auburn newspapers within days of the occurrence.[67] Although various versions of the story appeared, they all describe a period where Tubman was alone while the two men supposedly went to retrieve a key for the box of gold. During this time alone, Tubman became afraid and thought of "stories about ghosts haunting buried treasures."[68] Tubman reported that she thought she saw a ghost that turned out to be a cow. Although there was some suspicion among the Auburn community about whether Tubman and her brother were in on the heist, she was ultimately judged to be an "innocent pawn" based on her philanthropic track record and stature in the community.[69] Tubman scholars have speculated about whether Tubman's inclusion of ghosts in her story was a shrewd protective strategy. By playing into white stereotypes about superstitious Black people, she could solicit sympathy from the community rather than enduring contempt for what would be a serious crime.[70]

Tubman's inclusion of ghosts likewise aligns with an African-derived sense of the supernatural world inhabited by multiple entities that populated the Black "sacred imagination."[71] The former slave Nathaniel John Lewis, for example, explained that treasures are always accompanied by ghosts: "wheahevuh theah is money aw othuh treasure a ghos is put theah to gahd it."[72] As Tubman would have been well aware, ghosts were not just there to guard; they were also there to ward off treasure-seekers. Lewis claimed that one of the female ghosts he saw scared them off with a laugh: "The laugh that spirit gave went right through me. I nevuh tried to dig up the money again."[73] Stories like Lewis's and the bountiful body of Black American references to ghosts force us to take Tubman's reference to ghosts seriously.[74] Many Black women, like Tubman, believed in ghosts as strongly as they did in other supernatural events, such as dreams and visions. Mary Hunter, for example, asserted, "I sho does belieb in dreams an ghoses. Ef uh hab suttn dreams, dey sho comes true."[75] However useful ghost stories were for evading the scrutiny of her white audience, it is equally plausible that a Black woman during the nineteenth century who heard from God directly, had visions of the future, and was given to being overtaken by spirit power also believed in the existence of multiple spiritual entities. Ghosts, spirits, and hags are most often associated with Black traditions in conjuring, but many Christians, although opposed to Conjure or "Black magic" as Tubman might have been, held beliefs about the supernatural that were overlapping and complex. The historian of religion Yvonne Chireau notes that "from slavery days to the present, many African Americans have readily moved between Christianity, Conjure, and other forms of supernaturalism with little concern for their purported incompatibility."[76] However, like many Black Americans of her time, Tubman embodied a fusion of Christianity and African-derived cosmological orientations.[77] At the same time, Tubman is most closely associated with the various evangelical Protestant religious sects she encountered growing up on the Eastern Shore of Maryland, especially the African Methodist Episcopal Church, with which she worked extensively later in life. For Tubman, as well as many Blacks, religion served as a source of individual and communal empowerment amid the horrors of enslavement.[78] African-derived spiritual orientations came with an alternative set of perspectives on mental and physical illness that sometimes contrasted drastically with mainstream psychiatric and medical outlooks and treatment practices.

JOE'S SONG: TUBMAN'S CONCEPTIONS OF RELIGIOUS EXPRESSION AND MENTAL DISABILITY

Although there is no shortage of claims made about Tubman's sanity, records exist to explain what she herself thought about mental disability or its meaning in relation to her behavior or core beliefs. We may never know exactly what Tubman thought, but we are able to approximate whether there was a "method to Tubman's madness," as Sarah Bradford contended. In this section, I consider such ideas in a story Tubman told more than once about a fugitive named Joe (Josiah Benson), whom Tubman helped escape from slavery to Canada. An extended version of the story appeared in Bradford's biography, *Scenes in the Life of Harriet Tubman* (1868). A slightly different version can be found in Bradford's updated biography, *Harriet, the Moses of Her People* (1886). A shorter reference to Tubman telling Joe's story also appeared in the diary of the Black writer and educator Charlotte Forten. I read the stories using the tools of literary analysis to consider how language, genre, form, historical context, and the circumstances of the production of the texts shape the meaning that can be derived from them.

Bradford's biography was both a historical document with facts and a historical accounting of events and a work of literature with a particular form, set of themes, and literary style. The pocket book was intended to generate funds for the then-destitute Tubman, who was without a wartime pension and unable to pay the mortgage on her Auburn property. Bradford did not take royalties from the publication; she gave Tubman all twelve hundred dollars of the proceeds. Bradford continued to put out new editions to financially support Tubman, which coincided with Tubman's own fundraising efforts (figure 4.2). Bradford constructed *Scenes in the Life of Harriet Tubman* from informal interviews she conducted with Tubman.[79] In his study of Works Progress Administration narratives, which were based on interviews taken from some former slaves, John Blassingame argues that scholars have to be cognizant that such highly mediated texts always have "two authors," both of whose voices and perspectives exist at the same time.[80] Bradford was not an ideal biographer of Tubman for a range of reasons, including her poor interview skills, hasty production of the text, and her racial views.[81] The overall construction of the narrative was entirely invented by Bradford. Drawing on her

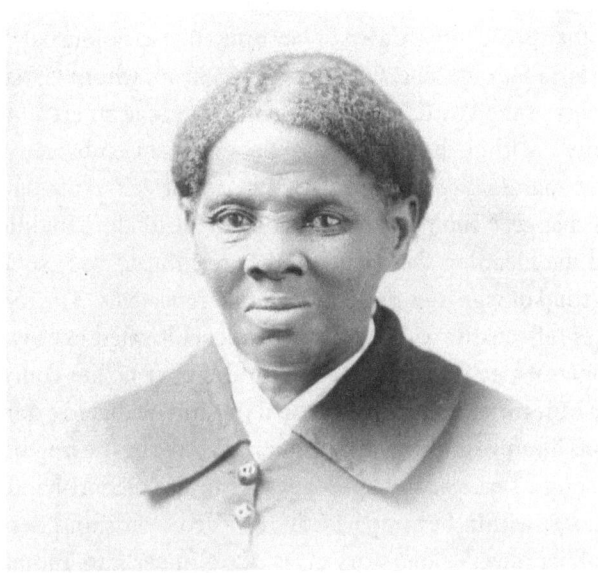

FIGURE 4.2 Harriet Tubman sat for this portrait while in Boston in 1886. She took the photo to help with the sales that could be generated from the new edition of her biography. The funds would go to support her Harriet Tubman Home for Aged and Indigent Negroes. The image appears in Franklin B Sanborn's book *Recollections of Seventy Years* (1909).

background as a children's author, she often chose modes of sentimentality over allowing space for Tubman's own humor and wittiness.[82] As much as she sought to build Tubman's image, Bradford was also concerned about her own reputation as a respectable mother and children's author.[83] Her narrative reflects her choices about how Tubman's dialect should be presented to her white middle-class audience.[84] Still, her biography is one of the most valuable sources of knowledge on Tubman's life.[85] Lois Horton affirms that Bradford's biography "established the heroic mythology that became Tubman the legend."[86] Despite the fact that Bradford's editorial hand is clearly at work in the biography, the power of Tubman's voice cannot be underestimated.

Tubman was a skilled orator who had experience narrating her life history to antislavery audiences as late as the 1850s and, into her elder years, in more intimate settings among the families of her Auburn friends.[87]

Tubman could not write; she used her oratorical skills to testify about her life. Like other preaching women of her time such as Sojourner Truth, Jarena Lee, Maria Stewart, and Rebecca Cox Jackson, whom Carla Peterson called "Doers of the Word," when Tubman spoke, she entered into "a state of liminality"; within this liminality, Black women embraced their race and gender marginality as it created a space for self-expression, power, and social change.[88] Tubman was operating in the folklore tradition, which structured the meaning she created in her retellings.[89] Joe's song was one among a group of vignettes that Tubman told repeatedly. The repetition of such stories reflects the way Tubman actively cultivated her own mythology.[90] Tubman's specific stories are key for deciphering her conceptualizations. Tiya Miles argues that even the sparsest and mediated extant cultural productions illuminate Tubman's viewpoints: "Among the fragments of her recorded songs, sayings, and speeches and in the second-hand accounts of her actions, within her imperfectly recorded words and deeds lay the imprints of her ideas."[91] Joe's story gives us a glimpse into Tubman's mind, where we find a counter-discourse about insanity and religious expression.

In the Bradford biography, Joe's story begins with a description of how Joe was such an exceptionally obedient and valuable laborer that he was frequently rented out by his enslaver. She writes that he became so essential to the person who rented him that the man eventually purchased him. His new master ordered that Joe be broken in through an inaugural beating. Joe reminded his master that he had never been a problem, but the man insisted, explaining that the beating was necessary to establish all his slaves' full submission. In Bradford's text, Joe resolved to run away to Canada with Tubman and a handful of others in November 1856 after quietly enduring the whipping. Black abolitionist William Still gave a different rendering of Joe's reason for running away. He referred to an interpersonal dispute with another slave rather than the harshness of the slave system.[92] By making the cause the whipping, Bradford's story amplified the wrongs of slavery, which evoked pity for Joe's plight and worked to aggrandize Tubman as a noble servant aiding in the fight against the institution.

Further along in Bradford's text, when the group arrived in New York, they were informed of runaway slave ads describing members of the party. Among the advertisements, Joe's offered the highest reward for capture—"$1,500," more than three times the price of others in the party. Although all the fugitives lived under the constant threat of recapture, especially in the aftermath of the chilling 1850 Fugitive Slave Act, learning of the reward had a crippling emotional effect on Joe. Upon hearing the news, his "heart sank." While the others sang and shouted as they journeyed closer and closer to the promised land, Joe sat "silent and sad." Singing had once sustained Joe on the perilous journey plagued with the constant risk of capture and exposure to the elements, but now he was filled with overwhelming dread: "He sang no more, he talked no more; he sat wid his head on his hand, and nobody could 'muse him or make him take any interest in anyting."[93] In her revised 1886 edition of Tubman's story, Bradford gave more details into Joe's distinct psychological response. It is not clear why the story changed, whether due to a new telling or pure fabrication. In the later version, Joe was "always thinking of the horrors that awaited him if recaptured."[94] In both versions, adjoined to the prose representation of Joe's story, Bradford included a line of spirituals the fugitives sang as they traveled. In Bradford's story the spiritual served as the lyrical articulation of Joe's plight.

The inclusion of the spiritual creates a place in the biographies where we see Tubman, the second author, breaking through Bradford's text. In oral retellings of her stories, Tubman often incorporated singing of hymns.[95] Particularly compelling in the account of Joe, the combination of music with speaking was demonstrative of Tubman's sermon-like storytelling style. The song about Joe's plight, like biblical psalms, captured in three stanzas both the personal narrative of the speaker and the psychological depth of their experience, something missing entirely in the diagnostic rubrics of psychiatry. In the first stanza of Joe's song, the speaker explains that they were on the way to Canada because they could no longer bear "the sad effects of slavery." Like Joe, whose decision to run was preceded by a vicious beating despite strenuous labor, the speaker laments working without reward and being forced to flee the "lash." The second stanza chronicles the psychological challenges of the escape itself. Behind every reward poster, the stanza reveals, are flesh-hungry captors: "The hounds are baying on my track, Ole master comes behind." At the end of the stanza, the speaker turns to the divine for help: "Oh, righteous Father, wilt thou not pity me, And aid me on to Canada where all the slaves are free."[96] The last stanza speaks of the promise of freedom associated with their destination, Canada, where they hope to find a peaceful home and leave behind lives of bondage.

In the final stanza, the story returns to prose form to end the tale. In the biography, none of the usual coping mechanisms—songs, community, prayer—were sufficient for Joe; only freedom would do. As they crossed the bridge into Canada, Harriet alerted Joe as to their location. At this news, Joe cried, sang, and shouted in "thrilling tones" the words "Glory to God and Jesus too." When they reached the suspension bridge that connected the United States to Canada, everyone was in awe of Niagara Falls. Harriet urged Joe to gaze on the cascading waterfalls, but he was preoccupied. Instead of being weighed down by his earthly troubles, he was transfixed in a celestial communion: "And can we doubt that the strain was taken up by angel voices, and that through the arches of Heaven echoed and reechoed the strain." Joe's singing was so loud and profound that others in the party tried to quiet him. They were afraid he would be read as mad. Joe's sorrow in the land of bondage was legible; it was a rational response to the turmoil they all faced. But this excess in expression in freedom was unsettling to all. Another member of the group, Peter, said "'Joe, stop your hollerin'! Folks'll think you're crazy.'"[97] Another man, William, made a similar plea, "Joe, stop your noise! [Y]ou act like a fool!" In her brief recounting of Tubman's 1863 retelling of the story full of "jubilant hymns," Charlotte Forten wrote in her diary that Tubman said that Joe appeared "'as if he were crazy.'" Forten helped to educate Blacks on the Sea Islands of South Carolina after Union troops occupied parts of the coastal Carolinas in 1861. While there, she met Tubman and was ecstatic about hearing her speak. She wrote, "How exciting it was to hear her tell the story. . . . My own eyes were full as I listened to her—the heroic woman!" In Forten's retelling, Tubman is rational and wise up against the "perfect delirium of Joe."[98] Both Bradford's and Forten's stories honored Tubman's spirituality and faith. She is represented as a powerful, heroic personality. Their portraits were not of an "insane" woman but of one especially blessed.

However, Tubman's characterization of Joe in the oral retellings likely spoke to her personal perspective on religious expression and sanity. In that moment of exaltation that seemingly took Joe beyond the physical world, Joe's story resembled that of Harriet herself. She, like Joe, had spiritual communion with a God who answered her prayers directly. Nineteenth-century spectators, whether Black or white, medical authority or lay person, had viewed Joe and Harriet's immovable exaltations as markers of insanity. In telling the story of Joe's ecstatic praise, Tubman signaled that she, like the Black people on the trip, was fully aware of the negative connotation and threat such accusations posed, which was reflected in the fact that others tried to quiet him. But Tubman's story does not end with the need for white psychiatric doctors or physicians or Joe's ostracization. For Tubman, such spiritual encounters protected and sustained her and her passengers on perilous journeys, safely delivering them from bondage. Milton Sernett discusses the utility of Tubman's religious outlook in his analysis of Tubman's mythology: "She seems to have believed that her trust in the Lord enabled her to meet all of life's exigencies with a confident foreknowledge of how things would turn out, a habit that others found impressive, or uncanny, as the case may be." Practicing a faith and spirituality that was visceral and demonstrative, Tubman, like Joe, was called a fool and crazy. Nonetheless, she held fast to the divine connection that she believed "saved her life often," in the words of her grandniece.[99] Tubman, like Joe, was impervious to charges of insanity. Perhaps, like Bradford, she conceded it as a foregone conclusion. Or maybe she felt her energy was best placed elsewhere. Her attention to matters of mental disability was not to publicly defend herself or quibble over theories regarding its etiology, but rather it was to care for those who bore the label without adequate support.

TUBMAN AND AFRICAN-DERIVED HEALING TRADITIONS

Rather than finding it a source of despair, Tubman made full use of some of the less painful lingering symptoms from her head injury, which fit within a larger paradigm of her devotion to tending to the needs of others. Her gifts amplified her caregiving practices, which were steeped in African-derived healing epistemologies such as the reliance on herbs and roots to treat ailments and manipulate bodily functions.[100] Tubman's contributions to the world thus went beyond the political realm to include her mastery of Black doctoring arts. Evidence of her practice appeared in four main arenas: in the Underground Railroad; in the US Army during the Civil War; in her own home; and in an infirmary she founded and named after John Brown.

Tubman likely acquired her skills and knowledge about healing through intergenerational oral lessons and from the enslaved people she continuously encountered on trips from the South. Many Black Americans learned how to use roots and herbs from American Indigenous cultures and older generations, including ancestors born on the African continent. Harriet Collins, who was born around 1870, recalled that she learned doctoring ways from her mother, who taught her "what she larnt from old folkses from Africy, and some de Indians larnt her."[101] Like many Black women, Tubman probably learned healing ways from her mother and grandmothers.[102] Tubman's first recorded use of substances was during her escape routes out of the South, especially on children and babies. Although usually they were not welcome, Tubman made it possible for babies to travel with her escape parties. She gave them laudanum, an opium tincture, to keep them quiet and evade capture. Tubman's use of substances along with roots and herbs continued long after her last rescue mission. She is known by popular audiences today for her bravery as a Civil War spy, but her service to the war also included another crucial role, that of nurse.

Tubman was famous for her treatment of the infectious diseases that ravaged soldiers, including pneumonia, typhoid fever, and dysentery. The journalist and novelist Samuel Hopkins Adams chronicles her efforts and clandestine curative methods in his story collection, *Grandfather Stories* (1947), most of which are set in the 1870s and 1880s, when he was a young boy: "In the hospital camps [Tubman] would nurse a case of scarlet fever or small-pox with as much indifference toward contagion as if it were chicken pox or stomach ache. For the latter, she had a sovereign remedy, a one-day 'yarb' cure, especially effective for dysentery. All her postwar life, she made trips to whatever woodland was adjacent, for the purpose of digging the root that was the basis of her remedy. The identity of the plant was her well-kept secret."[103] Adams captures both Tubman's fearless attitude toward sickness and her treatment methods. Like other Black women, her attitude about even the deadliest sickness was to view it not as something to be conquered or feared but instead as something to be faced strategically using wisdom and knowledge that had been passed down.[104] Tubman's superiors welcomed her tactics and concoctions. Henry Durant, an assistant surgeon in the Civil War, told Captain Warfield to "let 'Moses' have a little Bourbon whiskey for medicinal purposes."[105] Tubman was likely using the alcohol to treat malaria and other diseases.[106] Tubman was also known for her knowledge of treating dysentery (severe diarrhea). She "prepared from roots which grew near the waters" that were very effective.[107] Tubman's commitment to using her gifts and knowledge to help others did not wane over time. In her eighties, she founded an institution to help people who were discarded by society and liable to be categorized among the "colored insane" because of their physical and mental disabilities.

THE TUBMAN HOME

By the end of the nineteenth century, the revolutionary psychiatric project of curing the mentally disabled was in ruins. The asylums scattered across the states were in dire condition, plagued by overcrowding, underfunding, and staffing shortages. During this period of failure, called by historians of psychiatry a time of "custodial" care, Tubman was gearing up for her "last great ambition": to open an institution committed to caring for the most vulnerable of her community, including the deaf, blind, elderly, and "insane."[108] To my knowledge, scholars do not know a great deal about the institution, its inner workings, staffing, population, or fiscal operations. Only hints appear in extant historical records. After the publication of the 1901 edition of *Harriet, the Moses of Her People*, Bradford described visiting Tubman and witnessing Tubman's first efforts toward her goal in the form of an informal self-help community facilitated in Tubman's home. There, she cared for a group of Blacks; one newspaper report described the home as "a very plain little home which is an asylum for the poor people of her own color."[109] Tubman, who was often alleged to have been mentally disabled, had committed to meet the needs of what Bradford sympathetically called an "interesting and pathetic group": "the lame, the halt [sic], and the blind, the bruised and crippled little children, and one crazy woman."[110] By 1884, Tubman assigned tasks for growing fruits and vegetables and tending to animals so that the small group could support themselves.[111] For ten years, with meager means and an aging body, she cared for people in her home. In 1896, a newspaper writer described her humble efforts as follows: "She is very poor; but she devotes herself to the

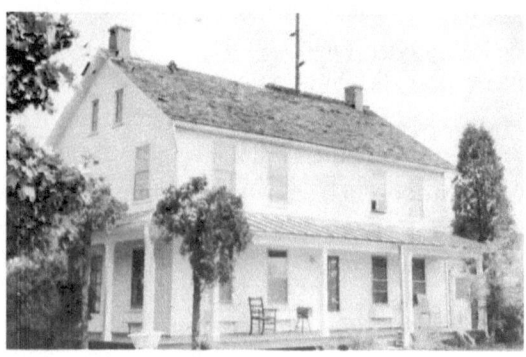

FIGURE 4.3 The Harriet Tubman Home for Aged and Indigent Negroes. New York State Park.

succor of colored men and women more aged and wretched than herself, and she cares for helpless children who are allied to her race. Her house is a hospital for the infirm and sick."[112] In 1908, Tubman institutionalized these efforts to care for the sick, elderly, and disabled by opening the Harriet Tubman Home for Aged and Indigent Negroes (figure 4.3).[113] She named the hall that served as the infirmary after John Brown.

In her book, Telford depicts the physical and mental conditions and disabilities to which Tubman herself tended, later aided by the nurses and matrons of John Brown Hall: "All these years the doors have been open to the needy, the most utterly friendless, and helpless of her race. The aged, forsaken by their own kith and kin, the babe deserted, the demented, the epileptic, the blind, the paralyzed, the consumptive all have found shelter and welcome. At no time can I recall the little home sheltered less than six or eight wrecks of humanity entirely dependent upon Harriet for their all."[114] Both Tubman and asylum superintendents needed more financial support than they received, the former depending on the charity of her well-to-do friends and the latter on cash-strapped state legislatures. Still, the care that the few mentally disabled Blacks received at Tubman's home contrasted drastically with what they encountered in "colored" wards or in the buildings of mental asylums.[115] Unlike men of medicine, white or Black, Tubman was not invested in cataloging her philosophies of caretaking in written form. But stories about Tubman's life reveal that she had an outlook on health and healing that diverged from the psychiatric authorities of her time. Tubman saw the needy who showed up on her doorstep as "blessings rather than burdens."[116] Although her means were small, Harriet Tubman had a special concern for the people who found their way to her. But most people with mental disabilities were not cared for in small homelike settings such as the one Tubman offered.

Some of the "colored insane" had complicated relationships with their families, who believed the asylum was the best place for their relatives to reside and receive care. As the next chapter will show, the emancipation of slavery ushered in a new era for asylums, which began to accept Black people in earnest. As a result, the numbers of Black people held in asylums, mostly in the South, quickly swelled to the thousands. The next chapter explores what it was like to not only be labeled the "colored insane" but also be housed in a nineteenth-century asylum. I provide a glimpse into the lives of the "colored insane" in one of the most infamous hospitals to treat Black people suffering from mental illness, the Georgia Lunatic Asylum. Black people who were sent to Georgia Lunatic Asylum faced racist psychiatric ideas and poor levels of care and often crude accommodations, a far cry from the intimate and welcoming vision of care available at the Harriet Tubman Home.

5

BLACK WOMEN'S PSYCHIATRIC INCARCERATION AT GEORGIA LUNATIC ASYLUM IN THE NINETEENTH CENTURY

In May 1897, Theophilus Powell gave a presidential address before the American Medico-Psychological Association, the nineteenth-century precursor to the American Psychiatric Association, regarding the progression of southern asylums (figure 5.1). He drew a reverential portrait of the self-sacrificing pioneers who courageously met the challenges of caring for the mentally disabled. But he went on to explain that these institutions had two distinct problems that northern ones did not: they had to manage the devastating economic and social destruction of the Civil War, and they had a "separate and peculiar problem"—caring for the "colored insane." Using language that recalled defenses of enslavement before the war, he declared, "What the race problem is to our whole section, so is the question of the colored insane to our specialty."[1] With this statement, Powell not only identified the number of the Black mentally disabled patients as a problem unique to the South but also distinguished himself and his southern colleagues as experts on issues associated with Black bodyminds.[2]

This chapter sets out to answer the following questions: What did it mean for Powell, as the administrator of the largest number of "colored insane" in the country, to "specialize" in their care? After emancipation, psychiatric hospitals began to accept Black patients in large numbers. How were they treated? What did it mean that their care was defined in

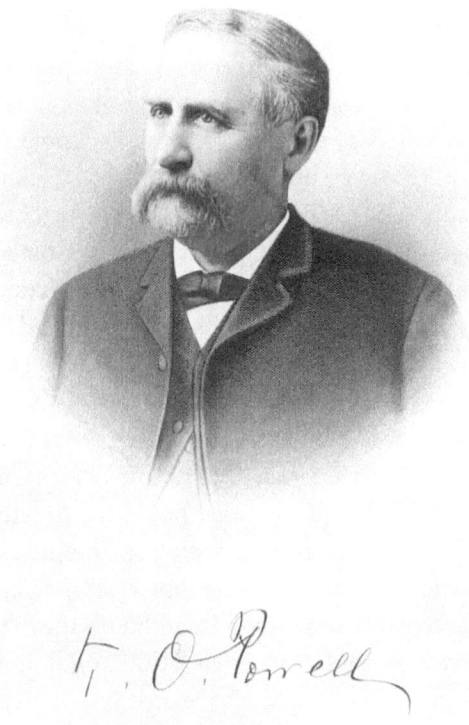

FIGURE 5.1 Theophilus Orgain Powell. This image appears in William J. Northen, *Men of Mark in Georgia: A Complete and Elaborate History of the State from Its Settlement to the Present Time, Chiefly Told in Biographies and Autobiographies of the Most Eminent Men of Each Period of Georgia's Progress and Development*. A. B. Caldwell, 1907–1912.

ways that recalled slavery? What was the effect on Black women in particular? At the end of the nineteenth century, various actors had competing definitions of the "race problem" and multiple approaches to solving it. Many Black intellectuals, such as W. E. B. Du Bois and Charles Chesnutt, framed it as the problem of the "color line," which I discuss in the next chapter. Figures such as Booker T. Washington argued that Black people should be seen as reliable and subservient, just as they had been during slavery. The Supreme Court judges who backed segregation in the *Plessy v. Ferguson* decision held that Black people could not integrate with the general population. The solution of segregating and systematically extracting Black labor is observable in the feminist and critic of psychiatry Charlotte Perkins Gilman's contention that Blacks should be assigned to detention centers where they could be put to work on public projects.[3] The southern white feminist Rebecca Ann Felton, who would become the nation's first woman senator, felt that Black men should be lynched "a thousand times a week if necessary" to protect white women.[4] Some race scientists thought Blacks were on the path to degeneration and extinction.[5]

Powell's sentiments reflect how psychiatrists identified Black mentally disabled people as a problem for southern white society. They pointed out that the race problem was evidenced in the high rates of insanity among Blacks and their increased admission to asylums. Psychiatrists saw these increases as proof that slavery was indeed a health-promoting institution for Blacks. The solution psychiatrists posed was to return Blacks to a curative environment defined by regimented daily routines, regular diet, healthy living quarters, therapeutic recreation and labor, and the promotion of socially acceptable behaviors. In addition, they treated "negro" minds, which were seen as distinct from "white" ones, in racially segregated facilities. Figures like Powell also leaned into hereditary explanations of mental disease and posed early eugenicist solutions to addressing the supposed postemancipation rise in insanity among Blacks.[6]

In the past decade, studies have begun to address related questions about the experiences of Black people in asylums. Moving the vast body of research on the history of psychiatry beyond a perfunctory documentation of discriminatory treatment in asylums, Wendy Gonaver, Elodie Edwards-Grossi, Mab Segrest, and Martin Summers have shown how the institution of slavery and postemancipation racial ideologies were integral to both the operation of asylums and the development of the field of psychiatry.[7] Notwithstanding, their studies leave room for more sustained examinations of Black peoples' lives before, during, and after their incarceration in asylums. In particular, there is little scholarship that focuses specifically on Black women's raced and gendered experiences. Although scholars of women's nineteenth-century asylum narratives have examined gender in the history of psychiatry, they have examined white insane women's lives, including how they wrote back to psychiatric authorities and presented counternarratives about confinement. But these studies have paid no attention to the lives of Black women.[8]

This chapter contextualizes and illuminates the complex experiences of nineteenth-century "insane" Black women. Although asylums were purported by experts like Powell to create environments of care, the experiences of Black women suggest instead that they endured precarious psychiatric incarceration. At the intersection of Black history, Black feminist theory, and the history of psychiatry, this chapter centers on the lives of Black women who were institutionalized at the Georgia Lunatic Asylum (GLA), one of the most infamous asylums in the US South as a result of the egregious conditions of the hospital across various time periods (figure 5.2).[9]

I have reconstructed the life narratives of five Black women—Viney W., Jane G., Olivia W., Alice M., and Amanda C.—working between various official documents. None of these women can speak for themselves, but their lives are evident in newspapers, asylum records, and police accounts. Throughout the chapter, I argue that postslavery psychiatric practices worked in tandem with a myriad of postbellum social realities, including cultural constructions of Black femininity, poverty, intimate

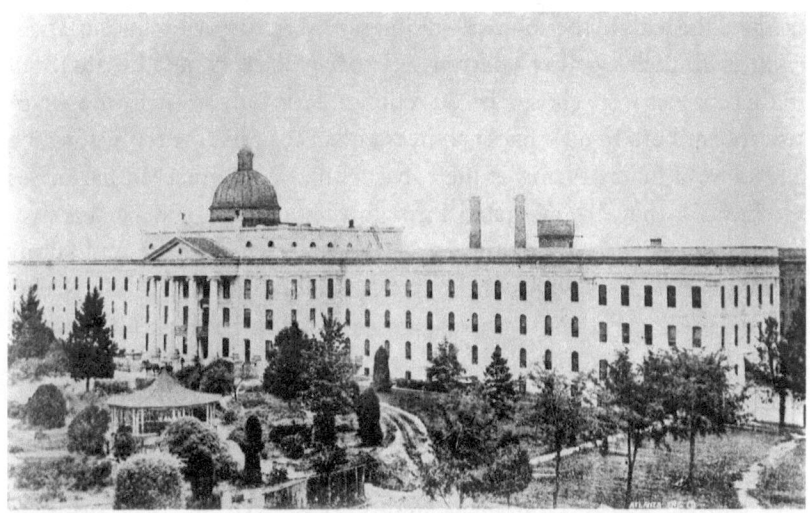

FIGURE 5.2 Milledgeville, 1894. Center Building at Georgia Lunatic Asylum, now known as Central State Hospital. Vanishing Georgia Collection, Georgia Archives.

partner violence, and racism, all of which serve to distinguish Black women's experiences of insanity and psychiatric incarceration from those of their white female counterparts and white and Black men.[10]

Recovering Black women's stories of psychiatric incarceration in the nineteenth century is challenging. Unlike asylum administrators' thoughts on the "colored insane," which were recorded in speeches, journals, and hospital annual reports, or the perspectives of white women, which were captured in published asylum narratives, psychiatrically incarcerated Black women's voices were not preserved. Rarely do the voices of Black people come into view in psychiatric archives. There are a few exceptions, of course. A sermon given by James Cossy, a free Black man held in the Eastern Lunatic Asylum in the 1820s, is included in the institution's records.[11] But more often patients were forced into silence. In the face of the silence of Black patients in general and Black women in particular, this chapter follows other studies in Black women's history by making informed and at times speculative conjectures about the women and their alleged illnesses to shine light on stories that were never meant to be told. The chapter relies on fragmented archival materials, including newspapers, brief GLA intake ledgers, and the writings of GLA superintendent Theophilus Powell, which together make it possible to glimpse the women's experiences. Although thousands of Black women trudged the halls of the colored buildings of GLA, only a few left sufficient records to stitch together a narrative. The five Black women I write about in this chapter were chosen because they are the only women whose stories appear both in newspaper sources and in the asylum archives, which allows for a fuller tracing of their lives. Still, the fragmented narratives are limited; they are mediated through the language and perspectives of doctors, judges, police officers, journalists, census takers, and family members. We do not hear the women's voices directly, if at all. Nevertheless, these particular women's stories contain the most information from which I could reconstruct narratives, and they offer a wellspring of knowledge about what it meant to be Black, female, and mentally disabled in the late nineteenth century. The following pages explain how postemancipation race- and gender-based medical discourses, in tandem with societal views on Black femininity, both shaped the category of insanity and justified Black women's distinct confinement to and treatment within a southern asylum.

BLACK WOMEN OF GLA

The main sources for the life stories of the women I examine in this chapter are newspaper articles and asylum intake ledgers.[12] The newspaper articles appeared in Atlanta-area publications from 1888 to 1894. Stories about Black women often were printed in a section called "In the Open Field: Short Stories of Minor Happenings Gathered from Many Sources, the City Briefly Mirrored." Consequently, newspapers printed their stories alongside other "minor happenings" in the lives of everyday people. For example, stories in this section mention such mundane occurrences as winning a spelling bee, new fruit imports from Cuba, and petty crimes. The proximity of Black women's stories to these everyday happenings suggests that the women were ordinary and their experiences commonplace. Further, it signals the ubiquity of racialized ideas about Black female insanity in the postemancipation South.

As asylum records show, the women go from being one among many mundane subjects in the public record to being a typical "case study" in the asylum. The asylum ledgers include a wide range of information about the women upon their arrival at GLA. They note demographic information such as county or state of origin, age, number of children, marital status, and occupation. The ledgers' overarching diagnostic categories are "lunatic," "idiot," and "epileptic." They also document various supposed precipitating causes of insanity, including "blow to the head," "menstrual derangement," and "ill treatment by her husband." The records chronicle people's past medical histories, which provided asylum keepers with information about the nature and degree of their insanity. Descriptions of past medical and personal histories include phrases like "homicidal or suicidal," "gets into a state of nudity," "destructive," "hereditary tendency," "duration of insanity," "eats and sleeps well," and "uses snuff." These descriptors were variously applied to all people. Prior to examining how these terms or diagnoses were mapped onto the five Black women discussed in this chapter, the women are introduced by citing the full transcripts of the articles and ledgers in which they appear. Together, these documents present a limited yet valuable portrait of each woman.

The narrative of Olivia W. is the most complete. Her census record indicates that in June 1880 she was twenty-one years old and worked as a housekeeper. The census taker made no notations about prior insanity in her case.[13] She lived with her husband Felix, a twenty-three-year-old farm laborer. Felix had been unemployed one month during the census year. Olivia's two children—John, who was three, and Anna, who was one—also lived in the household. The following decade, in July 1894, Olivia's life was less tranquil than what the census suggests. She appears in two newspaper articles, one from July 14, 1894, and the other from July 18, 1894:

> FOUR LUNATICS—The Fulton County jail has been converted into a lunatic asylum. There are now four lunatics inside its walls and they have been there for some time. Two of them are women, Olivia and Jane. The former is extremely violent and is kept in a darkened dungeon in the basement of the jail. Jane is the negress who shot the negro man out of the tree because she suspected him of conjuring her babe to death. A fifth lunatic, Amanda, was sent to the state lunatic asylum yesterday.[14]
>
> SENT TO THE ASYLUM—Two lunatics who have been inmates of the Fulton County jail for the past month were carried to the asylum yesterday. Olivia, a colored woman, was very violent and it was necessary to handcuff her. The other was a negro boy.[15]

At the GLA, Olivia's asylum narrative contains the following information:

> Olivia c/
> Lunatic from Fulton County. Native of Georgia. Age 28. Married. Cook. Baptist. First symptoms appeared about two months ago. Not hereditary. Cause—ill treatment by her husband. Not suicidal or homicidal but somewhat violent. Does not use tobacco. Received a violent blow on the jaw from her husband. Eats and sleeps well. Not dangerous with fire. Has been treated by city physician.
> Address: Harriet Foster, 436 Atlanta, GA.
> 52 Grady St.
> Received 16 July 1894.
> Died 10 Oct. 1896. Exhaustion.[16]

Amanda C., who appears in the July 14 article with Olivia, was also sent to GLA. Her asylum ledger reads as follows:

Amanda c/

Lunatic from Fulton County. Native of Georgia. Age 45. Widow six living children two deceased. Cook. Baptist. First symptoms appeared some months ago. Inclined to be violent. No hereditary tendency. Cause change of life. Probably had an attack previous to this one but not suicidal, homicidal or violent. Destructive. Uses snuff. Eats and sleeps well. Not dangerous with fire.

Received 12 July 1894
Discharged 23 Jan 1895
Restored
Address Missie Coursey 71 Plum St.
Atlanta, GA[17]

I have been unable to learn anything further about Amanda.

Viney W. entered the hospital in 1888. She appeared in the *Atlanta Constitution* on July 4, 1888: "Viney, a colored woman about forty years old, was so violent that her family had her arrested. In court she evidenced a dangerous type of insanity, and the jury quickly adjudged her to be crazy. Judge Calhoun committed her to the state lunatic asylum."[18] Her intake ledger reads as follows:

Lunatic from Fulton Co Ga. Age 30 years. Single—Occupation cook. Duration two or three months. Cause unknown. Not known as to whether she is homicidal or suicidal. Duration two or three months—will wander from home and get into a state of nudity. Nothing more could be furnished concerning her history by the person who brings her.

Received July 11, 1888
Died 31 April 1895
Dropsy
Address
Ordinary
Atlanta
Ga.[19]

According to the *Atlanta Constitution* article of July 14, Jane G. was sent to Milledgeville. However, there is no existing asylum ledger. The same is true for Alice M., who was declared "insane" by a police officer. Alice's story appeared on July 2, 1881, in the *Daily Constitution*:

> Alice, a negro woman, was found lying upon the sidewalk on Peachtree street yesterday by Officer Simmons. In her arms was a small deformed child, to which she was clinging. When approached by the patrolman Alice began calling loudly for help. To the officer it was apparent that she was either drunk or insane and an arrest was the result, but before reaching the station-house the latter was found to be the case. The child was taken from her and by direction of the county commissioners given to a colored woman. To-day [sic] Alice will be taken before a committee upon lunacy for an examination.[20]

In these archival traces, Black women are portrayed in one-dimensional and fatalistic ways, which results in discursive violence. Saidiya Hartman discusses how photographs of seemingly minor figures, urban Black girls, were intended to "classify, isolate, and differentiate" them according to prevailing notions of social deviance.[21] Black women's visibility, she reminds us, whether in photographs, words, or medical records, made Black women "target[s] for uplift or punishment, confinement or violence."[22] Although we only have secondary renderings of their stories, we are left to wonder whether these Black women would actually recognize themselves in public and medical records. Holding space for the possibility of fuller renderings of their lives, I read the records with a speculative openness to the concerns, issues, and desires that Black women might have had but that were elided from the medicalized representation of their bodyminds.

Rather than seeing silences in the archives as dead ends, I lean into them as sites of possibility for meaning. Ula Taylor urges scholars who examine the historical experiences of Black women to speak to the silences in the archives by employing a "historical imagination."[23] In this study, such a process requires critically evaluating the claims put forth by people with the power to comment on Black women's sanity while also theorizing notions of race, gender, and insanity to offer competing vantage points that more fully animate their lives. My analysis of the records is guided by various critical questions. For example, what does it mean to focus on violence allegedly perpetrated by insane Black women while ignoring the personal and political violences being levied against them? I also ground the women in the worlds they inhabited through deep historical contextualization and consideration of relevant cultural constructions of race and gender that inflected their experiences of mental disability. When slight echoes of their voices do appear, such as the screams of Alice, I pay attention to the significance they might have had for her as a postpartum mother rather than solely considering the views of the police officer who retained her or the newspaper editor who relayed the story. On the whole, this chapter juxtaposes the words and interests of authority figures with the various meanings these Black women might have assigned to any given aspect of their lives. Ultimately, I hope to show that these Black women cannot be reduced to the sparse portraits of insanity that outlived them.

SENT TO THE LUNATIC ASYLUM: BLACK WOMEN'S JOURNEYS TO GLA

Black women's distinct experiences at GLA correlated with their specific raced and gendered existence before they arrived at the asylum. Scholars have attended to women's sexuality as a site of management for psychiatric officials. Analyses about Black women in particular have converged around sexual lasciviousness as a concern of import.[24] Conceptions of Black female sanity were steeped in discourses about postbellum Black femininity and conceptions of insanity.

Postemancipation discourses of Black femininity that colored claims of Black female insanity were deeply connected to racial stereotypes. The figure of the Sapphire, which appeared in popular culture, was an offshoot of the Mammy and the Jezebel. Unlike the docile Mammy or the sexually loose Jezebel, the Sapphire was defiant toward whites and controlling toward Black men.[25] These stereotypes shaped the social expectations of Black women.

For these GLA narratives, the most salient theme is another preoccupation in the historical management of the insane—violence.[26] In a postemancipation southern society bent on reestablishing a white supremist social order, "dangerous" Black women posed a particularly grave threat. Jacqueline Jones describes that white observers often judged freed Black women as "aggressive": "Northern and foreign observers conveyed the distinct impression that Black women were particularly outspoken and aggressive (by implication relative to Black men) in their willingness to confront white authority figures."[27] Jones's argument suggests that the label of "violent" Black woman was not simply a reference to specific actions. The characterizations illuminate the ways that GLA women were viewed as always already potentially uncontrollable and therefore needing to be contained at the slightest evidence of deviance. Black women were "colored" violent *and* insane by being assertive. It is no surprise, then, that southern newspapers depicted Black "insane" women as violent, disruptive, or dangerous.

Newspapers rarely described white women in these negative terms. Unlike Black women, white "insane" women were depicted either as passive, fragile victims or as voices of protest. Mrs. King, a white woman at GLA, had the benefit of both. King was described as "unfortunate." Upon her release, she informed newspaper reporters about the "unjustness of her incarceration and the horrible way she was treated [at GLA]."[28]

The interplay between violence and perceived deviance among Black women surfaces in subtle ways in Alice's story. Alice is found to be insane by Fulton County police officer Simmons. The article indicates that she was to be "taken before a committee upon lunacy for an examination," which suggests that she would be subjected to the authority of the medical profession in addition to that of law enforcement. The non-medically trained officer's determination that Alice was "insane" rather than "drunk" even "before [they reached] the station-house" reveals how the authority of the law and that of the medical profession were compounding sources of domination and control over Black women.[29] Alice, like other Black women, would have likely been particularly vulnerable to the threat of Simmons's authority because of existing racial tensions. As the historian Tera Hunter contends, the atmosphere in Atlanta at the time was volatile: "Black Atlantans during Reconstruction were subjected to . . . physical violence, especially at the hands of white civilians and police."[30] In this hostile atmosphere, when Simmons approached Alice, who was "clinging" to her "small deformed child," she could have been calling for help as a result of fear for herself and her child or as a postpartum mother in distress. The record does not show that observers inquired about the source of her distress or fear. She had good reason to be afraid: once she was taken to the police station, Alice's child was taken from her.³¹ Alice's cry for help is the only hint of her voice available; we do not have fuller access to her perspective. Like many Black women in the aftermath of slavery, Alice likely feared the possibility of being separated from her child and suffered tremendous emotional pain when it occurred. In a postslavery world, being labeled insane opened Alice up to the violence of familial separation familiar to Black Americans. Of course, it is also possible that she called out to the policeman for help, but we cannot know. No matter how her encounter with the authorities occurred, she lost her child as a consequence of being deemed insane and subsequently committed to the GLA.

Although subtle forms of violence, such as those Alice experienced, were socially acceptable because of the allegation of insanity, the stories of Jane, Olivia, and Viney reveal that even the perception of Black female violence was not tolerated. Jane was sent to jail because she "shot [a] negro man out of the tree because she suspected him of conjuring her babe to death."³² Olivia was called "very violent" in one article and "extremely violent" in another, although there are no descriptions of her crimes or violent acts.³³ The record asserts, rather than demonstrates, a "violent" and "insane" Black woman, an easy construction during a period when many forms of self-assertion could be read as violence. Once judged violent, Olivia was locked "in a darkened dungeon in the basement of the [Fulton County] jail."³⁴ Viney was described as "so violent that her family had her arrested." The newspaper writer indicated that she evidenced such a "dangerous" kind of "insanity" that the jury "quickly adjudicated her to be crazy."³⁵ Although Viney was depicted as being the most violent of the women, her intake record makes no reference to violence. This inconsistency reflects the way in which social actors, including police officers, family members, and judges, measured Black women's sanity in relation to perceived standards and norms of femininity, most established by and for white women.

Black women not only dealt with the threat of violence from whites but were also subjected in many cases to intracommunity violence from Black men.³⁶ In the *Atlanta Constitution*, Viney's story appeared alongside a narrative about a Black man named Jake Collier, who also was sentenced by Judge John Calhoun. Like the average white southerner, Calhoun had a gendered and racialized conception of violence that excused, even condoned, violence against Black women. He found Collier guilty of "[giving] his wife a drubbing" and fined him "$15 and cost [sic] yesterday and bound him over to the city court for $100." Collier's violence against his wife was brutal: "Then he seized her about the waist and threw her from the window to the ground. She struck on her head, but before she could get to her feet Jake was in front with a pistol in her face." Undoubtedly, Judge Calhoun was privy to the details of Mrs. Collier's assault. Although he determined that Collier was not violent enough to be sent to GLA, he "quickly" judged Viney to be "insane." The Collier story exhibits the acceptability of violence inflicted upon Black women's bodyminds. In fact, considering Olivia's intake record, Mrs. Collier was more likely to end up in the asylum than her husband. The cause of Olivia's insanity, for example, was "ill treatment by her husband," who had given her "a violent blow on the jaw."[37] The historian Wendy Gonaver contends that such notations reveal that asylum physicians did not consider violence against women as a possible source of women's alleged aggression. The asylum, Gonaver argues, normalized domestic violence, making it possible to see excessive domestic brutality as a "medical pathology of individuals" rather than a broader societal ill in need of redress.[38] In the midst of a post-Reconstruction social climate that normalized state and domestic violence against them, the asylum was a potent and interlocking institutionalized threat for Black women.[39] Whether through perceptions of their violence or the acceptance of violence against them, conceptions of and assumptions about Black femininity worked to confine Black women in asylums. These conceptions operated in tandem with dominant constructions of insanity in the South that governed Black women's diagnoses and experiences of mental illness and psychiatric confinement.

LATE NINETEENTH-CENTURY MEDICALIZED THOUGHT ON BLACK MENTAL DISABILITY

Powell was the person directly responsible for the standards of care at the GLA that determined how Olivia, Amanda, and Viney were treated, but his ideas exist in the context of the major debates in late nineteenth-century psychiatry, medicine, and science in regard to the mental and physical capacity of Black people, their biological prospects for postslavery survival, and their suitability for full inclusion in the American body politic.[40] His ideas were formed against the backdrop of nineteenth-century men of medicine and science's relentless pursuit of knowledge about the existence of various "racial types" of mankind, the role of heredity versus environment in human development, and the concept of social evolution.[41]

Scientists, physicians, and psychiatrists pondered whether or not freedom from slavery was particularly injurious to Black mental health.[42] In 1869, the surgeon Sanford B. Hunt paired data from the US Sanitary Commission with prewar cranial measurements collected by polygenist Samuel Morton to propose that emancipated Black bodyminds evidenced deterioration. Hunt called for ongoing studies of postmortem Black brains to determine if they had been hindered by the environmental limitations of slavery or if biological determinism rendered governmental attempts to create opportunities for Black advancement futile.[43] "As between the two races," Hunt explained, "the problem is: Does the large brain by its own impulses create education, civilization and refinement, or do education, civilization and refinement create the large brain?"[44]

Psychiatrists primarily sided with those who believed that freedom from slavery harmed Black bodyminds. Innate group inferiority, associated with race rather than individuals, seemed to most white postbellum psychiatrists and physicians to be the cause of Black insanity; they argued that Black people's nervous systems failed to evolve, were prone to the excesses that led to insanity, and had an inability to handle the "mental strain" of freedom.[45] Psychiatrists blamed the rise in insanity on the loss of the structured daily living conditions that supposedly protected Black people's health during slavery.[46] Psychiatrists marshaled their own body of data, such as Black admission rates and census report data on the incidents of mental disabilities, to make their assertions about the deleterious effect of emancipation.[47] Prior to the Civil War, psychiatrists' discussions of race and mental disability decisively maintained that slavery protected Black bodyminds, although little research into either race or insanity was conducted and the conclusions were based more on prejudice than rigorous medical research or recorded case studies. After the Civil War, however, psychiatrists joined the new scientific fervor to collect data and produce research on Black Americans, and the questions of "insanity and physical degeneration" were especially important in the arena of ideas that were used to justify Jim Crow.

This was a question that interested all psychiatrists, but southern psychiatrists felt that because the Black population had long been higher in their region, they were best situated to contribute the new knowledge being produced about Black bodyminds.[48] J. F. Miller, superintendent of the only institution in North Carolina that catered exclusively to Black people, Eastern Hospital in Goldsboro, insisted that there were measurable increases in Black mental disabilities after emancipation. Like in early nineteenth-century discourses on mental disability, slavery remained the most critical factor in determining the causes, treatment, and etiology of insanity among Black patients.[49] Miller correlated the supposed explosion of cases of insanity in the postemancipation period to Black people's loss of the health-promoting environment of slavery:

> It is an undisputed fact, known to our Southern people that no race of men ever lived under better hygienic restraints or had governing their lives rules and regulations more conducive to physical health and mental repose. Their habits of life were regular, their food and clothing were substantial and sufficient, as a rule, and the edict of the master kept them indoors at night and restrained them from promiscuous sexual indulgence and the baneful influences of the liquor saloon. In sickness, he was promptly and properly cared for by physician and nurse. Freedom came to him and a change came over his entire life.[50]

Miller suggested that enslavement stamped out the rise of excessive desires and "sexual indulgence" among Black people even though cultural stereotypes of Black women as salacious Jezebels existed both during and after slavery. Echoing his antebellum predecessors, he also linked the supposed "mental repose" generated by slavery to the presumption that slaveholders forcibly regulated unhygienic social behaviors such as drinking and illicit sex.[51] Psychiatrists such as Miller were also convinced that slavery was not only good for creating the conditions for good health or a health-promoting environment but also kept at bay the grotesque and defective hereditary tendencies innate to the Black race.

Speaking to his colleagues at the Southern Medico-Psychological Association conference in Asheville, North Carolina, in 1896, Miller argued that freedom brought upon the former slave "a beautiful harvest of mental and physical degeneration and he is now becoming a martyr to an heredity thus established."[52] The "freed Negro," he contended, was particularly vulnerable to the overwhelming weight of heredity in the postemancipation period. Social scientists agreed that life after emancipation, compounded by the calamitous effects of the Civil War on the southern economy, stressed all southerners, but a subsection of the population, newly freed Black Americans, were unfit to weather such storms. As French anthropologist Paul Topinard argued, the excesses of "mania" and "idiocy" among Black southerners were pronounced because they were not equipped to "battle with the necessities of the social condition."[53] As freedmen, such experts concluded, Blacks would be unable to fend off their unrestrained sexual proclivities, emotional excess, and otherwise savage states. Social scientists used these data to argue that the population increase further threatened the mental, physical, and moral health of Black Americans. A member of the American Medical Association remarked that these innate attributes would eventually overtake the Black population, driving it to dwindle and disappear: "The increase in the defective classes will only hasten the final destruction of the race."[54] By 1903, the accepted belief in medical circles was that mental and physical deterioration was a constitutive feature of the Black community. The Atlanta National Conference of Charities warned that Blacks were "in danger of being destroyed by insanity."[55] When statistics showed that in fact the Black population was expanding, the purported inability of Black Americans to adapt to their new social conditions fueled white panic about the threat presented by their Black neighbors.

There were some mental conditions that seemed not to affect Black southerners. Some doctors argued that mental ailments that led to suicide in the general population, which was rampant among southern white women, men, and soldiers as a result of the financial, familial, and psychological toil and toll of war, were not evidenced in Blacks. Frederick Hoffman argued that Blacks had a infantile intellectual constitution, rendering them incapable of the "subtle motives" underlying suicide among whites.[56] Suicide among Black patients, he asserted, was only present as a result of their inclination to be consumed by passion. He also pointed to their supposed lack of self-control and inability to experience the kind of psychological distress that emerges from lamenting the past or worrying about future on account of the fact that Blacks had a "tendency to live wholly in the present."[57]

Although one strain of white scientific thinking was that Black Americans would go extinct, another was that Blacks only stood a chance at improving in a situation in which they freely battled with other races and gained equality through their own efforts.[58] Many social scientists believed that segregation and the suspension of white benevolence was the only path toward racial equality. Others, like the Dallas physician Dr. E. T. Easley, thought Blacks were hopeless and "notoriously incompetent" and not fit to live as equals in a free society. These collective medical, psychiatric, and scientific sentiments about Black postslavery physiological and psychological constitutions served as fodder in white nationalists' campaigns against Black full inclusion in American society, evidenced most notably in the suppression of Blacks through organized disenfranchisement, the destruction of Black-serving institutions, and grand enactments of violence such as the 1896 Wilmington massacre and coup, a subject of the next chapter.[59]

Powell's ideas about Black mental health are consistent with those prevalent at the time. His major extant writings span eleven years and consist of a special report in a GLA hospital annual report, two presidential addresses before medical associations, and a speech before the American Medical Association.[60] Although he was not a prolific writer, Powell's writings demonstrate a keen interest in the care of the "colored insane." All of his writing comments on the "colored insane," with one piece exclusively about them. These works reached both average readers, through local newspapers, and medical professionals, through prominent medical journals and the citations of other superintendents. Over the course of his twenty-eight-year tenure at GLA, he served simultaneously as the president of state, regional, and national medical associations. Despite his influence, especially among southern psychiatrists, few scholarly analyses of Powell's psychiatric thought exist.[61]

Undergirding Powell's psychiatric thought was his belief that two factors—heredity and environment—caused insanity.[62] His first standalone analysis of insanity was consistent with the general trend in nineteenth-century psychiatry toward emphasizing genetics in its etiology. Powell reasoned that people inherited tendencies, weaknesses, and predispositions that made them susceptible to a wide range of triggers, what he referred to as "exciting causes" of "insanity," which ranged from emotional upsets such as "disappointed affection" and "loss of wife, husband or children," to excessive behaviors and character flaws such as "over-work," "jealousy," and "religious excitement," to physiological changes or disruptions such as "blows to the head" or "menstrual dysfunction."[63] He argued that "structural and physiological defects of the central nervous system" led to inherited predispositions.[64] In his estimation, hereditary predispositions were at the root of all cases of insanity. In other words, even if put in a bad environment, someone could only develop insanity if they were already susceptible. His ideas evolved to the point that they were precursors for eugenics, most notably in an 1887 presidential address before the Medical Association of Georgia, "Heredity and Environment." In the speech, he offered his definition of heredity, "that biological law by which all beings endowed with life tend to repeat themselves in their descendants," coupling it with the claim that the best way to reduce insanity and other inherited traits such as criminality and juvenile degeneracy would be to control the proliferation of supposedly tainted offspring by ensuring that tainted people could only marry those who were "healthy" and "robust."[65] Because widespread degeneracy posed an imminent threat to the human race, he believed drastic measures needed to be taken to regulate reproduction, such as requiring medical approval for marriage licenses.

Although this emphasis on heredity was paramount in Powell's medical explanation of insanity, the role of environment was not trivial, especially because it served as clear justification for the utility of asylums. A person's environment or surroundings, he believed, could improve, modify, and even eradicate insanity. For Powell, environment entailed both hospital provisions, such as sanitary dwellings and nutritional diets, and behavioral regulations around sleep, leisure time, and moral education. Some extant images of the hospital reveal the overtly medicalized spaces that they included, such as operating rooms, whereas other spaces appear more domesticated and reflect the time that passed as people lived out their lives both separately and connected to others (figures 5.3 and 5.4). Superintendents believed that the asylum had the best chance of being curative if it regulated people's diet and sleep and provided a homelike environment, systematic employment, and plenty of opportunities to "divert the mind into normal channels," such as amusement halls, chapels, and libraries.[66]

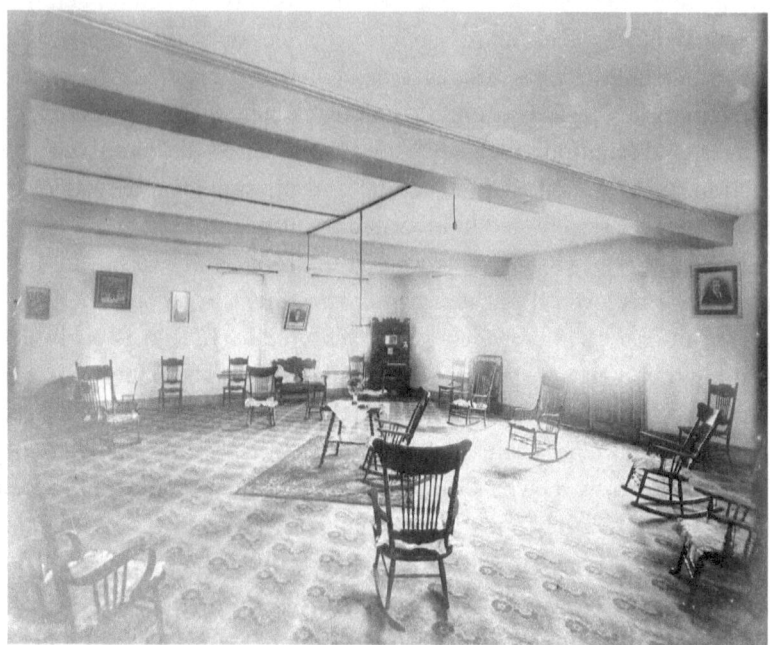

FIGURE 5.3 Milledgeville, ca. 1894. View of the day room at Georgia Lunatic Asylum, now known as Central State Hospital. Vanishing Georgia Collection, Georgia Archives.

The institution of slavery was an ever-present frame of reference in Powell's discussions of insanity among Black southerners. He believed that there had been few instances of insanity in the Black population during slavery because enslaved people's environments had been managed in favor of mental health. As did others in the period, he argued that slave masters had forced slaves to "obey the laws of health." In Powell's case, these laws included moral elements such as teaching "from infancy" habits of obedience and self-control and the limitation of excess and overindulgence in freedom, liberty, and alcohol; they also included easy access to sufficient nourishment, regular sleep, and rest, the latter two of which he believed were necessary for the "recuperation of the brain and nervous system." Slavery prevented group-based tendencies from being realized, and thus, among the freed people, the "colored insane" evidenced a greater possibility for individual degeneracy and debasement. For example, although an individual white person could pass down a vice such as

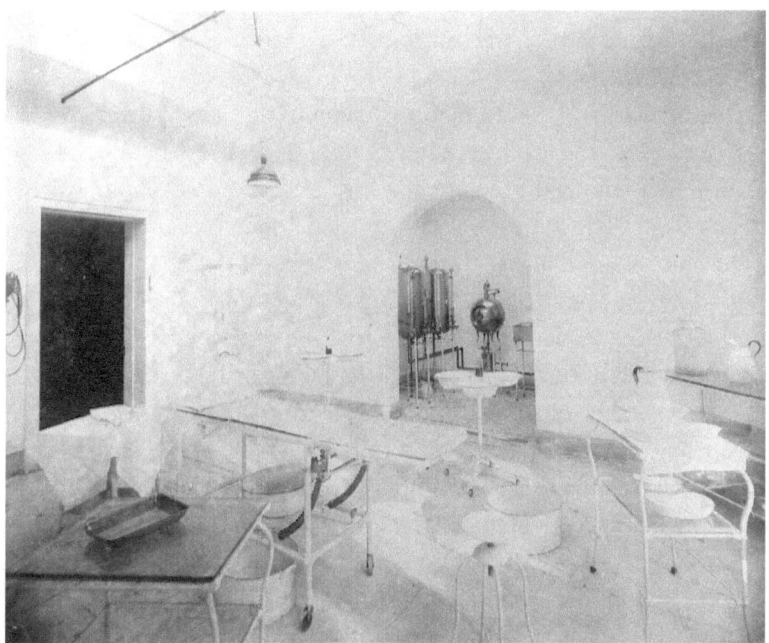

FIGURE 5.4 Milledgeville, ca. 1894. Interior of an operating room at Georgia Lunatic Asylum, now known as Central State Hospital. Vanishing Georgia Collection, Georgia Archives.

alcoholism, which Powell identified as the chief cause of insanity among all people, Black people as a race had an innate disposition toward alcoholism because of their "emotional nature." The "tendency to irregular habits" that "frequently led to excesses which produce insanity," Powell claimed, was a particular quality of Black people. He made a distinction between the heredity-based insanity witnessed among whites, or, as he put it, an "inherited tendency toward disease," and the postemancipation forms of insanity Blacks experienced that were the result of unchecked innate unhealthy tendencies.[67] More worrying to Powell, though, was the possibility that the postemancipation conditions of insanity that were spreading across the Black community would eventually become inherited tendencies, as he believed the first generation of children born after emancipation were already demonstrating. Some of the women discussed here were a part of the generation of Blacks that he was concerned about. Powell maintained the argument that emancipation was harmful to

Blacks, aligning himself with white supremacist political ideologies, and at the same time, he adhered to "scientific" theories about the etiology of mental disease.

After alcoholism, Powell held that syphilis and tuberculosis, or "consumption," were the leading causes of insanity in the general population but especially among the "colored insane." He elaborated on these diseases extensively in "The Increase of Insanity and Tuberculosis in the Southern Negro Since 1860, and Its Alliance, and Some of the Supposed Causes," read before the American Medical Association in 1896 and reprinted in the association's journal in December of the same year. Reasserting his previous stance about Black people's innate negative characteristics and the positive environmental conditions of slavery, he argued that many freed people had developed a "consumptive, syphilitic and alcoholic constitution," which made them easily susceptible to diseases to which slaves had been immune.[68] Interestingly, Powell universalized his race-based critiques by asserting that the fate of former slaves was broadly applicable: "Too much liberty and freedom, so far as the laws of health are concerned, is dangerous to the mental and physical integrity of any people."[69] Powell was echoing the widespread pathologization of Black freedom that occurred among medical authorities before emancipation.[70] In the postbellum period, it may appear curious that he would make this claim because, pushed to its logical conclusion, it offered a justification for the enslavement of whites. This certainly was never his aim. Rather, the claim supported his approach to asylum care that emphasized the central role of environment in treatment. Hygienic standards emphasizing the regulation of individuals' daily lives and sanitary surroundings, supposedly achieved during slavery, were desirable for combating syphilis, tuberculosis, and insanity in asylums. Although this explanation justified the practice of psychiatric incarceration, it also identified the asylum environment as a source of communicable diseases such as tuberculosis. Defending his institutional governance, Powell asserted that the "care and treatment is the same" for both whites and Blacks, so the higher tuberculosis death rates among Blacks could be attributed to the fact that many Black people came to the hospital already infected. Among all of Powell's beliefs about the "colored insane," his most persistent message was that their growing number was one of the most important challenges facing the broader community and the field of psychiatry.

Powell's writings exemplify how nineteenth-century psychiatric thought was shaped by the cultural climate in which it was practiced. Rather than objective scientific and medical discovery, his discussions of Black insanity were informed by and responded to the meaning of race in the post–Civil War US South. As Dorothy Roberts explains, "racial reclassifications did not occur in response to scientific advances in human biology, but in response to sociopolitical imperatives. They reveal that what is being defined, organized, and interpreted is a political relationship not an innate classification."[71] The political tensions of Powell's era were illuminated by Jim Crow practices of racial segregation and subjugation and the rhetoric of the Lost Cause movement, which longed for slavery-era racial hierarchies. Considering this racial climate, it is unsurprising that Powell's supposedly medical assertions about Blacks conveniently aligned with white supremacist social agendas. Like other psychiatrists, Powell held contradictory conclusions simultaneously about insanity among Black people. The "colored insane" were seen as the same as whites because of their mental ailments and, at the same time, as fundamentally different because of their race.[72] This tension is evident in Powell's explanations of the origins of insanity among Blacks, for which he fell back on racist ideas about Black innate inferiority. The most disturbing aspect of Powell's (and other superintendents') outlook is that it obscured many of the real health consequences of racism in the postemancipation South, including mental distress from racialized terror and violence; race-based systemic poverty associated with economic institutions such as debt peonage, sharecropping, and convict leasing; the proliferation of postwar illnesses; and the lack of access to healthcare. All of these factors compounded or created mental health crises among Black Americans in the period.

RACE, GENDER, AND BLACK WOMEN'S GLA NARRATIVES

Powell's references to the "colored insane" seldom distinguish between Black women and Black men. His conflation of male and female care suggests that race was the primary category of difference. To be sure, race figures importantly in Black women's GLA narratives. However, Powell's emphasis on race obscured the role gender played in their lives. Several themes emerge when we consider the ways race and gender simultaneously affected freedwomen's lives at GLA, including the significance of motherhood, marriage, and the racialized regulation of life at the asylum.

Motherhood had a distinct meaning for Black women during the postbellum period. It also complicated their experiences of psychiatric incarceration. Forty-five-year-old Amanda entered GLA on July 12, 1894. She had "six living children [and] two deceased."[73] Two days later, Olivia entered the hospital.[74] Her intake papers make no mention of her two children, John and Anna, who would now have been seventeen and fifteen, respectively.[75] Nearly half of the Black women entering the hospital the year Olivia and Amanda arrived were mothers.[76] The archival records provide us with these facts, but there are no extant asylum narratives that might communicate what motherhood meant for them. Surely, though, life in a society that was hostile to Black autonomy and communal survival shaped the meaning of motherhood for Olivia and Amanda.

For many enslaved Black women, one of the most devastating features of enslavement was their inability to fully mother their children. Unsurprisingly, then, the meaning of motherhood for postbellum Black women was deeply connected to their attainment of freedom. The historian Noralee Frankel argues that Black women "held definite opinions about what freedom meant.... It meant being allowed to live with their families without the threat of any of them being sold." The desire to be connected to their children drove thousands of freedwomen to search for children who had been torn from them during slavery. This desire also led many Black women to resist postemancipation working conditions that created a conflict between work and family: "Besides doing the cooking, washing, sewing, and gardening, freedwomen took charge of caring for their own children. Pregnant and nursing mothers wanted to give up outside work. Mothers sometimes argued with their employers about giving their babies more attention instead of working in the fields."[77] Freedwomen had to constantly negotiate the demands of labor with their desire to maintain their families.

Olivia and Amanda would have had to contend with a history of denied and constrained motherhood and an intensified desire to maintain bonds with children. Being incarcerated at GLA, however, brought about conditions akin to the institution of slavery with respect to familial ties. Powell adhered to the longstanding belief in separating people, Black and white, from their families. The treatment rationale was that people needed to be removed from the exciting circumstances that produced their insanity.[78] As a result of this practice, the asylum isolated Black mothers at GLA from their children, sometimes miles apart and often with no hope of visitation or expectation of seeing them again. Elevated mortality rates for Black women at GLA ensured that this was the case for many. Antebellum slave narratives offer compelling evidence that severed connections between mothers and their children were a source of great psychic wounding during slavery, and similar emotional pain surely existed among Black women at GLA. Some women's ages suggest that they would have experienced firsthand the despair of being torn from children or from their own mothers during slavery, which would have made their alienation particularly devastating.

Olivia and Amanda were mothers and were also among the 65 percent of Black women at GLA who were either married or widowed.[79] Like tens of thousands of freedwomen, Olivia and Amanda likely eagerly embraced their newfound civil liberties, which were deeply connected to their sense of what it meant to be free.[80] Although scant records prevent us from knowing the dates of their marriages, it is likely that they were like thousands of former bondspeople throughout the South who sought legal marriages after emancipation. For the first time, many were able to formalize familial bonds outside the specter, control, and interests of enslavers. Legalized marriage also carried with it the promise that children now belonged to their mother *and* father and thus could not be sold. These families could remain intact.[81]

Black Americans were enthusiastic about marriage after emancipation. However, the postwar political climate complicated Black women's pursuit of the institution. After an initial wave of white antagonism toward Black marriage, a set of new laws sprung up to criminalize and punish Black unions.[82] Some Black widows refused to marry again because doing so would jeopardize their government pensions.[83] As Baptists, Amanda and Olivia may have been obligated to marry in order to join the church.[84] Marriage for some was connected to communal participation, which was vital to survival after emancipation, and for others, it presented threats to economic security or the value of lived experiences. The asylum was yet another barrier to the fulfillment of the hopes and promises of communal uplift that marriage offered Black women in the late nineteenth century. When Amanda and Olivia arrived, they were forced to endure a protracted separation from their families. Powell disrupted hundreds of Black marital arrangements indefinitely. Out of the twenty-nine Black married women who entered the asylum with Amanda, only five others would join her in being deemed "restored" enough to be sent home to their families.[85]

Black women in the GLA not only had a unique set of issues to contend with when it came to motherhood and family ties but also experienced everyday life in the asylum differently than their white female or Black male counterparts. From the first line of the GLA asylum entry ledgers, we witness how race and gender shaped Black women's asylum experiences. The ledgers of Olivia, Amanda, and Viney all begin with their names but with no honorifics. White women's ledgers open with "Mrs.," "Ms.," or "Miss." These titles in white women's narratives symbolized their access to norms of womanhood that could be leveraged to support their claims of sanity and that influenced the extent to which the asylum could serve as a place of healing, comfort, and refuge.

Gender alone did not determine Black women's status or treatment at GLA. Black females were not only listed as female but also as "colored." This is reflected in the inclusion of the letter "c" above a dash, which is above two dots in their entries.[86] On the one hand, Black women's entry ledgers, like those of white women, abound with gendered forms of irregularity in the intake records: "womb disease," "menstrual derangement," "menstrual suppression," "menstrual irregularity," and "uterine disease." These significations reveal that the women were subjected to then-prevalent assumptions about madness and the female reproductive system. Powell, like his contemporaries, believed women were more susceptible to mental illness because they were inherently more "delicately constituted."[87] On the other hand, Black women's signification as "colored" meant that they were also subjected to Powell's belief that mental illness in Blacks was a "penalty" of being freed from slavery; it also indicated the fact of segregation.[88] Both sets of beliefs exposed Black women to race-based arrangements for labor and housing and influenced the kinds of health conditions from which they suffered.

A cornerstone of Powell's treatment protocol was assigning patients to "useful employments" in the asylum. His treatment philosophy involved redirecting people's thoughts away from the "morbid, self-contemplations, and insane delusions" and toward socially useful activity. For Powell, work was necessary for mental restoration: "Man's powers, mental and physical, were given to use; the development of those powers requires that they should be exercised to retain their integrity, and perform their proper functions."[89] In his estimation, regular and purposeful work, which was always gendered, sharpened the mental powers. Men performed labor on the farm, in the garden, or in the engine house, whereas women carried out domestic tasks such as sewing, cooking, or laundering. Later annual reports reveal that labor assignments were also racialized, as Black women worked in the laundry while white women were seamstresses.[90]

Labor had a distinct meaning for freedwomen like Viney, Olivia, and Amanda. By the 1890s, most white women's work in the domestic sphere was not wage-earning work, whereas poverty forced Black women, even those with spouses, into the workforce.[91] Black women were given more physically demanding work in the asylum, a reflection of racialized assumptions. Black women's status at GLA was similar to that in other segregated asylums where they, according to the historian Peter McCandless, "worked more and died faster than their white counterparts."[92] A history of unpaid labor informed why Black women in late nineteenth-century Atlanta defined freedom in part as control over their own labor.[93] They formed labor unions and trade organizations and organized protests to resist white attempts to reestablish a subservient labor pool.[94] Black women domestic workers were crucial to these labor struggles. Even if they similarly believed in the value of work, Black women and Powell differed in terms of what work meant. Black women's ideas about the significance of labor clashed with Powell's aim to provide "careful and systematic employment, indoors and out, shop and field." His use of free labor as a "means to divert and lead the mind into normal channels" was undoubtedly more oppressive than curative for postemancipation Black women.[95]

Black women's classification in the GLA also influenced both how and where they were treated. For Black people, race trumped diagnosis as a deciding factor in where they resided. Powell, like other superintendents, believed segregating people along racial lines was good for both

Blacks and whites. Northern physicians disingenuously promulgated the therapeutic merits of institutional segregation. Southern doctors were more pellucid in asserting that the advantage was not medically based but rather one of social conformity. Admitting that people were segregated based on "social reasons alone," Powell explains that it was the "unanimous . . . opinion" among southern practitioners that "the separation of white and colored patients is to the advantage of both races."[96] This view reflects the ways in which broader cultural norms were incorporated into psychiatric practice. Powell's belief in segregation, which had no objective scientific value, reinscribed external racial hierarchies in the hospital setting.

Racial hostility accompanied these social hierarchies both inside the GLA and outside. Across the later decades of the nineteenth century, white hostility and acts of terror against emancipated Black people proliferated across Georgia, driving many Black Georgians to flee in fear for their lives to Atlanta or Athens. The 1872 report of the Joint Select Committee to Inquire Into the Condition of Affairs in the Late Insurrectionary States brims with accounts of whippings, shootings, hangings, castrations, beatings, killings, harassment, voter intimidation, and burnings of Black homes, churches, and schools at the hands of individual white citizens and the "Ku Klux organization." There were also instances of gendered racial violence against Black women. For example, Black women were whipped based on perceived insubordinate behavior such as "talking saucily" to whites.[97] In addition to physical attacks, Black women were subject to rape and sexualized violence.[98] The common experience of mental disability did not dissipate racial attitudes white people brought with them into the asylum. Racial animosity stoked racial violence in many hospitals throughout the country despite attempts to segregate people.[99]

Although Powell did not record interracial conflicts, evidence of entrenched prejudices crept into asylum narratives. In January 1888, Miss Emma P., a white native of Greene County, one of the most violent in Georgia, was given a diagnosis that overlapped with Black patients at the GLA. She was diagnosed as a "lunatic," had "housework" as an occupation, and was even considered "violent." But her violence had a distinct, racial target: Emma was said to be violent "towards negroes only" as "the presence of negroes excit[ed] her." Similarly, Mrs. Sallie M. was described as "disposed to be violent toward negroes."[100] Even some people's paranoia was race based. Seventy-four-year-old Mary B. "fear[ed] negroes [would] kill her."[101] Mary was received in the hospital on June 19, 1879. A recent immigrant with experience living in Ireland and Scotland, she had only been in Georgia for five years but had quickly assimilated the racial hatreds of the South. Although Irish women faced exploitation at the hands of physicians, Mary's case record presents the classic narrative of ethnic white immigrants embracing American race conceptions.[102] Emma's, Sallie's, and Mary's racial views illuminate how asylum life for Olivia, Amanda, and Viney was potentially as hostile as life in southern culture outside the asylum's walls. Furthermore, if any mental distress arose from the sheer terror and violence Black women experienced before entering the asylum, such distress was never identified as a precipitating cause of insanity in the asylum ledgers. Given the racial animosities inside the GLA, Black women were never given the chance to escape the constricting grip of hatred.

SEGREGATION AND STANDARDS OF CARE

In 1867, the first Blacks were admitted to Georgia's state mental facility via the Freedmen's Bureau Hospital.[103] Alongside the white population, the number of "colored insane" rose dramatically over the decades. A building explicitly designed to house Black patients was erected to accommodate them. By 1870, the population of "colored insane" could no longer fit in its space and the existing building had to be enlarged.[104] It was expanded again in 1879 and 1881 yet was filled to capacity again by 1888.[105] Overcrowded segregated dwellings were a feature of the hospital at every stage.[106]

Black patients were housed in separate buildings from whites. Their buildings were less ornate than the main Powell building (figure 5.1 and figure 5.5). The differences on the outside extended to differential treatment inside the buildings. Segregated psychiatric treatment correlated with unequal standards of care. At GLA, Black women fared the worst.[107] Provisions were scarce for all patients, but Black women had even more limited access to feminine products, like bonnets, dresses, or hosiery, and sanitary products, including soap and slippers.[108] Subpar housing

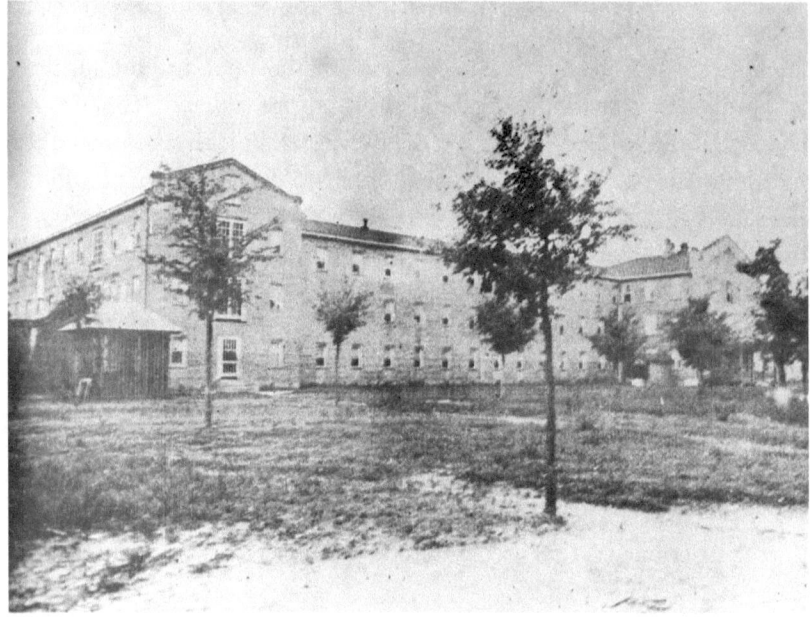

FIGURE 5.5 Colored building: Milledgeville, ca. 1894. View of part of the building used to house African Americans at Georgia Lunatic Asylum, now known as Central State Hospital. Vanishing Georgia Collection, Georgia Archives.

worsened in 1897, shortly after the women this chapter traces arrived, when the dilapidated so-called "Negro" building at GLA burned down as a result of a hospital worker's negligence. Nearly a thousand Black patients were left without shelter. In the aftermath of the fire, Viney, Amanda, and Olivia lived for several months with other Black women in tunnels with makeshift beds made from mattresses and blankets.[109] These unsanitary conditions undoubtedly worsened their prognoses.

Even after a new building was built, overcrowding, poor provisions, and unsanitary conditions persisted, posing serious health risks to Black women. Like Black patients in asylums throughout the South, Black sufferers at GLA died at a higher rate than whites.[110] By the time Olivia and Amanda arrived, Black women were dying at nearly twice the rate of their white female counterparts.[111] Olivia quickly added to the bleak statistics. Upon arrival, Olivia "[ate] and [slept] well" and was said not to "use tobacco."[112] Although seemingly in good health, twenty-eight-year-old Olivia died of "exhaustion" two years later.[113] Viney died of dropsy seven years after she entered GLA.[114] Compared to their white female counterparts, Black women died at higher rates of both exhaustion and dropsy, but those illnesses did not pose the gravest threat. Instead, diseases most closely tied to hospital provisions—consumption (tuberculosis) and marasmus (severe malnutrition)—were the most lethal. Tuberculosis, the deadliest disease of the nineteenth century, not only ravaged the Black population nationwide but also was the leading cause of death for Black women at GLA.[115] Current medical knowledge instructs that poor diet and sanitation do not cause tuberculosis, but they put Black women at significantly higher risk of succumbing to the disease. Black women were subject to asylum conditions that mirrored those of the antebellum slave quarters where the disease had previously wreaked havoc, thanks to nutrient-deficient diets, poor clothing, and overcrowded dwellings. The lethal combination devastated the Black female population. Black women's tuberculosis death rate in the hospital was higher than that of both white women and Black men, 2.3 percent compared to 1.5 percent and 0.6 percent, respectively.[116] Marasmus, often described as "wasting" because of the inability of the person to absorb nutrients, was the second leading cause of death for Black women, who died from it at four times the rate of their white female counterparts.[117] Although the death rates from marasmus were also high among Black men, when we consider the two illnesses combined, Black women had the worst outcomes: approximately 23 percent of Black male deaths, 34 percent of white female deaths, and 45 percent of Black female deaths were linked to these illnesses.[118]

Powell admitted publicly that tuberculosis affected Black women at higher rates and resolved that "isolation of tuberculosis cases [was] the most rational method at [his] command."[119] The German physician and microbiologist Robert Koch's 1882 revelation that bacteria caused tuberculosis set the course for what would become curative antibiotic therapies in the 1950s; however, during the 1880s, sanatoriums remained the main sites of treatment for the disease, where the focus was on isolation and hygiene. Yet, even Powell's proposed plan to isolate Black women with tuberculosis, which we now know would have slowed the spread, was undermined by the constant overcrowding of the colored building.[120] Not only was isolation not pursued, but no special efforts were made regarding nutrition and hygiene for Black women suffering from tuberculosis, worsening their odds of recovering. Black women's rates of tuberculosis and marasmus reveal how hospitals, which positioned themselves as places of mental health, created vulnerabilities and disabilities for Black women. Especially in the case of tuberculosis, even those who survived were susceptible to recurrence and lifelong debility. The conditions of the asylum, including familial separation, excessive labor, white hostility, poor provisions, health risks, and racial hostility, simultaneously echoed the horrors of enslavement and exacerbated postemancipation challenges to Black health and citizenship.

In sum, confinement at GLA exacerbated Blacks' existing wounds and created additional forms of sickness and vulnerability. Even without the first-person narratives of Olivia, Viney, Amanda, Alice, and Jane, we can imagine the issues they faced. The practice of psychiatry with respect to Black women was linked to the politics of race and gender. Their lives powerfully illuminate the fact that asylums like GLA perpetuated problems associated with years of social and institutionalized confinement rather than offering solutions to the challenges Black women faced in the years after emancipation. Furthermore, their experiences display an early episode in a broader American story: they were categorized as mentally inferior, subjected to myriad forms of systemic racism and sexism that compromised their mental health, and given subpar treatment practices that imperiled their health. All these practices continued well into the twentieth century.[121]

6

CHARLES CHESNUTT AND MENTAL DISABILITY IN THE AGE OF BLACK FREEDOM

The book is not a study in pessimism, for it is the writer's belief that the forces of progress will in the end prevail, and that in time a remedy may be found for every social ill.

—CHARLES W. CHESNUTT, "CHARLES W. CHESNUTT'S OWN VIEW OF HIS NEW STORY, *THE MARROW OF TRADITION*"

Charles Waddell Chesnutt (figure 6.1) was one of the most important Black American fiction writers in the late nineteenth century.[1] His acclaim was in no small part a result of his distinguished and expansive publishing record: he authored over fifty short stories, two plays, a biography of Frederick Douglass, six novels, and dozens of essays, speeches, poems, letters, and journals. He was also the first Black writer to cross the color line in publishing. His 1887 short story, "The Goophered Grapevine," was the first story by a Black writer to be published in the *Atlantic Monthly*, a prestigious periodical. His subsequent collection of short stories, *The Conjure Woman* (1889), solidified his place as one of the first major Black American literary writers.[2] His second novel, *The Marrow of Tradition* (1901), has become essential reading in the Black American literary canon.[3] Although Chesnutt is often known for the quality of his creative writing, I argue in this chapter that his work is also essential to the story of Black mental disability in the nineteenth century.

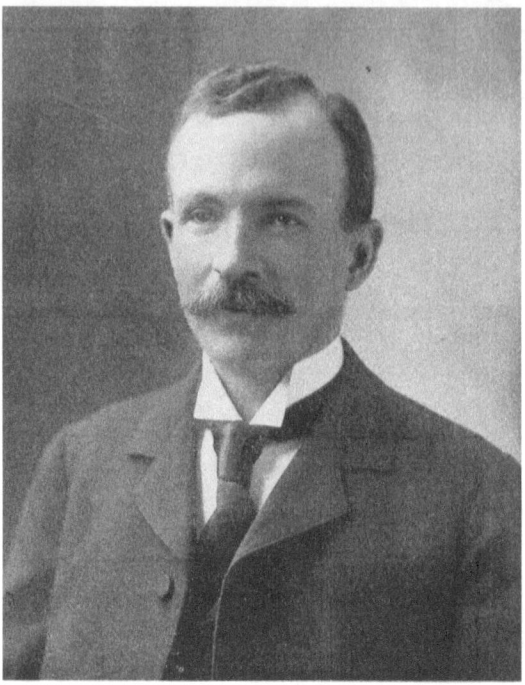

FIGURE 6.1 Charles W. Chesnutt. Schomburg Center for Research in Black Culture, Jean Blackwell Hutson Research and Reference Division.

The previous chapter featured nineteenth-century diagnostic formulations of mental disability and described alleged causes of mental conditions within the contours of medicalized discourses that were steeped in nineteenth-century cultural conceptualizations of race, gender, and mental disability. Unearthing the psychiatric rubrics, formulations, and logics that formed the basis of how mentally disabled Black people were treated inside asylums in southern communities is an indispensable part of the broader cultural history of mental disability; yet, it is hardly the whole story. Because that history focuses on documents in which Black voices are largely absent, the meaning of disability from the vantage point of Black people is also scant, limiting our understanding of the actual array of ideas circulating in the period. This chapter thus shifts the focus from conceptualizations about mental disability produced by psychiatric authorities to ideas that arise in literary fiction, a different realm of knowledge production that allows for deeper cultural context and more imaginative representations of mental disability. Fiction cannot directly replace the voices that are missing from medical archives, but it offers alternative sources of knowledge regarding mental disability that circulated during the period.

Like the famous Black poet Paul Lawrence Dunbar, Chesnutt enjoyed enthusiastic patronage from a leading American literary critic, the vocal anti-imperialist and NAACP advocate William Dean Howells.[4] After the publication of Chesnutt's first two collections of short stories, Howells praised the recent author and affirmed that he was on par with his white peers. He claimed that Chesnutt belonged to the "good school, the only school" of literary writers.[5] While Chesnutt was still writing *The Marrow of Tradition*, Howells published an article on representative Black men in which he praised Chesnutt alongside the most well-known and respected Black figures of the past and present, Frederick Douglass and Booker T. Washington.[6] Three months later, in October of 1901, *The Marrow of Tradition* was published—and three months after its release, Howells issued a damning (and oft-cited) review stating that the book was "bitter, bitter," ending both his professional support for Chesnutt and their acquaintanceship.[7] Howells at times challenged ideas about Black intellectual inferiority, saying there is "no colorline in the brain."[8] Yet, when presented with a novel that proved his point, Howells was oppositional. Chesnutt had misjudged the extent to which Howells and other northern progressive whites, whom he saw as the only "hope of the Negro," would remain invested in scientific and medical theories of Blackness.[9] Vann Woodward notes that during the 1880s and 1890s northern whites and former abolitionists commonly "mouthed the shibboleths of white supremacy regarding the Negro's innate inferiority, shiftlessness, and hopeless unfitness for full participation in the white man's civilization."[10] Even though northerners were opposed to race massacres such as the one portrayed in Chesnutt's novel, many readers were especially hostile to *The Marrow of Tradition*. They were not pleased with what Chesnutt saw as a hopeful portrait of racial unity, shared human vulnerability, and complete biological, social, and moral equality between the races.

In his writings, Charles Chesnutt provided his readers with formulations of mental disability that countered the medicalized conceptualizations about Black bodyminds that emanated from the scientific, medical, and psychiatric establishment. Chesnutt made several contributions to our understanding of mental disability in the nineteenth century. First, his representations of authoritative Black medical figures such as Aun' Peggy in *The Conjure Woman* and Dr. Miller in *The Marrow of Tradition* defied popular nineteenth-century notions of Blacks as innately mentally and physically deficient. Second, in contrast to psychiatrists who ignored the effect of racism on Black experiences of mental disability, Chesnutt presented stories that provided deep contextualization of the mental disability that resulted from the violence connected to slavery and postemancipation racial strife. Third, he unveiled the ways medicalized logics of Black innate inferiority were deployed in the broader culture and served as fodder for murder and destruction.[11] Fourth, he presented a mentally disabled character, Jerry, that defied the psychiatric logic that mental disabilities were race based rather than inherited on an individual basis. Finally, his works offered a new vision of the American future characterized by mental, physical, and moral equality between the races, cross-racial interconnectivity, and shared human vulnerability to disease and loss.

To create his vision of the American future, Chesnutt relied on anthropological theories about the heterogenous fusion of Americans into one nonracialized "American type." He hoped that the advent of the new "American type" would ameliorate racial distinctions that informed the culturally fabricated "Negro Problem." Drawing on his preferred anthropological theories, he directly engaged key debates in the psychiatric, medical, and scientific world about heredity, environmentalism, degeneracy, and social evolution. Chesnutt's arguments about racial amalgamation are important not only because they are an example of a Black response to the scientific, medical, and psychiatric doctrines laid out in other chapters but also because understanding them provides a crucial new perspective on one of the most important novels in the Black literary canon.

In what follows, I begin with a discussion of Chesnutt's theory of racial amalgamation, conveyed in a series of articles from *The Boston Transcript* in which he addressed racial theories of his time. The ideas he developed in these articles were reformulated in his literary works, as I will show in readings of *The Conjure Woman* and *The Marrow of Tradition*.

CHESNUTT'S THEORY OF RACIAL AMALGAMATION

Chesnutt intervened in medical, scientific, and psychiatric debates through his theory of racial amalgamation, a process of interbreeding, or as he also called it, "admixture." His writings about amalgamation reflect his self-conception as an intellectual whose chief affinity was with erudite men of letters not with white Americans or Blacks, whether poor or middle class (figure 6.2).[12] Chesnutt demonstrated an uncanny ability to diagnose Reconstruction-era problems with the precision of a social scientist.[13] Literary scholar William Andrews has recognized Chesnutt's scientific approach to writing about Black life, as well as his insistence that slavery's lingering effect had to be confronted to bring about racial equality: "Monitoring the social ills of the South consistently left Chesnutt the social student with one diagnosis—the patient suffered most profoundly

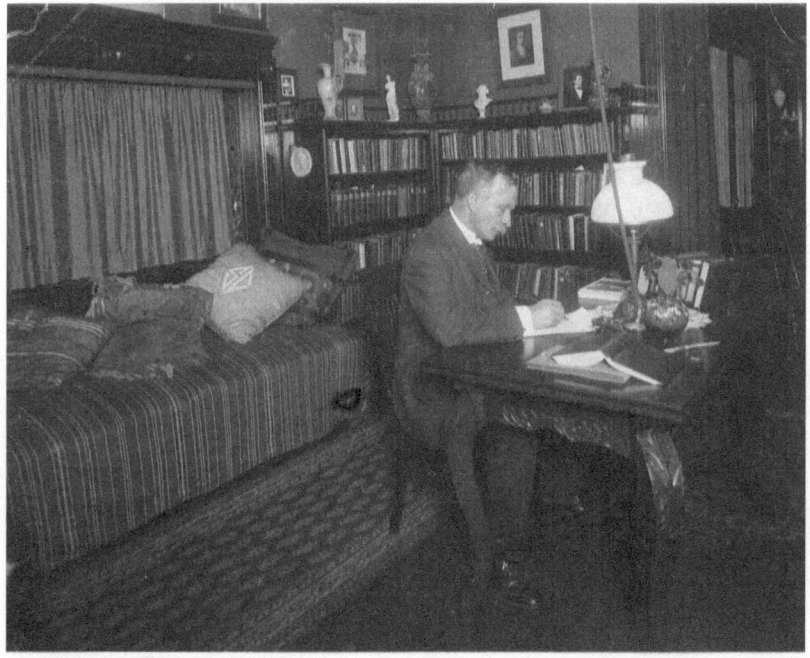

FIGURE 6.2 Chesnutt's library at 9719 Lamont Avenue. Cleveland Public Library Digital Gallery.

from the corruptive grip of the past upon the present."[14] After the publication of his first novel, *The House Behind the Cedars*, Chesnutt informed an editor at Houghton Mifflin that in his next literary project he would continue his discussion from the *Boston Transcript*, in which he laid out the social Darwinist idea of racial amalgamation.

The three articles in the *Boston Transcript* were published in 1900. In the first, "The Future American: What the Race Is Likely to Become in the Process of Time," Chesnutt situated his ideas in relation to germane scientific theories of the time. In the second, "The Future American: A Stream of Dark Blood in the Veins of the Southern Whites," he argued that racial mixing was already happening among Blacks, chiefly because of slavery, and to a lesser degree among whites. In a rhetorical performance of racial "outing," he gave several examples of famous white individuals and families that had a "dark ancestral strain."[15] In the third article, "The Future American: A Complete Race-Amalgamation Likely to Occur," he presented the "unnatural" obstacles to amalgamation, chiefly racial prejudice in the form of antimiscegenation laws, segregation, lynching, and massacres, with the Wilmington massacre being one of the most catastrophic incidents of the late nineteenth century.[16]

In the first article, Chesnutt positions himself as an intellectual authority before giving a synopsis on contemporary thought. He writes, "Before putting forward any theory upon the subject, it may be well enough to remark that recent scientific research has swept away many hoary anthropological fallacies," which is a rhetorical assertion that he has the intellectual acumen of a theorist and will demonstrate his grasp and conceptualizations of scientific arguments accordingly. Throughout the essays, Chesnutt denounces the anthropological claims of race scientists who rely on metrics like "the shape or size of the head" to determine the "average intelligence of a race." He assumes that northern readers accept the notion that environment is more impactful than any innate hereditary traits that appear among racial groups: "By modern research the unity of the human race has been proved (if it needed any proof to the careful or fair-minded observer), and the differentiation of races by selection and environment has been so stated as to prove itself. Greater emphasis has been placed upon environment as a factor in ethnic development, and what has been called 'the vulgar theory of race,' as accounting for progress and culture, has been relegated to the limbo of exploded dogmas."[17]

However, the "vulgar theory of race" was broadly accepted and flourishing.[18] The year before Chesnutt published his trilogy of essays, W. S. McCurley made an argument against amalgamation, which he also called racial "fusion." He argued against fusion both on the grounds that cultural norms in the North and South prevented it from happening and on the basis that dissolving the environmental limitations inherent to slavery had no effect on the hereditary qualities of Blacks. Racial mixing, he asserted, makes for defective humans: "The negro is not, and never can be, the equal of the caucasian. . . . It is an unnatural production; and instead of a superior race, it brings into the world beings neither white nor black, with physical and mental defects."[19] Two years after Chesnutt published his "Future American" articles, influential American economist Joseph Alexander Tillinghast published his work "The Negro in Africa and America," in which he argued that Blacks were deficient based on both heredity and environment. He argued that the worst attributes of Blacks, including excesses of passion, deception, indolence, carelessness, and brutality, were rooted in their African origin. Their undesirable traits were, he argues, "an integral part of the West African's nature long before [slavery]."[20] He felt that Black freedom and access to education in the decades following slavery had proved that environment gave way to hereditary influences: "No ethnic group, with its inborn nature moulded for ages in an undisturbed environment, can be radically transformed within ten or twenty generations."[21]

Chesnutt was inspired by the social Darwinist theories of William Ripley. Unlike those committed to the "vulgar theory of race," Ripley afforded strong credence to the role of social factors like tradition and socialization.[22] Ripley also argued that the natural course of human development was based on heterogeneous fusion: "The European races, as a whole, show signs of a secondary or derived origin."[23] Chesnutt believed that the process of heterogeneous mixing that Ripley discovered among Europeans was also inevitable among Americans. He writes, "the formation of the new American race type will take place slowly and obscurely for some time to come, after the manner of all healthy changes in nature."[24]

Chesnutt's vision of racial amalgamation had several conceptual key points. He directly refuted theories that people of mixed racial heritage would be sterile, prone to extinction, or otherwise constitute inferior human beings. Instead, he suggests that racial mixing would likely result in a superior product: "Any theory of sterility due to race crossing may as well be abandoned; it is founded mainly on prejudice and cannot be proved by the facts.... My own observation is that in a majority of cases people of mixed blood are very prolific and very-long lived."[25] The American racial type would not be a "pure white race" but rather a white race (in color and name) that came from a mixture of white, Black, Indigenous, and other races swept up in the American expansionist efforts.[26] Cherise Pollard argues that his prediction of the end of the white race is a radical proposition: "These acts are revolutionary: white purity is no longer an issue, and the black body is no longer a threat to the American body politic."[27]

Among the groups to be included in this "strange alchemy," he contended, Black Americans would be the hardest to incorporate on account of the deep-seated racial animus present in US society. Chesnutt thought this difficulty would eventually be overcome, but it required a change in perspective among white Americans. Despite the social element of race, Chesnutt saw the visible markers of difference as particularly troublesome.[28] He maps out how a systematic pursuit of racial mixing would solve the race problem:

> The mechanical mixture would be complete; as it would probably be put, the white race would have absorbed the black. There would be no inferior race to domineer over; there would be no superior race to oppress those who differed from them in racial externals. The inevitable social struggle, which in one form or another, seems to be one of the conditions of progress, would proceed along other lines than those of race.... From a Negroid nation, which ours is already, we would have become a composite and homogenous people, and the elements of racial discord which have troubled our civil life so gravely and still threaten our free institutions, would have been entirely eliminated.[29]

Rather than assuming that one race is inherently superior, he notes that both Black and white Americans, like immigrants from Europe, have "undesirable traits," although he does not detail them.[30] Still, he asserts that the American type will be only as good as the parts that make it up: "The white race is still susceptible of some improvement; and if, in time, the more objectionable Negro traits are eliminated, and his better qualities correspondingly developed, his part in the future American race may well be an important and valuable one."[31]

Chesnutt believed that both whites and Blacks, the masses and the middle class alike, needed to prepare for racial amalgamation.[32] He thought Blacks needed to capitalize on the role of the environment in human development and ready themselves for absorption, mainly through education and the acquisition of the key elements of middle-class respectability, characterized by "wealth and culture and social efficiency."[33] His message to white Americans was that they should refrain from the practices that would prevent or delay racial fusion. They needed to relinquish theories of Black mental and physical inferiority and adopt both a more sympathetic view of Blacks and a vision of human unity. He also wanted to compel whites to recognize that they needed Blacks to create a better American society and more evolved human beings. His utopian antiessentialist vision of race never materialized. As Dean McWilliams argues, Chesnutt's "fictions capture the problems of his present more accurately than his essay predicted the future."[34] Nevertheless, he sought to translate his spirit of hope and path toward amalgamation into his literary writings.

MENTAL DISABILITY IN *THE CONJURE WOMAN*

The Conjure Woman is known for displaying the richness of Black folklore traditions without demeaning and stereotypical images of Black people and their dialects (figure 6.3). It revised romanticized views of the southern landscape and race relations under slavery that proliferated in the popular plantation fiction of white southern writers such as Thomas Nelson Page and Joel Chandler Harris. A collection of seven short stories woven together in a complicated narrative structure, *The Conjure Woman* operates on three levels. The first level centers on a northern white couple, John and Annie, who migrate to the South to escape the northern climate (which has been unfavorable to Annie's health). They hope to exploit cheap land and labor and to pursue opportunities for enterprise; they are carpetbaggers. They hire a formerly enslaved man, Uncle Julius, to work on their newly acquired land, and they also benefit from his insider knowledge about the people who once occupied the

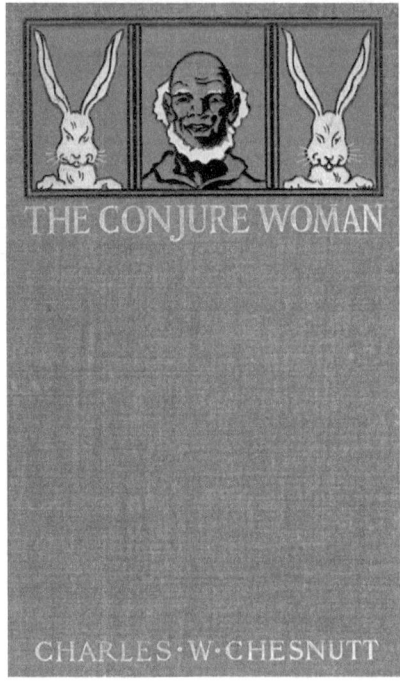

FIGURE 6.3 *The Conjure Woman* 1899 cover. Documenting the American South.

space. Their story offers an opportunity for the reader to approach southern race relations from a fresh and impressionable standpoint that is partial to social harmony and inclusivity. In the first story in the collection, "The Goophered Grapevine," John tells Uncle Julius that he does not have to move away when the couple approaches him because "there is plenty of room for us all."[35]

The framing stories often begin with a discussion between Uncle Julius and the couple concerning their plans to pursue personal or business interests on the land. This prompts Uncle Julius to tell them a story about the antebellum past. A trickster figure, Uncle Julius tells the story in a way that sometimes jolts the couple into taking actions that conveniently align with Julius's own desires. Contrary to plantation fiction wherein the "Uncle" figure simply mouths stories, Julius uses irony and makes judgments about the northerners, whose mental acuity he openly questions. He cannot understand their desire to buy a dilapidated plantation with haunted grapevines: "Well, suh, you is a stranger ter me, en I is a stranger ter you, en we is bofe strangers ter one anudder, but 'f I 'uz in yo' place, I wouldn' buy dis vim ya'd." The couple does not heed his advice, partly because John suspects that Uncle Julius benefits financially from the neglected grapevines. This highlights Uncle Julius's independence of thought and action, which is critical to the various insights he imparts.

The Black folkloric stories that Uncle Julius tells the couple form the collection's second narrative level. These stories elucidate the inner workings of life during slavery, the psychological ramifications of the violent institution, and the function of Black magic in mediating its harsh conditions. The third level is the connection between all of the short stories, which is reflected in their shared main characters such as the white couple, Uncle Julius, and a Conjure woman named Aun' Peggy. The final level creates a cohesive life world that the couple comes to understand. Their familiarity ultimately causes them to sympathize with the mental conditions of its inhabitants and descendants. In "Dave's Neckliss," an uncollected short story that shares characters with *The Conjure Woman*, John sees Uncle Julius as both a person and the product of historical circumstances: "[We] were able to study, through the medium of his recollection, the simple but intensely human nature of the inner life of slavery. . . . [He] presented to us the curious psychological spectacle of a mind enslaved long after the shackles had been struck off from the limbs of its possessor."[36]

Although mental disability figures prominently in the corpus of Chesnutt's fiction, in this chapter, I focus primarily on "Mars Jeems's Nightmare" because it features a provocative look at the ways mental instability appeared among Blacks and whites through the character of a harsh slave master.[37] The representations of mental disability in *The Conjure Woman* exist outside the limiting realm of psychiatry's medicalized model of disease. As previous chapters have shown, most postbellum psychiatrists theorized that Black insanity arose from innate racial deficiencies, a tendency to sexual and emotional excess that easily gave way to mental instability, and an inability to handle the "mental strain" of freedom. In *The Conjure Woman*, mental disability is neither inherent to the nature of Black people nor a consequence of freedom. Rather, mental disability is tied to various forms of cultural violence that are wielded against Black bodyminds. In "Po Sandy," for example, Chesnutt describes how the bodymind of an enslaved woman named Tenie deteriorates after she witnesses the death of her love interest Sandy. In a discussion about Tenie's role in the plantation economy, the narrator exclaims, "ain' much room in dis worl' fer crazy w'ite folks, let 'lone a crazy nigger."[38] Chesnutt draws on this idea indirectly in "Mars Jeems's Nightmare" by referring to the lack of accommodation around disability as the most damning example of a master's excessive cruelty.

Beyond a consequence of brutality, mental disability in "Mars Jeems's Nightmare" functions as the conduit for the possibility of a new world in which social relations between Black and white individuals are transformed; the two racialized groups are interdependent, and the Black Americans are not only powerful but also use their authority to the benefit of the white Americans who are subject to it. In this imaginative world, Black people are granted the opportunity to not only improve their own lives or save themselves but also restore the morality of white characters.

Chesnutt circumvented Western concepts of psychiatry primarily by telling his stories through the prism of the supernatural, particularly Black American Conjure traditions. He did not write from the standpoint of a Conjure practitioner or even a well-trained anthropologist. In his literature, readers encounter a palatable depiction of Conjure traditions from the perspective of someone who learned of Conjure from amateur observations of communities in the US South. His stories retain the broad concepts of Conjure that he believed were necessary to bring about a paradigm shift in his white northern readership. Within the sacred imagination of Conjure, mental health issues indicate communal or interpersonal disruption requiring spiritual intercession by someone with expertise—a Conjure man or woman. Conjure was used during slavery as a tool to combat the master's ability to inflict harm on enslaved people. Indeed, the need for respite from unbearable conditions on a plantation provides the impetus for Solomon, a main character in "Mars Jeems's Nightmare," to seek out the Conjure woman Aun' Peggy.

The major conflict in the frame story for "Mars Jeems's Nightmare" concerns an opportunity for Uncle Julius's grandson Tom, a representative of the first generation born outside of slavery. At the outset of the story, the white northern couple fires Tom because of his poor performance. To make the point that the couple should grant sympathy to his kinfolk, Uncle Julius tells a story about an enslaver, Mars Jeems, who is made more sympathetic to the slaves on his plantation by the force of a Conjure spell. Julius's story begins with Solomon's lament that he cannot see his lover because Mars Jeems forbids Black unions on his plantation. He even sells Solomon's love interest away to another plantation. Mars Jeems is cruel in many ways. In addition to exceptionally brutal beatings, his callousness extends to exhausting work conditions, forcing people to work from dawn into the night (as opposed to sunup to sundown). He also proscribes their social outlets and forms of reprieve such as dancing, singing, or listening to music, which likely helped enslaved people cope with the emotional toll of slavery.

To drive home just how untenable this situation was, the narrator bemoans that Mars Jeems was equally cruel to enslaved people in their most vulnerable and involuntary states, including "nachul bawn laz'ness," "sickness," and "trouble in de min.'"[39] The narrator does not further detail what "trouble in the min'" consists of, but this elision makes the reference to mental disability profound. It is also a notable departure from nineteenth-century psychiatric attempts to locate disability in clearly defined (and heavily policed) disease categories. "Trouble in the min'" stands in as a reservoir for mental conditions that fall outside an individual's usual or perhaps desirable mental functioning. In Chesnutt's story, the emphasis is not on making a condition legible but rather on making room for its existence within communities, even those with the most stringent profit-driven labor imperatives.

Chesnutt's effort to generate a sense of sympathy in the reader for his Black characters is most powerfully achieved, paradoxically, through his depiction of mental disability in the white antagonist Mars Jeems, rather than the Black characters. When Solomon secures help from Aun' Peggy to reestablish his love connection, Mars Jeems experiences mental instability that manifests fully outside Western medical models of disease, appearing instead according to the epistemological logics of the Black sacred tradition. Aun' Peggy instructs Solomon to put a goopher concoction in Jeems's okra soup, which the slave master unknowingly ingests. The goopher is symbolic of the mythical creatures in the Black sacred imagination, such as the moonack, which was said to cause physical or mental disability in anyone unfortunate enough to encounter it in southern woods, caves, or trees. True to custom, the elixir transforms Mars

Jeems into a mysterious and confused slave, referred to as the "noo nigger," who is lent to Mars Jeems's plantation. The spellbound "new" slave has no recollection of his name, origins, or work skills. When the overseer presses him on his background, the baffled new slave replies, "My head is all kin' er mix' up." Just like slaves with "trouble in de min," the new slave's altered mental state warrants no sympathy; instead he is subject to brutal beatings, meager rations, and prolonged solitary confinement in a barn.[40] Because he is so difficult to break in, the new slave is eventually set to be sent down river to New Orleans. Before the sale is complete, however, Solomon, following Aun' Peggy's instructions, feeds the new slave a sweet potato as he sleeps in his holding cell. The next day, Mars Jeems appears in the woods complaining about a nightmare, the signature symptom of consuming the goopher soup. He also emerges with a better attitude—giving money freely, firing the brutal overseer, reducing working hours, allowing dancing, and even granting marriages.

In this story, mental disability is not a marker of abnormality in need of medical scrutiny; instead, it is a conduit for positive transformation both for the white enslaver, who becomes more altruistic, and for the Black community, which gains some reprieve from slavery's exploitation and repression. The story challenges visions of the past in which there were fixed power dynamics and distance between whites and Blacks. In the story, a slave master is intimately connected to Blacks and, in fact, becomes a slave through conjuring. Further toppling assumptions about power among whites during slavery, Mars Jeems is not omnipotent; rather, Aun' Peggy is the most formidable figure. The Conjure woman figure suggests that enslaved people had recourse to advisors with special spiritual skills that are superior to the "rational" traditions of science, medicine, and psychiatry. In the tales, the Conjure woman levels the playing field for everyone in the community because she is the figure to which everyone can go for help precisely because she has the power to shape the lives of both enslaved people and their masters. She is a foil to the medical doctor or psychiatrist who vociferously claimed to *know* the Black bodymind.

Chesnutt's compelling story also brings about a change in the narrative present, acting on the white couple hearing the story. The couple decides to give Tom a second chance. Unlike the docile Black narrator iconic of white plantation fiction, Uncle Julius is a truth teller in reciting the moral of the story. Chesnutt forces his readers to be aware that the descendants of enslaved people dealt with not only physiological harm but also social conditions such as poverty and illiteracy through no fault of their own and therefore deserved opportunities for self-improvement. He also claims that Black Americans are not the only ones who stand to gain because white people who heed the lesson will "prosper en git 'long in the worl'"; that is, they will gain access to indelible personal betterment. The lesson Uncle Julius offers, however, is not just an appeal: Uncle Julius channels the Conjure woman's power through his warning that if his white auditors do not take this more contextualized view of Blacks, then they will be "li'ble ter hab bad dreams."[41] Chesnutt leaves unanswered whether the couple's change of heart is the result of the appeal or the threat; either way, it leaves intact the power of Black Conjure and everyone's possible (if unwitting) subjection to it.

The stakes of this conceptual shift were high. If white audiences became desensitized to Black people's authority or viewed it as potentially beneficial, then maybe they would not fear the prospect of Black Americans rising in the social world. Or better yet, they might help put an end to the virulent violence being levied against Black people in cities and towns across the US South. One of the most devastating examples of such violence was the 1898 Wilmington massacre and coup.

FICTION AS A MODE OF SOCIAL CHANGE IN
THE MARROW OF TRADITION

The Marrow of Tradition focuses on the life of an optimistic Black physician, William Miller, and his family's entanglement with a former Confederate soldier and editor of a local white supremacist newspaper, Major Philip Carteret (figure 6.4). Carteret's wife Olivia is also the unacknowledged half-sister of Miller's Black wife, Janet Miller. The setting of the novel is the fictional town of Wellington, a stand-in for the Black-majority city of Wilmington, North Carolina.[42] The story was written on the heels of the bloody 1898 massacre and coup in the prosperous

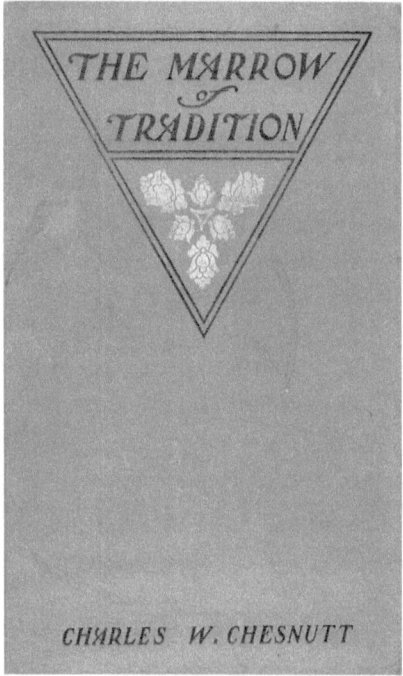

FIGURE 6.4 *The Marrow of Tradition* cover. Collection of the Smithsonian National Museum of African American History and Culture.

port city. The massacre and coup were initiated by white segregationist Democrats who violently opposed Black suffrage and civil rights.[43] At the end of the nineteenth century, Wilmington was the largest city in North Carolina and the home of many successful Black citizens, a significant number of whom were prosperous business owners, doctors, lawyers, and politicians. The Democrats violently rejected what they perceived as Black domination. An armed mob of two thousand white vigilantes was enraged by the rise in political power of the city's Black Republicans, which they gained via widespread voting and their alliance with white Populists.[44] Both white business leaders and working-class men massacred and deposed the city's elected Black leaders. Infuriated by the ongoing success of biracial government, former Confederate soldier Colonel Alfred Moore Waddell exclaimed to an excitable crowd of disgruntled white citizens, "We shall never surrender to a ragged raffle of negroes, even if we have to choke the Cape Fear river with carcasses."⁴⁵

Chesnutt did not simply depict the infamous Wilmington massacre in *The Marrow of Tradition*; he also used the creative space of the novel as a site in which the world could be made anew.⁴⁶ The value of *The Marrow of Tradition* did not rest solely in its ability to "set the record straight" by offering an alternative narrative, one less encumbered by the nineteenth-century Democratic hold on the narrative recounting of the Wilmington massacre and coup. Chesnutt furnished a story that sought to change the culture of the society from which it was produced. Unlike newspaper accounts of the incident, for example, Chesnutt's novel offered possibilities that were either beneath the surface or seemingly impossible during the historical moment. Chesnutt remained steadfast in his aim to change the minds of his white readership, but with *The Marrow of Tradition*, he took a more confrontational approach. Matthew Wilson argues that he sought to "elevate his white readers" through "presenting them with a counterhistory that he hoped would help them remember what they had been taught to forget."⁴⁷

Chesnutt was not alone in recognizing the power of the creative pen for bringing about social change. The racial justice activist Mary Church Terrell lamented that ending her creative writing career was a missed opportunity for meaningful social justice: "I have thought for years that the Race Problem could be solved more swiftly and more surely through the instrumentality of the short story or novel than in any other way."⁴⁸ Victoria Earl Matthews posited that Black writings should challenge negative depictions of Black people as they appeared in public newspapers, books, pamphlets, and other print outlets. Black writings, in her estimation, needed to serve as "counter-irritants against all such writing."⁴⁹ Chesnutt's pursuit of social change, then, was not limited to readily apparent and often physical sites of resistance, such as hospitals, schools, the polls, or the picket line; his preferred terrain was the battlefield of ideas, where he sought to bring about a change in the American public's opinion about Black citizens. While physicians and psychiatrists were making Black people into objects of study and bodies on which social meanings about race, gender, and disability were inscribed, often violently, Chesnutt's creative works worked to undo such discourses and replace them with others less mired in subjugation.

PSYCHOLOGICAL SCARS OF POSTEMANCIPATION RACIAL VIOLENCE

In the chapter in which Chesnutt renders the most detailed description of the day of the Wilmington massacre, he signals to the reader that his account offers more than historical facts (figure 6.5). The picture white newspapers painted was of heroic white men who were able to fight off and suppress a raging Black uprising that was led by misguided white Republicans who supported the spread of "Negro domination" in the South. White southerners first used the terminology of "race riot" to describe the events, which belied the actual events in which a mob of angry whites terrorized the Black citizenry.[50] On November 10, 1898, thousands of Black Wilmingtonians fled in horror, pleading with their God to be spared an encounter with all groups of white men, whether it was the bloodthirsty Red Shirts, a pack of angry militia men, or equally frightful, a group of drunken vigilantes. They hid desperately in swamps and the Pine Forest Cemetery, grateful for the cover their dead loved ones provided,

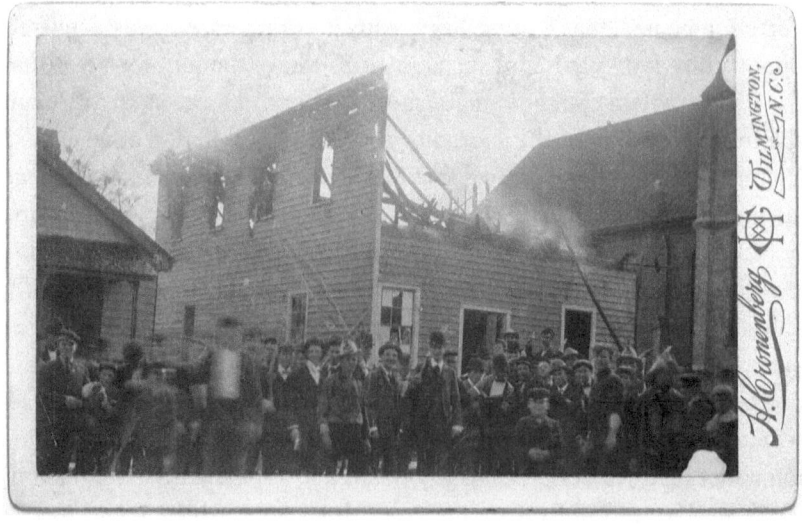

FIGURE 6.5 A mob celebrates in front of the building that housed the black-owned and -edited newspaper, *The Daily Record*. Courtesy of New Hanover County Public Library.

and clasped tightly their children and kin. These mothers, fathers, children, grandparents, cousins, aunts, and uncles who had once embraced each other tenderly, did so that day in trembling fear. Even as late as the twenty-first century, researchers, descendants, and government officials have tried to cobble together numbers to quantify the devastation: death toll estimates range from dozens to hundreds; 2,000 Black residents fled; the number of Black voters fell from 126,000 to 6,100; and it would be eighty years before another Black official was elected.[51] Chesnutt's portrait forced readers to confront the limitations of historical renderings of tragic events. People, places, and buildings should all be included in revisionist histories, but Chesnutt suggests that they must also capture the records that Wilmington Blacks kept on their bodyminds.

Psychiatrists and physicians ignored these physiological records of mental distress in their assessments of postslavery Black bodyminds. Chesnutt's description included the usual truths of the massacre—Black people being stopped repeatedly by armed groups, being searched, and then fleeing for safety. But the regular script of Black Wilmingtonians' harassment turning into murder, the burning of buildings, and the expulsion of Black elected officials is cut short in favor of a description of the unacknowledged psychological toll of the event: "If he [a Black Wilmingtonian] resisted any demand of those who halted him—But the records of the day are historical; they may be found in the newspapers of the following date, but they are more firmly engraved upon the hearts and memories of the people of Wellington. For many months there were negro families in the town whose children screamed with fear and ran to their mothers for protection at the mere sight of a white man."[52] In this moment in the novel, Chesnutt's use of the dash disrupts his usually graceful prose and the grammatical perfection of the English language. His interruption of the logical flow of the sentence and imagery simultaneously compel the reader to mentally fill in the familiar events and redirect their attention to postmassacre realities. Although the concept of posttraumatic stress would not be defined for decades, Chesnutt details how the lingering psychological effect of terror resurfaced repeatedly.

For Chesnutt, the phenomenon of recurring distress was familiar and almost instinctive to the descendants of slavery. When Dr. Miller is trying to make sense of what he is witnessing in the streets of Wilmington, still ignorant that a massacre is unfolding, he becomes unsettled, a feeling that the narrator explains as historically informed:" 'What on earth can be the matter?' he muttered, struck with a vague feeling of alarm. A psychologist, seeking to trace the effects of slavery upon the human mind, might find in the South many a curious illustration of this curse, abiding long after the actual physical bondage had terminated."[53] As this passage shows, Dr. Miller does not reflect on the origins or modes of transmission of his subtle emotional response; it is the third-person narrator who explains the heightened emotional moment in the story. The narrator's omniscience offers outside, rational, and objective instruction to the reader about the source of Dr. Miller's uneasiness. Switching abruptly to a more scholarly tone, he conveys that a *good* psychologist or any truly astute medical or scientific thinker could ascertain that mental suffering was transmittable and unbound by time, will, or death. The expert should also be aware, this passage suggests, that the almost instinctive fear Black people endured was an added layer of harm. It was not simply a benign scientific phenomenon; being overcome with fear was an undesirable and metaphysical "curse" that haunted Black people.

Chesnutt's argument for the psychic wounding of postslavery violence comes through powerfully in his portrayal of Silly Milly, a mentally broken character and mother of Black resistance leader Josh Green. Contrary to hereditarian perspectives on postemancipation Black mental health, Chesnutt shows that innate debasement or ill preparation for freedom was not the source of Black mental instability; it was Black experiences of extreme violence.[54] Silly Milly became mentally unstable after witnessing the lynching of her husband by the Ku Klux Klan, led by Captain McBane, a former overseer newly rich off his convict leasing business. Green describes the atrocities from the perspective of an agonized child: "'One night a crowd er w'ite men come ter ou' house an' tuck my daddy out an' shot 'im ter death, an' skeered my mammy so she ain' be'n herse'f f'm dat day ter dis.'" After seeing the effect of the lynching of his mother, Green vowed to kill McBane; he guessed rightly that avenging his family would cost him his life. Chesnutt also offers commentary on Silly Milly from the vantage point of Dr. Miller, a representative of medicine and science, who situates her in the community and presents her as a case study of cruelty and victimization: "He [Dr. Miller] had often seen Josh's mother, old Aunt Milly,—"Silly Milly," the children called her,—wandering aimlessly about the street, muttering to herself incoherently. He had felt a certain childish awe at the sight of one of God's creatures who had lost the light of reason, and he had always vaguely understood that she was the victim of human cruelty, though he had dated it farther back into the past. This was his first knowledge of the real facts of the case." Silly Milly also serves as a reminder for Miller that racial terror during the postslavery era was especially hard on women and children. In the midst of the murderous riot, Miller hurries to ensure his wife and child's safety. En route, he considers the worst that might happen to them, and Silly Milly comes to mind as a grave possibility: "Then there flashed into his mind Josh Green's story of his 'silly' mother, who for twenty years had walked the earth as a child, as the result of one night's terror, and his heart sank within him."[55] Miller's fears reflect that his own efforts for self-betterment do not shield him or his family from the mental and physical harms that accompany racial violence. The reflections of this logical man of medicine also affirm that Silly Milly was not in fact silly at all; her response to brutality was not only understandable but also expected.

INTERROGATIONS OF BLACK COGNITIVE AND INTELLECTUAL CAPABILITIES

Chesnutt achieves a radical reconfiguration of social relations in part by exposing the fallacy of claims about Black mental deficiency in terms of both mental disease and intelligence. In the second chapter, Major Carteret attends his son Theodore's (nicknamed Dodie) christening, at which the guests engage in debates about the supposedly innate characteristics of their Black neighbors. The attendees move from a conversation about whether or not Black people are trustworthy to Carteret's revelation of his deeper racial logic. Major Carteret is a staunch Democrat who resents the fact that Dr. Miller occupies his ancestral home. His family lost their money after the war, but he was fortunate enough to be able to use his wife's wealth to found and run a newspaper, *The Morning Chronicle*. He uses his platform to stir up anti-Black racial sentiments, yet he thinks of himself as too much of a gentleman to commit violent acts himself. In the novel, his white nationalist views about Black economic, educational, and political success are attached to disdainful remarks about Black inferiority:

"'I merely object to being governed by an inferior and servile race.'"[56] This outlook is shared by other leaders in Wellington, including Captain McBane and former confederate soldier General Belmont. The men discuss strategies to "escape from the domination of a weak and incompetent electorate" and to "confine the negro to that inferior condition for which nature had evidently designed him."[57] Here, the Wellington massacre and coup leaders reassert that "weakness" and "incompetence" are attributes supposedly apparent in all Black people. Rather than challenging this outlook through explicit counter-dialogue, Chesnutt undermines this biologically deterministic logic through his literary characterization of the competent Dr. Miller.

Chesnutt depicts Dr. Miller as a respected professional and ambitious physician who is an embodied contradiction to the three white men's claims of Black inferiority.[58] Miller is motivated by a sincere belief that if Blacks prove themselves worthy, they will be accepted by whites eventually. Dr. Miller symbolizes the possibilities for Black communities given the right opportunities for educational, financial, and career advancement. For a Black audience, Chesnutt presents an aspirational figure, someone they could potentially be if they take advantage of every opportunity afforded them. The doctor is a second-generation son of the Miller family, who through their hard work, financial responsibility, and moral respectability achieved in less than thirty years the quintessential American quest of pulling themselves up by their bootstraps. Mr. Delamere, a relic of southern aristocracy, a frail but honorable old man with "white hair" and "painfully weak" legs, paints this picture of Dr. Miller's family in response to Major Carteret's "hostile" remarks at the christening[59]: "'I think they have done very well, considering what they started from, and their limited opportunities. There was Adam Miller, for instance, who left a comfortable estate. His son George carries on the business, and the younger boy, William, is a good doctor and stands well with his profession. His hospital is a good thing, and if my estate were clear, I should like to do something for it.'"[60]

Dr. Miller's opportunities led him to the field of medicine. He is an exceptional doctor whose publications demonstrate his mastery of the very fields that are used to subjugate Black people.[61] Miller is a revered protege of the white physician Dr. Burns, a Philadelphia surgeon Major Carteret solicits when Dodie accidentally swallows a piece of a toy rattle, threatening his life.⁶² Dr. Miller not only has received medical knowledge through his formal training abroad but also is a cocreator in the development of medical fields; he opened a hospital to provide medical care and aspired to train nurses, pharmacists, and physicians. Dr. Miller's efforts to expand the healthcare infrastructure in Wellington also capture the spirit of the respectability politics of Black elites who aimed not only for individual betterment but also to improve the conditions of the Black masses, exemplified most famously by the slogan "lifting as we climb." The credulous Dr. Miller holds the ardent belief that Blacks' personal betterment efforts will usher in social equality: "He [Dr. Miller] was now offered a further confirmation of his theory: having recognized his skill, the white people were now ready to take advantage of it."⁶³ Dr. Miller's acumen is further amplified through the admiration of Dr. Burns, a white physician who has garnered the respect of the white Wellingtonians. When Dr. Burns requests that Dr. Miller assist him in an operation, he considers him a colleague with whom he can share an appreciation of managing novel medical cases.⁶⁴ Dr. Burns's gesture is one of reciprocation; Dr. Burns previously assisted the Black doctor on a case about which Dr. Miller published in a medical journal.⁶⁵

In addition to the highly intelligent character of Dr. Miller, Chesnutt offered an alternative to the hereditarian idea that Blacks, as a race, were predisposed to cognitive deficiency through his depiction of Jerry, a Black porter at *The Morning Chronicle*.⁶⁶ The militant Josh Green is the most apparent foil to the assimilationist Dr. Miller.⁶⁷ However, when considering medicalized discourses of the Black bodymind, Jerry is also a striking foil to cognitively gifted Dr. Miller. Jerry is the grandson of the devoted Mammy figure, Mammy Jane, who worked for two generations of the Carteret family even after the end of her compulsory care during slavery. Jerry shares her quiet servitude to Wellington whites and poses little threat to their feelings of racial superiority. The narrator remarks that Jerry could not fully comprehend the white riot conspirators' initial conversations because of "certain limitations which nature had placed in the way of [his] understanding [of] anything very difficult or abstruse."⁶⁸ Here "nature" refers to the notion that Jerry was born with a finite and limited set of inherited mental aptitudes over which he has no conscious control. Chesnutt toys with the idea of whether Jerry's heredity is based on his ancestors as a race or on his individual, biologically connected kin.[69] White psychiatrists in the period claimed that individual whites could have and inherit isolated traits of mental deficiency; they did not extend that medical rubric to their Black patients. Chesnutt's inclusion of these divergent Black characters, with contrasting mental capacities, effectively levels the differences attributed by race in terms of the potential for variability in mental disposition. By having one Black person who is limited by nature and one who is able to advance, he demonstrates that the principles that are applicable to whites are also suitable for Blacks. Chesnutt's depictions reveal that he did not simply reject scientific and medical principles altogether. Chesnutt embraced medicine and psychiatry's basic etiological claims about the hereditary causes of mental disability, but he did away with the most racist elements of racialized medical thought. Chesnutt called for an equal application of what was seen as the best scientific knowledge regarding mental disability of the time, which he believed reinforced Blacks' equal humanity. Even the embodied corrective Dr. Miller presents as a model of peak intellectual aptitude is not enough to change the racial attitudes of the white characters in the novel. Carteret, Belmont, and McBane regard Dr. Miller and his fellow businessmen and elected leaders as uppity troublemakers in need of discipline, punishment, or eradication, which they believe will teach the Black masses a lesson about the fatal consequences of trying to rise above their station in life.

CHESNUTT'S VISION OF THE AMERICAN FUTURE

Chesnutt's novel reflects both his own relatives' stories of survival during the Wilmington incident and Black fictional representations of white mob violence during and after Reconstruction, which centered how such tragedies shattered Black people's intimate familial bonds.[70] Chesnutt's novel takes a unique turn because it meditates on how such tragedies imperil both a white *and* a Black family in the wake of the massacre. *The Marrow of Tradition*'s final plot twist introduces the new social order that Chesnutt saw as hopeful and that perhaps his critics rejected.

The family's concerns over mental and physical health are the catalyst through which several remarkable changes occur: white and Black characters are bound together, white characters experience a change in perspective, and they pursue an unexpected course of action rooted in Chesnutt's concept of human unity. Chesnutt entangles Dr. Miller's family's overwhelming grief at the loss of their son in the massacre with the emotional distress the Carterets suffer as their son lies near death. In the midst of the massacre, Miller's son is killed by a stray bullet and Dodie suffers with the croup in the Carteret home. Having achieved his goal of destroying Black prospects for equality, Major Carteret returns home to his sick child. However, as a result of the very massacre he incited, he is unable to find help for his son. The town's physicians and surgical specialists are absent; others are reluctant to travel to the town because of the commotion. Even the pharmacies have closed early on account of the incident, leaving the Carteret family with no other option than to solicit the help of Dr. Miller. Mrs. Carteret literally begs on her knees for Dr. Miller's help: "The next moment, with a sudden revulsion of feeling, she had thrown herself at his feet,—at the feet of a negro, this proud white woman,—and was clasping his knees wildly."[71] A Black doctor's medical care of a sick white child was a radical proposition not because Blacks lacked magnanimity but because southern whites of Major Carteret's ilk shunned the notion of being subjected to Black authority of any kind. This new positionality, in which white southerners needed the expertise of Black professionals, toppled the social order in which Black individuals were seen as innately suitable for subservient roles only, a proposition readers likely rejected.

The final chapter, entitled "Sisters," opens with Dr. Miller answering the door to a distraught Mrs. Carteret. Dr. Miller is struck by the half-sisters' resemblances, both phenotypical and audible.[72] Mrs. Carteret, he thinks is "so near the image of his own wife." Even the women's cries for help are identical; Mrs. Carteret, the narrator notes, cries "with [Dr. Miller's] wife's voice."[73] These mirroring traits assure Dr. Miller that the two are related by blood. Following his logical assessment of the clear similarities between the two, the narrator writes from the vantage point of Dr. Miller, emphasizing that Mrs. Carteret "*was* his wife's sister." Dr. Miller is reluctant to help Mrs. Carteret because he is consumed with anger and sorrow as his son has been murdered in the massacre initiated by Major Carteret. Yet, the fact of the biological heredity softens Dr. Miller to Mrs. Carteret's appeals; Dr. Miller reflects, "Yet, after all . . . [Mrs. Carteret] was his child's kinswoman." Despite this reference to biological bonds, what finally persuades Dr. Miller to help Mrs. Carteret, on the condition that his wife agrees, is a recognition of her shared experience of mental precarity: "She was a fellow creature, too, and in distress." At that moment, Mrs. Carteret is not standing before him as a white woman with superior social status and power but as an equal to his own wife; both are emotionally distraught over a child, a dying one for the white sister and a recently perished one for the Black.

Because Dr. Miller decides he will only grant Mrs. Carteret's wish if his wife agrees, Mrs. Carteret takes her plea to her half-sister hoping that their shared status as mothers will make Janet sympathetic to her. In the exchanges between the two mothers, the reader observes this vulnerability that is bound neither by racial heritage nor by hatred:

> Standing thus face to face, each under the stress of the deepest emotions, the resemblance between them was even more striking than it had seemed to Miller when he had admitted Mrs. Carteret to the house. But Death, the great leveler, striking upon the one hand and threatening upon the other, had wrought a marvelous transformation in the bearing of the two women. The sad-eyed Janet towered erect, with menacing aspect, like an avenging goddess. The other, whose pride had been her life, stood in the attitude of a trembling suppliant.[74]

This portrait of vulnerability in both women had different import for the various readers of the novel. For Black readers, it served as an acknowledgment of the disturbance that events such as race massacres inflicted on the family unit and the intimate ties that were disrupted. But it was also a signal regarding Chesnutt's political strategy around Black people's paths toward racial harmony and equality. Although vengeance was an emotional state that Chesnutt wanted the white reader to understand and the Black reader to have affirmed, he did not offer it as a good path for Black Americans (easing the fears of whites and directing/instructing the efforts of Blacks). Janet eventually grants the request of her sister, takes no revenge, and even refuses her share of the inheritance from Samual Merkell's estate. This vow of forgiveness and foregoing of retaliation reflects Chesnutt's general stance against militant forms of resistance to racial injustice in favor of less disruptive and disturbing courses of racial harmony. Here Chesnutt's novel contrasts drastically with other representations during the period.

Saving Dodie, the central concern of the chapter, has meaning beyond saving the literal life of the Carterets' child. Dodie is symbolic of the future of American society. The conflict in the chapter over whether or not Dr. Miller will save Dodie suggests that the future is undetermined and contingent on the actions of those to whom it is connected. References to the hope and precarity of the future of the nation appear early in the novel as Mammy Jane, Dodie's nurse, observes that the child has a mole on his left ear, a terrible omen; she is sure that he was "born for bad luck."[75] This observation foreshadows the life-threatening sickness that Dodie battles at the end of the novel. A revelation of the other possible fate of the nation surfaces six months after Dodie's birth, when Mammy Jane declares that child is "the largest, finest, smartest, and altogether most remarkable baby that had ever lived in Wellington."[76] Dodie's life-threatening sickness, then, is a moment in which an open question is posed to the reader about which fate will prevail.

The story ends with a cliffhanger. Dodie's survival becomes possible and with it a possible choice between the dual futures he has offered—one that suggests the nation could flourish and the other that suggests it will founder. For Chesnutt, it was a future dependent on whether it incorporated the best version of all races, which Dr. Miller embodied, to create a better American racial type. He was keen on exposing the ideological barriers to true racial fusion. In a candid moment in the midst of the terror, the narrator gives insight into the emotions behind white resentment and terrorization of Blacks; it is not white anger but fear that drives their actions:

> In the olden time the white South labored under the constant fear of negro insurrections. Knowing that they themselves, if in the negroes' place, would have risen in the effort to throw off the yoke, all their reiterated theories of negro subordination and inferiority could not remove that lurking fear, founded upon the obscure consciousness that the slaves ought to have risen. Conscience, it has been said, makes cowards of us all. There was never, on the continent of America, a successful slave revolt, nor one which lasted more than a few hours, or resulted in the loss of more than a few white lives; yet never was the planter quite free from the fear that there might be one.[77]

Chesnutt believed that the internal psychological state of fear was the motivating force behind white atrocities in the past slave society and the postslavery era. This fear, Chesnutt suggests, could be assuaged through a recognition of cross-racial connectivity. For some white characters, connectivity translates to support for Black self-help efforts. Mr. Delamere, for example, leaves three thousand dollars to his servant "as a mark of [his] appreciation of services rendered and sufferings endured by Sandy." To further relieve his conscience or "take a load off [his] mind," he allocates the remainder of his estate to the Wellington Black community, entrusting Dr. Miller to use the assets to fund the "hospital and training-school for nurses."[78] Chesnutt was in favor of such endeavors, but his novel suggests that they fell short in bringing about true social change.

Chesnutt showed that the new American future also required a philosophical shift. Having chosen forgiveness, Doctor Miller races to save Dodie's life and inquires about Dodie's status. After a confirmation from Major Carteret that the boy is alive yet "nearly gone," the white apprentice doctor, whose skill level is inadequate to save Dodie, calls out to the Black doctor: "Come on up, Dr. Miller. . . . There's time enough, but none to spare."[79] For Chesnutt, the future of America depended not only on Black people exercising forgiveness but also on the honing of Black intellectual and mental capacity. Much to the disdain of late nineteenth-century whites, Chesnutt's future called for an acceptance that Black Americans were physically and mentally equal. But most thorny, whites needed Black people and they had to be willing to submit to, even embrace, Black prowess and authority.

CODA

In the fall of 2024, I had captivating exchanges with colleagues at the University of Michigan Medical School about twenty-first-century Black maternal mental health in Michigan, specifically the rates of perinatal mood and anxiety disorder (PMAD) diagnoses. A conundrum arose when researchers compared two different sets of data, one focused on clinical diagnoses documented by medical professionals and another focused on responses to a mental health screening questionnaire—Michigan Medicaid administrative claims and the Phase 7 Michigan Pregnancy Risk Assessment Monitoring System (MI-PRAMS) survey, respectively. Although Black and white women often gave responses on the survey that are usually associated with PMADs, there was a discrepancy in the rates of clinical diagnosis across the two populations. Self-reporting of PMAD symptoms and clinical diagnoses of PMADs were better correlated among white women than Black women. In other words, Black women reported symptoms of mental health conditions at similar rates as white women but were less likely to be diagnosed with mental health conditions. This quantitative research is meaningful for drawing our attention to Black women's embodied experiences of mental health. Yet, it also elicits more questions about their bodyminds than it answers.

As a humanist, I am curious about what knowledge, narratives, and insights lie within and between the quantitative and qualitative data. What cultural archetypes inform the way physicians *see* or *do not see*

Black women's mental distress?[1] Are physicians' pharmaceutical solutions to mental health problems at odds with the therapeutic orientations of Black women?[2] How might Black women's attempts at self-definition and naming be illegible in medical spaces? Perhaps most elusive, what is the role of the everyday knowledge that circulates within Black women's communities about the *harm* of medicine, harm that they are aware is tri-temporal—past, present, and future—and multilevel—individual, familial, and communal?[3] Many of these queries cannot be answered by medical research alone; that is, *more* data, variables, and calculations may not prove more enlightening. Qualitative research by social scientists could probe the lives of Black women in areas that evade quantitative medical data. Different types of data, perhaps interviews with doctors and Black women, could fill in some of the gaps. Yet, even social scientists cannot capture the sometimes underlying and unacknowledged conceptions of Black female subjects or medical doctors.

Like James McCune Smith, Harriet Tubman, Harriet Jacobs, and Charles Chesnutt, for answers to these questions, I turn to lyrical traditions for their truths and revelations and the various ways that they tap into the commingling and ethereal echoes of American cultural narratives. Consider, for example, the following stanzas from a poem by Bettina Judd:

> I must have been found guilty of something. I don't *feel*
> Innocent here lurking with ghosts. See it happens like
> That. I start at a thought that is quite benign and end up
> peccant, debased.
>
> I had an ordeal with medicine and was found innocent
> or guilty. It feels the same because I live in a haunted
> house. A house can be a dynasty, a bloodline, a body.
>
> There was punishment. Like the way the body is
> Murdered by its own weight when lynched. Not that I
> was wrong but that verdicts come in a bloodline.
>
> In 2006, I had an ordeal with medicine. To recover, I
> learn why ghosts come to me. The research question is:
> Why am I patient?[4]

Judd forces us to confront the fact that for Black women being a patient is steeped in histories of past and present violences. The speaker asks us to linger on the ways that Black women refuse to wait for medicine to treat them with dignity and respect. The poem's last lines are a question about the nature of medical experiences and a call for justice. Like the speaker of the poem, I am enthralled by the historical ghosts and cultural recitals that reverberate across time. As this book attempted to show, I am best suited to tell similar origin stories of Black mental health discourses in the United States. Embedded in a historical moment that saw the birth of the field of psychiatry and vibrant articulations of mental disability from a multivocal group of Black people, *Colored Insane* is a rumination on the people, places, and ideas that constitute the collective, competing, and conflicting meanings of mental disability in the lives of Black people in the United States. Yet, the book also conveys both the promise and perils of conducting research at the intersection of various fields and relying on a wide range of source material. I offer it in part as a subtle call for more intersectional research conducted more broadly across the humanities, social sciences, and hard sciences, and more directly within the humanistic fields. In the paragraphs that follow, I suggest how it might prove a launching point for a discussion of the kinds of interventions that are possible when we bring together often siloed disciplines and disparate data.

At its foundation, *Colored Insane* is an example of applied Black feminist theory. Before writing a word, the drive to search for meaning at the seams is a Black feminist inclination. Black women and other women of color have often found themselves outside and between groups, fields, and nations. Black women, for example, are often invisible in spaces dominated by white women and equally so in those dominated by Black men. The position Black women occupy between these two groups opens up a simultaneously personal and political space, by necessity and choice, where they find courage, resistance, respite, self-definition, power, and pleasure.[5] I am guided by the idea that there is always knowledge in the *in-between* that is likely missed, omitted, and overlooked. With the same understanding, Black feminist thinkers, writers, and activists have often created new genres for their meaning making in which they combine various modes of expression—memoir, song, poetry, and autobiography.[6] Thus, our starting place should be to sit at the crossroads of various figures, fields, and genres of the past *and listen*. Upon hearing, there is also accountability. Black feminist scholars unremittingly ask ourselves, would the people about whom we write see themselves in the pages of our research? Would they find their voices, desires, yearnings, contentions, and laments represented at all, and if so, how well?

Research guided by Black feminist theoretical principles can make major interventions: historiographical, archival, and methodological. Regarding historiography, telling a new historical story about Black mental health requires a renarration of nineteenth-century medical discourses. Studies in the history of psychiatry have discussed the writings, speeches, and publications of medical figures who evoke discourses of race and slavery, yet these historical events had not been identified as a unified intellectual project (albeit unacknowledged). This work gives a name to the psychiatric, medical, political, and scientific intellectual trend of pathologizing Black bodyminds, especially "proslavery psychiatry." In the process of naming, outlining, and giving shape to racialized discourses, Black people's previously unacknowledged counter-discourses can better come into view. Naming discourses like proslavery psychiatry reminds us they are never static; they are built both across time periods and during given historical moments. Thomas Jefferson's musings about the racial differences in intellectual and emotional capacities between whites and Blacks did not just spur scientific research during his lifetime; his views outlived him. The idea that there might be measurable differences between racial groups was taken up by anthropologists, ethnographers, scientists, physicians, and psychiatrists and, at the same time, by political figures and other cultural actors. When we see how all of these figures debated and postulated about race, slavery, and the mental states of Black people, we better understand why and how Black figures like James McCune Smith responded so robustly to them. The outcome of putting previously unnamed discourses and related counter-discourses in conversation is a new historical story.

Part of the reason new stories about the past do not come into view is that we fail to recognize which texts are valuable for understanding them. Medical and scientific records are important for understanding embodied experiences of health, yet they prove insufficient for accessing Black life. James McCune Smith's life work is instructive in this regard. He was a published medical physician who also knew that medical data and research were of limited use for unveiling Black people's lives and health. As much as he defended the merits of objective scientific research, accurate and adequate statistics, and controlled medical studies, Smith knew that the most textured stories about the lives of Black people and their health did not come from documentary facts but were best articulated in fiction. Smith might have recognized that medicine's linguistic structures are often too constraining to fully understand or articulate the nature of mental disability among Black people. Audre Lorde famously noted the need to imagine ways of being outside constraining systems: "For the master's tools will never dismantle the master's house."[7]

Creating a new story means bringing together often-siloed interlocutors, some of whom are familiar but have not been looked to as sites of knowledge about Black mental health. No Black woman in history is as well known to the American public as Harriet Tubman. She is the only Black person and only woman who has come close to appearing on US currency. Tubman joins many other Black women figures—Anna Julia Cooper, Sojourner Truth, Frances Watkins Harper, and Ida B. Wells, to name a few—whose names, stories, and even voices have been recovered. With figures who are so well-known, we can fall into the trap of thinking that there is nothing new about them to say. Future studies of Black women need to appreciate not just the lives of Black women but also their ideas. Yet any full appreciation of their ideas means recognizing their own distinct ways of delivering them. Examining Tubman's thought, unlike that of other women whose ideas have been recovered, is difficult because she did not author first-person written texts and no transcripts of her speeches exist. Future research should not be discouraged by such seeming dead ends. This book opens the door to maneuvering through archival gaps to learn about topics such as mental health that were immensely important to figures but that went unrecorded. We may never know what Tubman thought exactly or how it might have changed over time, but in some ways, there is much to learn about what her positions were on topics like mental disability even without direct statements from her. They will be approximations, hopefully good ones, that provide a sense of the worldview of a woman of her stature, background, and experiences. Even a sense of her sentiments helps flesh out a story about mental health that we previously ignored or failed to even glimpse. To develop it further will require reading secondary renditions of her life and speeches carefully with an eye toward the multiple layers of interpretation and bias that are at play, which is true even of the most explicitly articulated autobiographical works. New discoveries will also depend on close attention to the discourses that circulated around iconic figures like Tubman.

Harriet Jacobs, who was literate, offers an example of a Black woman's embodied theorization on the page. As Brittney Cooper reminds us, Black women made the choice to "write their bodies into texts and to use Black female embodiment as the zero point of their theorizing."[8] Tubman and Jacobs, using different registers, thought deeply, systematically, and categorically about Black mental suffering, and they used their embodied experiences as a source of embodied knowledge. They declared then—and show us now—that white male psychiatrists, the recognized theorists, were not the authorities on their mental health. They had their own formulations about how, why, and when mental disability arose and how it should be understood in the context of Black people's lives.

When new archives are assembled, scholars must determine how they are best read. For example, it means considering the ways mental asylums' diagnostic records are laden with unspoken assumptions, suppressed meanings, and ideological underpinnings. As Michel Foucault would admonish, discourses of power are at work.[9] The asylum's examinations of Black women's lives on the page is an exercise of power. Disability scholar Ellen Samuels argues that the language and narrative conventions present within psychiatric documents are a reflection of medicine's "fantasies of identification," a joint process of documentation, medicalization, and marginalization.[10] Psychiatry repeatedly identified, measured, and assessed what constituted the "normal" mind and body and subsequently contained, managed, and regulated people accordingly. Attention to these meta-discourses helps us understand how and why silences in medical archives are created and sustained. Exposing psychiatry's making and remaking of mental disability leaves an opening for thinking outside its ideological fictions and barricades. Reading medical documents with silences of marginalized subjects in particular often requires reading with a speculative openness to what is missing. Future studies must use deep speculation to colorfully tell stories about which there are few traces of existence.[11]

For the task of reading into silences, the conventions of literary studies are particularly generative. Words, language, speech, turns of phrase, and even punctuation all *mean something*. All historical documents are *types* of creative texts no matter how seemingly uninventive or pedestrian. Texts exist only through the linguistic, written, and oral traditions of their creation. The written texts scholars often rely on also fit into specific genres—newspapers, census records, patient ledgers—that have particular forms and narrative conventions. Like all texts, they are products of the social, political, and historical circumstances in which they were produced. These layers together constitute specific meaning. Regardless of the types of text we encounter in the archives, scholars can read creatively. Although reading texts in new ways is promising, rarely do these types of practices fully furnish the revisions they beckon.[12] Here is where art in general and literature in particular may prove fruitful.

Cataloging instances of mental disability outside the pathologizing specter of medicine is a worthy venture because the history of mental health in the United States is in need of a broader body of data to understand psychiatry and society's historical handling of mental disability. Yet slave narratives, novels, short stories, essays, and sketches are valuable beyond their use as sources of documentary evidence.[13]

Following the lead of late Black feminist critic Barbara Christian, future scholarship should continue to look to Black literature for its theorizing power.[14] Theory, with a capital "T," has been associated with intellectual schools of thought, most notably structuralism and poststructuralism, often dominated by white men. Black theorizing practices are recognized only when conducted within those traditions. Barbara Smith made a case that theory, with a lowercase "t," could happen outside those traditions. By claiming that Black writers theorize in their creative works, she opened up the possibility that literary writing could stand up against and parallel with texts that set out to theorize about the world. Theri Pickens reflects on this possibility of seeing literary texts as theoretical: "They speak back to critics. And, if critics do not listen, we (ma) linger in thinking of them as having value because they solely illuminate a topic we have already decided to discuss. What happens when we view them as the drivers of these conversations? What solipsism do we avoid when we view them as theoretical sources that change the conversations critics are already having? This not only alters our engagement with primary sources but also fundamentally changes our relationship to secondary and theoretical sources."[15] Although I argue in this book that writers like James McCune Smith, Harriet Jacobs, and Charles Chesnutt engaged directly and intentionally with both literary and medical theorists, sources of deep conceptualization could also be found in places that did not set out purposely to iterate theoretical concepts. Literary texts, after all, are objects in themselves.

Most white postbellum psychiatrists and physicians theorized that Black insanity arose from innate racial inferiority, their inability to handle the "mental strain" of freedom, and the loss of the daily living conditions that supposedly protected Black people's health during slavery.[16] Black physicians conceded that there were rising rates of insanity, but they were more likely to locate the source of disease in the social, political, and economic realities of Black life.[17]

Postbellum Black creative writings such as those of Charles Chesnutt, however, demonstrate alternative formulations of mental disability that existed outside the diminishing and harmful medical models of disease present in nineteenth-century psychiatric documents.[18] These authors wrote from a vantage point that was more forthright in its subjectivity and less invested in epistemological omniscience. The creative writer's evidentiary power differed wildly from the cases, histories, observations, or experiments of the psychiatrist.

But literary writings warrant the same scrutiny and caution as any other subject material. Unlike medicalized sources, creative works do not set out to have direct and sustained conversations about health, nor are they respected by authorities on health or by the professions of their times. Furthermore, readers do not seek health advice or counsel from writers. Many nineteenth-century readers looked to literature for pleasure not prescriptions. In addition, literary writings operate within their own personal and professional traditions and economic motivations. Perhaps most exigent, their conceptual novelty is rarely apparent. Nuanced meaning has to be mined from literature. As a literary scholar, I approach these texts with an interest in language and the function of literary form, techniques, and tropes. Literary texts come with their own sets of historical and cultural contexts, authorial perspectives, and circumstances of production, all of which shape meaning about mental disability.

Doing research about mental disability, mental suffering especially, is hard not only because of the need to navigate the archives but also because the material itself often reflects histories of violence. As careful as I tried to be to honor my subjects, to some extent, this book represents the harm that was done to Black women and their communities. Reproducing the violence done to Black women not only runs the risk of reproducing violence in the terms Saidiya Hartman draws our attention to in her discussion of Frederick Douglass's portraits of Aunt Hester but also has a powerful and, at times, terrible impact on readers and writers.

When I began this project, I was a graduate student, but by the time I completed it, I was a faculty member and a mother of three children under the age of four. When I began writing the book, I was sure that as a scholar I did not have to occupy the subject position of the people I wrote about to passionately research or write about them, and I still believe this. Yet as a mother who suffered from postpartum depression, I find that the lines *hit differently*. Writing about the story of Alice, a woman clearly suffering emotionally as she cradled her newborn child, was bone-chilling. I had read the newspaper articles so many times, but after my first child was born, I reread them, and one day, I just wept. When I read the lines again about Jacobs peering at her children from her attic for seven years in order to save them, I understood it in a new way and my heart sank. I continued my research, however, because I was driven by the fact that *I* needed these stories and because of the reassurance I gained when I talked about my research, especially with everyday people, that *we all* need them.

ACKNOWLEDGMENTS

An academic book is never written in isolation. Truly, I am because we are. I am indebted to the kindness and generosity I have received along the way from financial institutions, colleagues, strangers, archivists, students, research assistants, reviewers, mentors, administrative and building staff, strangers, medical teams, doulas, nannies, ancestors, friends, and family.

Funding for this project came from the Institute for Citizens and Scholars (formerly the Woodrow Wilson Foundation), the Mellon Foundation, Summer Institute for Tenure and Professional Advancement Fellowship at Duke University, University of Michigan Institute for the Humanities, Institute for Research on Women and Gender, University of Michigan Center for Engaged Pedagogy, University of Michigan ADVANCE Program, University of Michigan Research Catalyst and Innovation Block Grant for Arts and Humanities, James William Richardson Dissertation Completion Fellowship, Emory University Race and Difference Initiative Travel and Research Grant, Consortium for the History of Science, Medicine, and Technology, and Laney Graduate School Travel and Research Grant.

I traveled to and hunkered down in many archives to conduct research for this project. I visited Barbados; Washington, DC; Georgia; Virginia; and Philadelphia. I am grateful for the archivists and librarians at Library Company of Philadelphia; the College of Physicians of Philadelphia;

Library of Virginia State Archives; College of William and Mary Swem Special Collections; William L. Clements Library; Georgia Historical Society; Georgia State Archives; Stuart A. Rose Manuscript, Archives, and Rare Book Library; Barbados National Archives; and the National Archives in Washington, DC.

The editorial team at Columbia University Press, especially Stephen Wesley and Alex Gupta, was exceptional in their attentiveness to the project and investment in its success. I am honored to be a part of the special series Race, Inequality, and Health, coedited by Samuel Roberts and Michael Yudell. I am truly grateful for the thoughtful and enriching comments from the editors and anonymous reviewers.

This project would not have been possible without my research assistants and independent editors. Some of my students volunteered their time to help me organize and transcribe nineteenth-century materials, including Amber Wei, Anna Hart, Ciara Madden, Diana Curtis, Kaitlyn Plummer, Vicky Wang, Kayla Clark, Danielle Clark, and Kylie Schafer. My University of Michigan Undergraduate Research Opportunity Program student, Kyle Spence, also contributed to the project. I am especially indebted to Elizabeth Duquette, Danielle LaVaque-Manty, and Brittany Jerzowski.

My love for research was first nurtured when I was a high school sophomore in the Telluride Association Sophomore Seminar. The six-week seminar on the campus of Indiana University is where I discovered that I loved research as much as teaching and that, as a professor, I could do both. I am grateful for my first academic role models, Iris Rosa and Daniel Walker, and all the faculty I watched and learned from through the Telluride Association, including Audrey McCluskey, Natasha Vaubel, Rubi Tapia, and Joshua Miller. As a college student, I learned what it meant to live a life of the mind. I am so grateful for my professors who inspired me, held long office hours, and taught me the fundamentals of doing research, including James Turner, Michele Wallace, Eric Cheyfitz, Locksley Edmondson, Nicole Waligora Davis, and Sandra Green. Darlene Evans spent countless hours helping me hone my writing skills and became a friend. Outside of the classroom, the women and friends of Wanawake Wa Wari, a Black women's cooperative living house, stayed up late with me discussing all the new ideas we were learning. It is a blessing to have learned, laughed, and cried with Sakeena Everett, TaMar Baptiste,

Abena Sackey, Monique Gilliam, Tracey Martin, Kristina Weems, and Ivy McCottry. The Mellon Mays Undergraduate Fellowship Program was instrumental in preparing me for the academy. All the conferences, workshops, and mentoring were critical in my journey. The Institute for the Recruitment of Teachers was pivotal in preparing me for graduate school. I am grateful for Kelly Wise, the founder, and Denise Salarza Sepulveda, Reginald Jackson, Clemente White, and Kelechi Ajunwa, mentors who took me under their wings.

This project was born in a graduate seminar at Emory University taught by Mab Segrest, who paved the road for my work. I was fortunate to have a dissertation committee that embraced an interdisciplinary project: Benjamin Reiss, Mark Sanders, and Lawrence Jackson. Other scholars who made a mark on my academic life during graduate school include Carol Anderson, Diane Stewart, Rudolf Byrd, Sander Gilman, Kimberly Wallace-Sanders, and Beverly Guy Sheftall.

Some community and intellectual space has to be built. I am grateful for those who helped me found and run the African American Studies Collective at Emory University, especially Alexis Wells-Oghoghomeh, Asha French, Jessie Dunbar, Alphonso Saville, Dominick Rolle, Michael Hall, Shively Smith, and Derrick Cohens.

Many colleagues have helped me develop the ideas in this book. I am grateful for all the feedback, conversations, writing groups, panels, and workshops that have strengthened this project during my time in graduate school, as a postdoc at the Center for Research on Race and Ethnicity in Society (CRRES) at Indiana University, and as an assistant professor at the University of Michigan with colleagues including Beau Gaitors, Mashadi Matabane, Michael Hall, Arika Easley-Houser, Walton Muyumba, Stephanie Li, Amrita Chakrabarti Myers, Jakobi Williams, Michelle Moyd, Valerie Grim, Phoebe Wolfskill, Theri Pickens, Andrea Williams, Courtney Marshall, Ayesha Hardison, Margaret Price, John Stauffer, Courtney Marshall, Myrna Garcia, Martha Jones, Lakisha Simmons, Victor Mendoza, Scotti Parrish, Jim Downs, Rana Hogarth, Susana Morris, Valerie Traub, Rubi Tapia, Rosario Ceballo, Abigail Stewart, Sara McClelland, Sandra Gunning, Anna Kirkland, Alex Stern, Peggy McCracken, Earl Lewis, Stephen Berrey, Aida Levy-Hussen, Jennifer Jones, Ava Purkiss, Megan Sweeney, Andrea Bolivar, Allison Alexy, and Charlotte Karem. The University of Michigan Women and Gender Studies administrative and building staff including

Donna Ainsworth, Sarah Ellerholz, and Archie Criglar also supported me in ways that were often invisible.

I'm thankful to the medical team that cared for my bodymind in the process of writing this book, including Jason Hesselberg, Kim Montz, Meagan Bretz, Lauren Mooney Jones, Dorthyrose Vowels, Nancy Boyd, and Sean Zagar.

I had three children in the process of writing this book, a singleton and then twins. Childbearing, childbirth, postpartum, and childrearing (sans stable childcare) brought this project to many halts. I owe more than I will ever have to all the midwives, physicians, doulas, and nannies who stepped into my life and helped care for me and my family. I'm especially grateful for Karen Hatch and Dana Hatch, who became family. My community of moms in Michigan, Demita Pursell, Brandie Schultz, Monica Scott, Yolanda Doster Wilkins, Raechel Rodgers, Alaina Jackson, Monica Goedert, Anti' Shay Thurman, and Kelle Tatum, steadied me along the journey.

I am upheld by the prayers of my mother, Mary Louis, and other mothers Yolanda Clarke, Nancy Toussaint, Marion Brown, and Angel. I am lost without the guidance of my late grandmother Martha Taylor and other grandmothers Linda Bufford and Ruthie Bufford. I am showered by the love of my late father Daniel Louis; other father, the late Derrick Bufford; grandfather Clinton Bufford; and uncle Olga Maddy. I'm thankful for my siblings, Monique Louis, Annette Louis, Jessica Louis, and Ardis Milton, and my sister/brother friends Chanel Tanner, Shermaine Jones, Sheree-Ann Denton, Angel Brown, Crystal Brown, and Erin Ferguson. My children are my best motivators. "Go mama go!!!" was the soundtrack of the last leg of the project. I am immensely grateful for my love, Dr. Blake Bufford, whose support had no bounds.

I was raised in Delray Beach, Florida. Where I'm from, they call me "Dee Dee." I cherish those who know me by that name. Without them, there would be no Dr. Diana Martha Louis.

NOTES

INTRODUCTION

1. Harriet Ann Jacobs, *Incidents in the Life of a Slave Girl, Written by Herself*, ed. L. Maria Child, 2nd ed. (Published for the author, 1861), 286–87. Located in Documenting the American South, University Library, the University of North Carolina at Chapel Hill, 2003.
2. Jacobs, *Incidents*, 289.
3. For more on the internal slave trade, see Ira Berlin, *The Making of African America: The Four Great Migrations* (Viking Adult, 2010).
4. Geoffrey Reaume, "Mad People's History," *Radical History Review*, no. 94 (2006): 182. The invention of contemporary terms associated with mental health, such as "brain disease" and "behavioral health," is a reminder that even the most acceptable terms in the present may be seen as disturbing in the future.
5. Margaret Price, *Mad at School: Rhetorics of Mental Disability and Academic Life* (University of Michigan Press, 2011), 9.
6. Brenda A. LeFrançois, Robert Menzies, and Geoffrey Reaume, eds., *Mad Matters: A Critical Reader in Canadian Mad Studies* (Canadian Scholars' Press, 2013), 10.
7. Disability scholars identify two approaches to disability: a medical model and a social model of disease. In medical models of disability, it is a misfortune, abnormality, or dysfunction located in individual bodies in need of fixing, cure, or eradication. In a social model of disability, theorists posit that disability is a social construction based on social and cultural systems that exclude, degrade, and withhold or deny disabled people access, status, resources, and power. For more on the medical and social models of disability, see Zosia Zaks, "Changing the Medical Model of Disability to the Normalization Model of Disability: Clarifying the Past to Create a New Future Direction," *Disability and Society* 39, no. 12 (2024): 3233–60; Richard K. Scotch, "Medical Model of Disability," in *Encyclopedia of American Disability History*, ed. Susan Burch (Facts on File, 2009), 602–3;

Eli Clare, *Brilliant Imperfection: Grappling with Cure* (Duke University Press, 2017); Kim E. Nielsen, *A Disability History of the United States* (Beacon, 2012); Catherine Jean Kudlick, "Social History of Medicine and Disability History," in *The Oxford Handbook of Disability History*, ed. Michael A. Rembis, Catherine Jean Kudlick, and Kim Nielsen (Oxford University Press, 2018), 105–24; Catherine Jean Kudlick, "Comment: On the Borderland of Medical and Disability History," *Bulletin of the History of Medicine* 87, no. 4 (2013): 540–59; Justin Anthony Haegele and Samuel Hodge, "Disability Discourse: Overview and Critiques of the Medical and Social Models," *Quest* 68, no. 2, (2016): 193–206; Tom Shakespeare, "The Social Model of Disability," in *The Disability Studies Reader*, 3rd ed., ed. Lennard J. Davis (Routledge 2010), 266–73; Lennard J. Davis, "Constructing Normalcy," in Davis, ed., *The Disability Studies Reader*; Rosemarie Garland-Thomson, "Feminist Disability Studies," *Signs* 30, no. 2 (2005): 1557–87.

8. Psychiatry as a field has played a significant role in pathologizing people along the lines of gender, race, sexuality, and class across time. See Jonathan Metzl, *The Protest Psychosis: How Schizophrenia Became a Black Disease* (Beacon, 2009); Maria Ramas, "Freud's Dora, Dora's Hysteria: The Negation of a Woman's Rebellion," *Feminist Studies* 6, no. 3 (1980): 472; Cecilia Dhejne, Roy Van Vlerken, Gunter Heylens, and Jon Arcelus, "Mental Health and Gender Dysphoria: A Review of the Literature," *International Review of Psychiatry* 28, no. 1 (2016): 44–57; Ronald Bayer, *Homosexuality and American Psychiatry: The Politics of Diagnosis* (Princeton University Press, 1987); Mical Raz, *What's Wrong with the Poor? Psychiatry, Race, and the War on Poverty* (University of North Carolina Press, 2013).

9. The anonymous reviewer wrote: "During her bondage she does not appear to have suffered any great amount of physical hardship. But the bitterness of *mental suffering* and enforced degradation which she was compelled to endure from her master's vices and the hatred of her mistress—and which she was utterly helpless to prevent—is fearful to contemplate." Reprinted in Charles T. Davis and Henry Louis Gates Jr., eds., *The Slave's Narrative* (Oxford University Press, 1990), 33; emphasis mine.

10. Elizabeth J. Donaldson, "Revisiting the Corpus of the Madwoman: Further Notes Toward a Feminist Disability Studies Theory of Mental Illness" in *Feminist Disability Studies*, ed. Kim Hall (Indiana University Press, 2011), 106. Other works of disability scholarship that consider mental disability include Andrea A. Nicki, "The Abused Mind: Feminist Theory, Psychiatric Disability, and Trauma," *Hypatia* 16, no. 4 (2001): 80–104; and Anna Mollow, "'When Black Women Start Going on Prozac: Race, Gender, and Mental Illness in Meri Nana-Ama Danquah's 'Willow Weep for Me,'" *Melus* 31, no. 3 (2006): 67–99.

11. See Linda Joy Morrison, *Talking Back to Psychiatry: The Psychiatric Consumer/Survivor/Ex-Patient Movement* (Routledge, 2005).

12. Here I take a cue from Susan Burch's study on asylums and Native Americans. Susan Burch, *Committed: Remembering Native Kinship in and Beyond Institutions* (University of North Carolina Press, 2021).

13. Other scholars who use the term include Burch, *Committed*; Alison Kafer, *Feminist, Queer, Crip* (Indiana University Press, 2013); Clare, *Brilliant Imperfection*; Samantha Dawn Schalk, *Bodyminds Reimagined: (Dis)ability, Race, and Gender in Black Women's*

Speculative Fiction (Duke University Press, 2018); Adria L. Imada, "A Decolonial Disability Studies?," *Disability Studies Quarterly* 37, no. 3 (2017).

14. Margaret Price, "The Bodymind Problem and the Possibilities of Pain," *Hypatia* 30, no. 1 (2015): 271. Price is drawing on the conceptualizations of the body from Nirmala Erevelles. Nirmala Erevelles, "Race," in *Keywords for Disability Studies*, ed. Rachel Adams, Benjamin Reiss, and David Serlin (New York University Press, 2015): 145–48.

15. Michel Foucault, *Psychiatric Power: Lectures at the Collège de France, 1973–1974*, ed. Jacques Lagrange (Palgrave Macmillan, 2006).

16. For a detailed discussion of the ways in which medical actors and scientists of the nineteenth century engaged in a practice of fictive identifications of the disabled body and mind, see Ellen Samuels, *Fantasies of Identification: Disability, Gender, Race* (New York University Press, 2014).

17. Black feminist literary critic Barbara Christian contended that Black Americans theorize about American culture, society, and life in their cultural productions. For the purposes of this book, their ideas about mental disability can be found in hundreds of nineteenth-century songs, plays, poems, folktales, and especially the most popular genres of the period, such as slave narratives, novels, journalism, and short stories. Barbara Christian, "The Race for Theory," *Cultural Critique*, no. 6 (Spring 1987): 51–63. Contemporary Black feminist scholars also make a convincing claim for seeing Black works as sites for theoretical conceptualizations of race, gender, and mental disability. See Brittney Cooper, *Beyond Respectability: The Intellectual Thought of Race Women* (University of Illinois Press, 2017), and Therí A. Pickens, *Black Madness: Mad Blackness* (Duke University Press, 2019).

18. Jacqueline Goldsby, *A Spectacular Secret: Lynching in American Life and Literature* (University of Chicago Press, 2006), 21.

19. Key early works in the development of disability studies include Lennard J. Davis, *Enforcing Normalcy: Disability, Deafness, and the Body* (Verso, 1995); Adrienne Asch, "Recognizing Death While Affirming Life: Can End of Life Reform Uphold a Disabled Person's Interest in Continued Life?," *The Hastings Center Report* 35, no. 7 (2005): S31–36; Douglas Baynton, "Slaves, Immigrants, and Suffragists: The Uses of Disability in Citizenship Debates," *PMLA* 120, no. 2 (2005): 562–67; Lennard J. Davis, "Crips Strike Back: The Rise of Disability Studies," *American Literary History* 11, no. 3 (1999): 500–512; Elizabeth J. Donaldson, "The Corpus of the Madwoman: Toward a Feminist Disability Studies Theory of Embodiment and Mental Illness," *NWSA* 14, no. 3 (2002): 99–119; Rosemarie Garland-Thomson, *Extraordinary Bodies: Figuring Physical Disability in American Culture and Literature* (Columbia University Press, 1997); Sharon Snyder and David T. Mitchell, *Narrative Prosthesis: Disability and the Dependencies of Discourse* (University of Michigan Press, 2000); Robert McRuer, "Crip Eye for the Normate Guy: Queer Theory and the Disciplining of Disability Studies," *PMLA* 120, no. 2 (2005): 586–92.

20. Christopher Bell, "Is Disability Studies Actually White Disability Studies?," in *The Disability Studies Reader*, ed. Lennard J. Davis (Routledge, 1997), 374–82. Other scholars have also challenged the absence of a serious critique of race in the field. See Jennifer C. James and Cynthia Wu, "Editors' Introduction: Race, Ethnicity, Disability, and Literature:

Intersections and Interventions," *Melus* 31, no. 3 (2006): 3–13. Other significant contributions on race and disability studies include Nirmala Erevelles, "Race," and Therí A. Pickens, "Blue Blackness, Black Blueness: Making Sense of Blackness and Disability," *African American Review* 50, no. 2 (2017): 93–103. Although Bell is a noteworthy figure in the genesis of Black disability studies, Black thinkers have been carrying out serious analysis of disability outside of and predating disability studies. See Anna Hinton, "On Fits, Starts, and Entry Points: The Rise of Black Disability Studies," *CLA* 64, no. 1 (2021): 11–29.

21. Schalk, *Bodyminds Reimagined*; Pickens, *Black Madness: Mad Blackness*; La Marr Jurelle Bruce, *How to Go Mad Without Losing Your Mind: Madness and Black Radical Creativity* (Duke University Press, 2021). Another key work on madness and literature includes Elizabeth J. Donaldson, ed., *Literatures of Madness: Disability Studies and Mental Health* (Springer, 2018).

22. John W. Blassingame, *The Slave Community: Plantation Life in the Antebellum South* (Oxford University Press, 1979); Orlando Patterson, *Slavery and Social Death: A Comparative Study* (Harvard University Press, 1982); Frances Smith Foster, *Witnessing Slavery: The Development of Ante-Bellum Slave Narratives* (Greenwood, 1979).

23. Deborah Gray White, *Ar'n't I a Woman: Female Slaves in the Plantation South* (Norton, 1999), 10.

24. Tyler D. Parry, "'How Much More Must I Suffer?': Post-Traumatic Stress and the Lingering Impact of Violence Upon Enslaved People," *Slavery and Abolition* 42, no. 2 (2021): 184–200; Kidada E. Williams, "The Wounds That Cried Out: Reckoning with African Americans' Testimonies of Trauma and Suffering from Night Riding," in *The World the Civil War Made*, ed. Gregory Downs and Kate Masur (University of North Carolina Press, 2015); Diane Miller Sommerville, *Aberration of Mind: Suicide and Suffering in the Civil War-Era South* (University of North Carolina Press, 2018), 85–119; David Silkenat, *Moments of Despair: Suicide, Divorce and Debt in Civil War Era North Carolina* (University of North Carolina Press, 2011); Nell Irvin Painter, *Soul Murder and Slavery* (Markham Press Fund, 1995); Terri L. Snyder, *The Power to Die: Slavery and Suicide in British North America* (University of Chicago Press, 2015), 150–51. Disability studies scholars have written about the disabling feature of slavery; see Jennifer Barclay, *The Mark of Slavery: Disability, Race, and Gender in Antebellum America* (University of Illinois Press, 2021); Dea H. Boster, *African American Slavery and Disability: Bodies, Property, and Power in the Antebellum South, 1800–1860* (Routledge, 2013); Stefanie Hunt-Kennedy, *Between Fitness and Death: Disability and Slavery in the Caribbean* (University of Illinois Press, 2020); Jim Downs, *Sick from Freedom: African-American Illness and Suffering During the Civil War and Reconstruction* (Oxford University Press, 2012).

25. Gerald N. Grob, *The State and the Mentally Ill: A History of Worcester State Hospital in Massachusetts, 1830–1920* (University of North Carolina Press, 1966); Gerald N. Grob, *Mental Institutions in America: Social Policy to 1875* (Free Press, 1972; reprint, Transaction, 2009); Gerald N. Grob, *Mental Illness and American Society, 1875–1940* (Princeton University Press, 2019); Gerald N. Grob, *The Mad Among Us: A History of the Care of America's Mentally Ill* (Maxwell Macmillan, 1994); Norman Dain, *Concepts of Insanity in the United States, 1789–1865* (Rutgers University Press, 1964); David Rothman, *The*

Discovery of the Asylum: Social Order and Disorder in the New Republic, revised ed. (Aldine de Gruyter, 2002); Andrew T. Scull, "Madness and Segregative Control: The Rise of the Insane Asylum," *Social Problems* 24, no. 3 (February 1977): 337–51; Andrew T. Scull, "Psychiatry and Social Control in the Nineteenth and Twentieth Centuries," *History of Psychiatry* 2, no. 6 (1991): 149–69; Robert Castel, "Moral Treatment: Mental Therapy and Social Control in the Nineteenth Century," trans. Peter Miller, in *Social Control and the State: Historical and Comparative Essays*, ed. Stanley Cohen and Andrew Scull (Robertson, 1983), 248–66; Michel Foucault, *Madness and Civilization: A History of Insanity in the Age of Reason*, trans. Richard Howard (Random House, 1965); Michel Foucault, *Discipline and Punish: The Birth of the Prison*, trans. Alan Sheridan (Random House, 1977); Constance M. McGovern, "The Myths of Social Control and Custodial Oppression: Patterns of Psychiatric Medicine in Late Nineteenth-Century Institutions," *Journal of Social History* 20, no. 1 (Fall 1986): 3–23; Ellen Dwyer, *Homes for the Mad: Life Inside Two Nineteenth-Century Asylums* (Rutgers University Press, 1987); Nancy Tomes, *A Generous Confidence: Thomas Story Kirkbride and the Art of Asylum-Keeping, 1840–1883* (Cambridge University Press, 1983); Thomas E. Brown, "Dance of the Dialectic? Some Reflections (Polemic and Otherwise) on the Present State of Nineteenth-Century Asylum Studies," *Canadian Bulletin of Medical History* 11, no. 2 (1994): 267–95; Norman Dain, *Disordered Minds: The First Century of Eastern State Hospital in Williamsburg, Virginia, 1766–1866* (Colonial Williamsburg Foundation, 1971), 108–13; Gerald N. Grob, "Class, Ethnicity, and Race in American Mental Hospitals, 1830–75," *Journal of the History of Medicine and Allied Sciences* 28, no. 3 (July 1973): 207–29; Leland Bell, *Treating the Mentally Ill: From Colonial Times to the Present* (Praeger, 1980), 58–73; Steven Noll, "Southern Strategies for Handling the Black Feeble-Minded: From Social Control to Profound Indifference," *Journal of Policy History* 3, no. 2 (1991): 130–51.

26. These works include Elaine Showalter, *The Female Malady: Women, Madness and English Culture, 1830–1980* (Pantheon, 1985); Phyllis Chesler, *Women and Madness*, revised ed. (Palgrave Macmillan, 2005); Peter McCandless, *Moonlight, Magnolias and Madness: Insanity in South Carolina from the Colonial Period to the Progressive Era* (University of North Carolina Press, 1996); Todd L. Savitt, *Medicine and Slavery: The Diseases and Health Care of Blacks in Antebellum Virginia* (University of Illinois Press, 1978); and Benjamin Reiss, *Theaters of Madness: Insane Asylums and Nineteenth-Century American Culture* (University of Chicago Press, 2008).

27. Élodie Edwards-Grossi, *Mad with Freedom: The Political Economy of Blackness, Insanity, and Civil Rights in the U.S South, 1840–1940* (Louisiana State University Press, 2022); Wendy Gonaver, *The Peculiar Institution and the Making of Modern Psychiatry, 1840–1880* (University of North Carolina Press, 2018); Mab Segrest, *Administrations of Lunacy: Racism and the Haunting of American Psychiatry at the Milledgeville Asylum* (New Press, 2020); and Martin Summers, *Madness in the City of Magnificent Intentions: A History of Race and Mental Illness in the Nation's Capital* (Oxford University Press, 2019). Several significant studies on race, psychiatry, and asylums focus mainly on the twentieth century, including Dennis A. Doyle, *Psychiatry and Racial Liberalism in Harlem, 1936–1968* (University of Rochester Press, 2016); Gabriel N. Mendes, *Under the Strain of Color:*

Harlem's Lafargue Clinic and the Promise of an Antiracist Psychiatry (Cornell University Press, 2015); and Mical Raz, *What's Wrong with the Poor?: Psychiatry, Race, and the War on Poverty* (University of North Carolina Press, 2013).

28. Critical studies that look to Black people for their own conceptualizations of science and health include Britt Rusert, *Fugitive Science: Empiricism and Freedom in Early African American Culture* (New York: New York University Press, 2017); and Sharla M. Fett, *Working Cures: Healing, Health, and Power on Southern Slave Plantations* (University of North Carolina Press, 2002).

29. Smith has recently been recovered as an important figure in Black history. The most comprehensive analysis of Smith's works is a collection by John Stauffer. John Stauffer, ed., *The Works of James McCune Smith: Black Intellectual and Abolitionist* (Oxford University Press, 2006). Much of the other recovery scholarship on Smith has been produced by medical historians.

1. ANTEBELLUM PSYCHIATRIC AND MEDICAL DISCOURSES ON THE BLACK BODYMIND

1. Foundational asylum studies that discuss the moral treatment include Norman Dain, *Concepts of Insanity in the United States, 1789–1865* (Rutgers University Press, 1964); David Rothman, *The Discovery of the Asylum: Social Order and Disorder in the New Republic*, rev. ed. (Aldine de Gruyter, 2002); J. Sanbourne Bockoven, *Moral Treatment in American Psychiatry* (Springer, 1963); Eric Carlson and Norman Dain, "The Psychotherapy That Was Moral Treatment," *American Journal of Psychiatry* 117, no. 6 (1960): 519–24; Nancy Tomes, *A Generous Confidence: Thomas Story Kirkbride and the Art of Asylum-Keeping, 1840–1883* (Cambridge University Press, 1983); Constance M. McGovern, *Masters of Madness: Social Origins of the American Psychiatric Profession* (University of Vermont by University Press of New England, 1985); Gerald N. Grob, *The Mad Among Us: A History of the Care of America's Mentally Ill* (Maxwell Macmillan, 1994); Gerald N. Grob, *Mental Institutions in America: Social Policy to 1875* (Free Press, 1972; Transaction, 2009); Gerald N. Grob, *Mental Illness and American Society, 1875–1940* (Princeton University Press, 2019); Lawrence B. Goodheart, *Mad Yankees: The Hartford Retreat for the Insane and Nineteenth-Century Psychiatry* (University of Massachusetts Press, 2003). For discussion of Foucauldian-informed interpretation of the moral treatment as a form of social control of patients and as a method of forcing their adoption of moral and social values of bourgeois society, see Gerald N. Grob, *From Asylum to Community: Mental Health Policy in Modern America* (Princeton University Press, 1991), 287–88.

2. For most of the seventeenth century, the general public in Western societies across the globe believed that mental disabilities had supernatural origins. People saw an individual's condition as divine punishment for evil or the result of sinful misdeeds. During this time, people with mental disabilities were often subject to exorcisms performed by clergymen. The mentally disabled, who were seen as dangerous or shameful, lived torturous lives; they were bound by physical restraints, locked away in homes and jails, or wandered aimlessly. Toward the end of the eighteenth century, ideas about the etiology of mental

1. ANTEBELLUM PSYCHIATRIC AND MEDICAL DISCOURSES 219

disability shifted. Rather than being the result of supernatural possession, physicians claimed that mental disability was the result of physiological or somatic disease in the body; "insanity," they proclaimed, had natural, not supernatural, origins. Despite the period's more scientific stance, mentally disabled people's lives improved little. Treatments for insanity were harsh because the techniques were borrowed from the medical practices of "heroic medicine," "solidism," and "humor theory," which were characterized by bleeding, purging, endemics, corporal punishments, and gagging, among other practices. Practitioners believed that mental health conditions were manageable but not curable. In the wake of the Enlightenment, the world witnessed a fresh excitement about the curability of mental illness. This optimism about reforming social institutions and medicine came as a product of both humanitarian fervor and new perspectives that mental disability was impacted significantly by not just somatic dysfunction but also psychological issues. For a fuller discussion of the state of medicine in the eighteenth century, see Roy Porter, *The Cambridge Illustrated History of Medicine* (Cambridge University Press, 2001).

3. Although debates about terminology were mostly contained in psychiatric professional spaces, journals, and books, various terms made their way into the field of medicine more broadly. By 1817, there were over three dozen medical terms related to distinct mental health conditions. John Redman Coxe, *The Philadelphia Medical Dictionary*, 2nd ed. (Thomas Dobson and Son, 1817).

4. Nancy Tomes, *A Generous Confidence: Thomas Story Kirkbride and the Art of Asylum-Keeping, 1840–1883* (Cambridge University Press, 1983), xv.

5. Benjamin Rush had an environmentalist approach to mental disability and did some of the first theorizing on race and Black bodyminds. With respect to race, he believed that Blacks exhibited irrational behavior such as dirt eating. He also believed that Blacks developed some forms of madness as a result of being enslaved. He saw Black people's skin color as a form of leprosy. Élodie Edwards-Grossi, *Mad with Freedom: The Political Economy of Blackness, Insanity, and Civil Rights in the U. S. South, 1840–1940* (Louisiana State University Press, 2022), 21–22.

6. For more on gradual freedom, see Eric Foner, *The Fiery Trial: Abraham Lincoln and American Slavery* (Norton, 2011); Robin Bernstein, *Freeman's Challenge: The Murder That Shook America's Original Prison for Profit* (University of Chicago Press, 2024); Joanne Pope Melish, *Disowning Slavery: Gradual Emancipation and "Race" in New England, 1780–1860* (Cornell University Press, 1998); Manisha Sinha, *The Slave's Cause: A History of Abolition* (Yale University Press, 2016).

7. Slaveholders also consulted nonmainstream healers and homeopathic doctors. For more on treatment of the "colored insane" before slavery, see Todd Savitt, *Medicine and Slavery: The Diseases and Health Care of Blacks in Antebellum Virginia* (University of Illinois Press, 1978), 247–79; William Postell, *The Health of Slaves on Southern Plantations* (Louisiana State University Press, 1951), 86–87; Peter McCandless, *Moonlight, Magnolias, and Madness: Insanity in South Carolina from the Colonial Period to the Progressive Era* (University of North Carolina Press, 1996), 195–204; Sharla Fett, *Working Cures: Healing, Health, and Power on Southern Slave Plantations* (University of North Carolina Press, 2002), 94, 96.

8. Jefferson's views were in concert with European speculations on the intellectual capacity of Africans and Negroes. In the section "Anthropology" in his *Lectures on Philosophy of*

the Spirit (1827), Georg Wilhelm Friedrich Hegel discusses the linkages between racial features or characteristics and cognitive capacity. He contends that one way to measure where racial groups fall on the scale of human capacity is to consider their relationship to nature. Based on the premise that animals are distinct from humans because of their union with nature, he argues that the connections between man and nature are more pronounced in less civilized nations such as those in Africa. According to Hegel, because of their lack of civilization, Africans are not only less physiologically and mentally developed but also more accustomed to slavery because they lack the ability to be free conscious thinkers. In *Lectures on the Philosophy of World History* (1837), he makes another notable charge. Hegel argues that in addition to lacking an ethical or rational capacity, Africans lack a communal existence, which proves for him that they are not a part of social or human history. Immanuel Kant takes Hegel's articulations regarding collective history a step further when he claims that Blacks are linked to pasts that did not "prepare them for either democracy or citizenly practices because they [African pasts] are not based upon the development of reason in public life." Quoted in Dipesh Chakrabarty, *Provincializing Europe: Postcolonial Thought and Historical Difference* (Princeton University Press, 2000), 51.

9. Thomas Jefferson, *Notes on the State of Virginia* (Prichard and Hall, 1788), 153, 150. Located in Documenting the American South, University Library, the University of North Carolina at Chapel Hill, 2006.

10. Although Jefferson believed that Blacks were inferior, he did not approve of the institution of slavery even as he held slaves. Though his distaste for slavery was not picked up by proslavery advocates, they did use his assumptions about the inherent differences between races.

11. For an extended discussion of the use of scientific studies for proslavery and antislavery arguments, see Winthrop Jordan, *White Over Black: American Attitudes Toward the Negro 1550–1812* (University of North Carolina Press, 1968).

12. Savitt, *Medicine and Slavery*, 277; Wendy Gonaver argues that some of the first people admitted to asylums in the South were Black but that the practice was quickly abandoned. Wendy Gonaver, *The Peculiar Institution and the Making of Modern Psychiatry, 1840–1880* (University of North Carolina Press, 2018), 4.

13. McCandless, *Moonlight, Magnolias, and Madness*, 15–16.

14. For a thorough study on Black American experiences in St. Elizabeth's Asylum, see Martin Summers, *Madness in the City of Magnificent Intentions: A History of Race and Mental Illness in the Nation's Capital* (Oxford University Press, 2019). For a discussion of various legislative actions and debates cornering the opening of the first Black hospitals for the treatment of Blacks with mental disabilities in southern states, including Virginia, North Carolina, and Louisiana, see Edwards-Grossi, *Mad with Freedom*. For a discussion of the impact of slavery on antebellum asylums before the Civil War, see Mab Segrest, *Administrations of Lunacy: Racism and the Haunting of American Psychiatry at the Milledgeville Asylum* (New Press, 2020), 30–39.

15. The foremost study on race and slavery at Eastern Lunatic Asylum is Gonaver, *The Peculiar Institution*. Also see Edwards-Grossi, *Mad with Freedom*, 37–43; and Savitt, *Medicine and Slavery*, 258–79.

1. ANTEBELLUM PSYCHIATRIC AND MEDICAL DISCOURSES 221

16. Savitt, *Medicine and Slavery*, 258-99, 264. Dr. Francis T. Stribling, who was the superintendent of the Western Lunatic Asylum, was opposed to enslaved or free Blacks entering his asylum. He thought accepting slaves would diminish the perception of the hospital as one for paupers and would make it unattractive to paying customers.
17. Records of Eastern State Hospital, 1770-2009, Accession 44812, State Government Records Collection, the Library of Virginia, Richmond, Virginia.
18. Records of Eastern State Hospital, 1770-2009, Accession 44812, State Government Records Collection, the Library of Virginia, Richmond, Virginia. For a discussion of gender and psychiatry, see Elaine Showalter, *The Female Malady: Women, Madness, and Culture in England, 1830-1980* (Pantheon, 1985); Phyllis Chesler, *Women and Madness* (Doubleday, 1972); Nérée St-Amand and Eugène LeBlanc, "Women in 19th-Century Asylums: Three Exemplary Women; a New Brunswick Hero," in *Mad Matters: A Critical Reader in Canadian Mad Studies*, ed. Robert J. Menzies, Geoffrey Reaume, and Brenda A. LeFrançois (Canadian Scholars' Press, 2013).
19. Virginia, *Acts of the General Assembly of Virginia*, 1845-1846 (J.E. Goode, 1846), 18. Also quoted in Savitt, *Medicine and Slavery*, 278.
20. Quoted in Summers, *Madness in the City of Magnificent Intentions*, 2. Summers provides a capacious historical study of the various racial dynamics that impacted the thinking of administrators and race-informed practices of care throughout the nineteenth century and into the mid-twentieth century.
21. Summers, *Madness in the City of Magnificent Intentions*, 3, 5.
22. Blacks with mental disabilities were also treated at the Georgia Infirmary Hospital and the New Orleans Charity Hospital.
23. Edwards-Grossi, *Mad with Freedom*, 44.
24. Savitt, *Medicine and Slavery*, 252.
25. Juriah Harriss, "What Constitutes Unsoundness in the Negro?" *Savannah Journal of Medicine* 1, no. 3 (September 1858): 145-52.
26. Fett, *Working Cures*.
27. Summers, *Madness in the City of Magnificent Intentions*, 3-4.
28. Frederick Douglass, "The Colored Insane," *Frederick Douglass' Paper*, April 1, 1852.
29. Douglass, "The Colored Insane."
30. "General Intelligence," *Christian Recorder*, June 9, 1866.
31. For a discussion of Black people with disabilities during slavery, see Dea H. Boster, *African American Slavery and Disability: Bodies, Property and Power in the Antebellum South, 1800-1860*, (Routledge, 2013); Jenifer L. Barclay, *The Mark of Slavery: Disability, Race, and Gender in Antebellum America* (University of Illinois Press, 2021); Kidada E. Williams, *They Left Great Marks on Me: African American Testimonies of Racial Violence from Emancipation to World War I* (New York University Press, 2012).
32. Theodore Dwight Weld, *American Slavery as It Is: Testimony of a Thousand Witnesses* (American Anti-Slavery Society, 1839), 135. Located in Documenting the American South, University Library, the University of North Carolina at Chapel Hill, 2000.
33. Weld, *American Slavery as It Is*, 136. Using the testimony of Hartford, Connecticut's American Asylum for the Deaf and Dumb, he reasoned that there were sixteen hundred "deaf and dumb" slaves in the South.

34. The enchanted universe is Yvonne Chireau's term that refers to the spiritual world that African Americans believed they inhabited alongside the natural world. Yvonne P. Chireau, "Conjure and Christianity in the Nineteenth Century: Religious Elements in African American Magic," *Religion and American Culture: A Journal of Interpretation* 7, no. 2 (Summer 1997): 239. For more on Black religious traditions, see Theophus H. Smith, *Conjuring Culture: Biblical Formations of Black America* (Oxford University Press, 1994); Elliot Gorn, "Black Magic: Folk Beliefs of the Slave Community," in *Science and Medicine in the Old South*, ed. Ronald L. Numbers and Todd Savitt (Louisiana State University Press, 1989); Albert J. Raboteau, *Slave Religion: The "Invisible Institution" in the Antebellum South* (Oxford University Press, 1978); Margaret Washington Creel, *A Peculiar People: Slave Religion and Community Culture Among the Gullahs* (New York University Press, 1988); Charles Joyner, *Down by the Riverside: A South Carolina Slave Community* (University of Illinois Press, 1984).
35. Fett, *Working Cures*, 140.
36. Smith, *Conjuring Culture*, 5. Despite psychiatrists' and physicians' desire to untether religious faith from disease, Blacks and whites continued to view their health as deeply tied to their religious state.
37. Thaddeus Norris, "Negro Superstitions," in *The Negro and His Folklore in Nineteenth-Century Periodicals*, ed. Bruce Jackson (University of Texas Press, 1967), 138.
38. Georgia Writers' Project, *Drums and Shadows: Survival Studies Among the Georgia Coastal Negroes* (University of Georgia Press, 1940), 25. Conjure was often seen as the culprit in unexplained disease or when someone was not responsive to medical treatment. E. Geddings, "Case of Extraordinary Enlargement and Ossific Transformation of the Ovaria," *Southern Medical and Surgical Journal* 2, no. 10 (May 1838): 579–85.
39. Geddings, "Case of Extraordinary Enlargement," 580.
40. Fett, *Working Cures*, 94.
41. Georgia Writers' Project, *Drums and Shadows*, 102.
42. Theodore Rosengarten, *Tombee: Portrait of a Cotton Planter* (Morrow, 1986), 20. See also Fett, *Working Cures*, 94. Whites had a range of attitudes regarding conjure. Some whites believed in the power of conjure doctors and sought them out.
43. In conjuring traditions, insanity and death were consequences of not addressing the supernatural power being wielded against an individual. Fett, *Working Cures*, 95.
44. "Durham's Voodoo Doctor," Box A661, folder: North Carolina, Witchcraft, WPA Folklore Project, LC, as cited in Fett, *Working Cures*, 95.
45. Fett, *Working Cures*, 95.
46. Samuel A. Cartwright, "The Diseases of Negroes: Pulmonary Congestions, Pneumonia, & c., No. II," *De Bow's Review of the Southern and Western States* 11 (1851): 213.
47. Samuel A. Cartwright, "Dr. Cartwright on the Caucasians and the Africans," *De Bow's Review and Industrial Resources, Statistics, etc.* 25 (1858): 45–56.
48. Samuel A. Cartwright, "Remarks on Dysentery Among Negroes," *New Orleans Medical and Surgical Journal* 11, no. 2 (September 1854): 163.
49. W. S. Forwood, "Serpent Worship Among the Negroes," *De Bow's Review: Agricultural, Commercial, Industrial Progress and Resources* 6, no. 1 (1861): 98. For other physician

1. ANTEBELLUM PSYCHIATRIC AND MEDICAL DISCOURSES   223

   references to belief in the supernatural in cases of disease among Blacks and occasionally whites, see Sir William Burnett, "On the Effects Produced by Poisonous Fish on the Human Frame," *Southern Medical and Surgical Journal* 2, no. 12 (December 1846): 730–31; K. G. Holloway, "Remarkable Case of Fibro-Schirro Cartilaginous Enlargement of the Ovaria," *Southern Medical and Surgical Journal* 2, no. 12 (July 1838): 714–20; H. R. Casey, "Contribution to the History of Typhoid Fever," *Southern Medical and Surgical Journal* 7, no. 12 (December 1851): 707–18.

50. A. P. Merrill, "An Essay on Some of the Distinctive Peculiarities of the Negro Race," *Southern Medical and Surgical Journal* 12, no. 2 (February 1856): 88.

51. Ambrose McCoy, "Voodooism in the South," *Louisville Medical News*, December 13, 1884, 380, 381. This argument was also made by Merrill, "An Essay on Some of the Distinctive Peculiarities of the Negro Race." Also see David G. Cox, "Race, Reconstruction, and the Invention of 'Negro Superstition,' 1862–1877," *Journal of American Studies* 55, no. 5 (2021): 1125–52.

52. Although earlier censuses collected basic data on population, the 1840 census added several categories, including literacy rates, the number of educational institutions, and the sum of "deaf and dumb," "blind," and "insane" persons under private and state-funded care. The national census is a product of the Constitutional Convention of 1787, when statesmen decided that congressional representation was to be dependent upon each state's population. Thus, enumeration of the citizenry was necessary for fulfilling the constitutional mandate. This is also the convention that settled on the infamous three-fifths compromise, which in effect disregarded Black humanity by considering slavery in terms of representation and taxation. The census also represented the nation's keen interest in the use of social statistics to support a nationalistic sentiment. As Gerald Grob puts it, the census "seemed to offer proof that America was destined to become the predominant world power." The way in which the 1840 census was used to reinforce racism showed how comfortably slavery was etched into America's imagination of itself. Gerald N. Grob, *Edward Jarvis and the Medical World of Nineteenth-Century America* (University of Tennessee Press, 1978), 70. For historical background on the census, see W. Stull Holt, *The Bureau of the Census: Its History, Activities, and Organization* (Brookings Institution, 1929), 1–92; Carroll D. Wright and William C. Hunt, *The History and Growth of the United States Census*, 56th Congress, 1st Session, No. 239 (Government Printing Office, 1900), passim.

53. For a discussion of the political life of the 1840 census, see Edwards-Grossi, *Mad with Freedom*, 45–56. For a discussion of the international response to the census, see pages 53–55.

54. These ratios appear in Edward Jarvis, "Insanity Among the Coloured Population of the Free States," *American Journal of the Medical Sciences* 7, no. 13 (January 1844): 72–73. The raw census data can be found in the Compendium of the Enumeration of the Inhabitants and Statistics of the United States, as Obtained at the Department of State, from the Return of the Sixth Census (Washington, DC, 1841), 4–103. Grob, *Edward Jarvis*, 70–72. Although studies of the census beginning in the 1970s pointed to the racial bias inherent in the census numbers, later studies showed that the racial discrepancies were a matter

of human error and incompetence, not deliberate manipulations and racial propaganda. See Edwards-Grossi, *Mad with Freedom*, 46–47.

55. His findings first appeared in Edward Jarvis, "Statistics of Insanity in the United States," *Boston Medical and Surgical Journal* 27, no. 7 (September 1842): 116.

56. See Sander Gilman, *Difference and Pathology: Stereotypes of Sexuality, Race, and Madness* (Cornell University Press, 1985), 137, 139–42. The physician played a key role in the development of a good and healthy citizenry. Thus, after the release of the 1840 census, physicians and scientists produced a body of publications containing interpretations of the data along with policy recommendations. Grob, *Edward Jarvis*, 38. For a discussion of how census data was used before and after emancipation to support research on the mental and physical health and mortality rates of Blacks, see John S. Haller, *Outcasts from Evolution: Scientific Attitudes of Racial Inferiority, 1859–1900* (McGraw-Hill, 1971), 40–68.

57. For background on the state of nineteenth-century medicine, see Charles E. Rosenberg, "The American Medical Profession: Mid-Nineteenth Century," *Mid America* 44 (July 1962), 163–71; Joseph F. Kett, *The Formation of the American Medical Profession: The Role of Institutions, 1780–1860* (Yale University Press, 1968); Richard H. Shryock, *Medicine and Society in America, 1660–1860* (New York University Press, 1960); William Rothstein, *American Physicians in the Nineteenth Century: From Sects to Science* (Johns Hopkins University Press, 1972).

58. For more on the state of nineteenth-century psychiatry, see Norman Dain, *Concepts of Insanity in the United States, 1789–1865* (Rutgers University Press, 1964); Gerald N. Grob, *Mental Institutions in America: Social Policy to 1875* (Free Press, 1973); and Gerald N. Grob, *The State and the Mentally Ill: A History of Worcester State Hospital in Massachusetts, 1830–1920* (University of North Carolina, 1966). For an extended discussion of the transition from moral treatment to custodial care, see Grob, *The State and the Mentally Ill*.

59. In this formulation, psychiatrists thought Africans to be less prone to mental disability because of their less-developed state of civilization. See Benjamin Reiss, *Theaters of Madness: Insane Asylums and Nineteenth-Century American Culture* (University of Chicago Press, 2008), 69–70.

60. Jarvis, "Statistics of Insanity in the United States," 116–21.

61. Edward Jarvis had complicated views on slavery. Upon seeing slaves in the northeast, he noted that slaves were "a lazy, idle unprofitable race, doing not half the work a white can do . . . caring nothing for his owner's interests." He continued, "It would be a blessing to this country to transport the whole to Africa." Quoted in Grob, *Edward Jarvis*, 25. These lines reflect his general attitude toward Blacks as lacking in moral character. He abhorred slavery, but he thought involuntary servitude prevented the development of physical and moral senses. Quoted in Grob, *Edward Jarvis*, 45, 53.

62. Jarvis, "Statistics of Insanity in the United States," 121.

63. It should be noted that this conception was held throughout European psychiatry as well.

64. For a more detailed discussion of Jacksonian society and insanity, as well as prominent psychiatrists during the era who subscribed to this idea, see chapter 3, "Insanity and the Social Order," of Rothman, *Discovery of the Asylum*, 109–29. Although the Whigs

opposed Jackson's laissez-faire economics and the extension of suffrage (to all white men), the one matter that the Jacksonians and the opposing Whigs agreed upon was to avoid quarrels over slavery.

65. Janet Miron, *Prisons, Asylums, and the Public: Institutional Visiting in the Nineteenth Century* (University of Toronto Press, 2011), 4, 65; Dain, *Concepts of Insanity*, 8.

66. Dorothea Lynde Dix and US Congress, House, and Senate, *Memorial of D.L. Dix: Praying a Grant of Land for the Relief and Support of the Indigent Curable and Incurable Insane in the United States*, 30th Cong., 1st sess., Misc. No. 150 (Tippin & Streeper, 1848), 2. Her statement dovetails with her lack of sympathy for slaves, whose condition she viewed as less severe than that of the mentally disabled. While working for mental health reform, she "turned her back on the prejudice, hate, and violence of the slave system." Quoted in David Gollaher, *Voice for the Mad: The Life of Dorothea Dix* (Free Press, 1995), 265.

67. Quoted in Norman Dain, *Disordered Minds: The First Century of Eastern State Hospital in Williamsburg, Virginia 1766-1866* (Colonial Williamsburg Foundation, 1971), 112.

68. Early scientific studies on differences between the races contributed to social and cultural perceptions of race. They supported claims of Black inferiority and justified slavery. Chapter 2 provides an analysis of how proslavery arguments were intertwined with medical and scientific racist claims. For works on the use of scientific studies for proslavery and antislavery arguments, see Jordan, *White Over Black*. For a discussion of the use of various scientific strains of thought such as monogenism, polygenism, and naturalism in the slavery debates, see Stephen Jay Gould, *The Mismeasure of Man* (Norton, 1996), 63–104; for an extended study on the American school of thought on polygeny as support for slavery, see William Stanton, *The Leopard's Spots: Scientific Attitudes Toward Race in America, 1815-59* (University of Chicago Press, 1960).

69. Richard Hofstadter, "From Calhoun to the Dixiecrats," *Social Research* 82, no. 1 (2015): 245–61.

70. John C. Calhoun, *The Works of John C. Calhoun*, ed. Richard Cralle, 6 vols. (D. Appleton, 1863–1867), 5:337.

71. Edwards-Grossi, *Mad with Freedom*, 51; Paul Finkelman, *Defending Slavery: Proslavery Thought in the Old South: A Brief History with Documents* (Bedford/St. Martin's, 2003).

72. Hayden was not alone in his assertions. Under the banner of medical science, other physicians made similar claims. See Samuel Forry, "Vital Statistics Furnished by the Sixth Census of the United States, Bearing Upon the Question of the Human Race," *New York Journal of Medicine and the Collateral Sciences* 1, no. 2 (1843): 151–67; and Samuel Forry, "On the Relative Proportion of Centenarians, of Deaf and Dumb, of Blind, and of Insane, in the Races of European and African Origin, as Shown by the Censuses of the United States," *New York Journal of Medicine and the Collateral Sciences* 2, no. 6 (1844): 310–20. For historical reflections on the faulty use of the census, see Benjamin Pasamanick, "Myths Regarding Prevalence of Mental Disease in the American Negro: A Century of Misuse of Mental Hospital Data and Some New Findings," *Journal of National Medical Association* 56, no. 1 (1964): 6–17; and Thomas S. Szasz, "The Sane Slave: An Historical Note on the Use of Medical Diagnosis as Justificatory Rhetoric," *American Journal of Psychotherapy* 25, no. 2 (1971): 228–39.

73. C. B. Hayden, "On the Distribution of Insanity Among the Coloured Population of the Free States," *Southern Literary Messenger* 10 (1844): 180.
74. Edwards-Grossi, *Mad with Freedom*, 55–56.
75. Edwards-Grossi, *Mad with Freedom*, 24–35.
76. Samuel A. Cartwright, "Report on the Diseases and Physical Peculiarities of the Negro Race," *New Orleans Medical and Surgical Journal* 7 (1851): 691–715.
77. Although extreme in his views, Cartwright, along with men like Josiah Clark Nott, was among the many southern physicians to argue for physical and mental differences between races. For more on the ideas of these physicians, see John Haller, "The Negro and the Southern Physician: A Study of Medical and Racial Attitudes, 1800–1860," *Medical History* 16, no. 3 (1972), 238–53.
78. Cartwright, "Report," 691.
79. Cartwright, "Report," 692, 694, 693, 694.
80. Cartwright, "Report," 693. For Cartwright, the term "civilization" referred to progress in the form of industry; arts and sciences; complex language systems; a government structure with separate legislative, judicial, and executive branches (as opposed to an omnipotent chief or king); and structural developments such as roads, buildings, and monuments.
81. Reiss, *Theaters of Madness*, 69–70.
82. Cartwright, "Report," 694.
83. Cartwright, "Report," 694, 696.
84. George Fitzhugh, *Sociology for the South, or the Failure of Free Society* (A. Morris, 1854), 82–83.
85. Cartwright, "Report," 707
86. Cartwright, "Report," 708.
87. He indicated that dysaesthesia *aethiopis*, unlike drapetomania, affected "both mind and body." Cartwright, "Report," 709.
88. Cartwright, "Report," 712, 709, 710–11, 713.
89. For a discussion of superintendents' use of Shakespeare, see Reiss, *Theaters of Madness*, 79–102.
90. Herbert Gutman, *The Black Family in Slavery and Freedom, 1750–1925* (Vintage, 1976), 293.
91. Conceptions of Black women after slavery were largely influenced by stereotypes about them. Black women were excluded from notions of respectable womanhood during slavery. After emancipation, figures like the Mammy and Jezebel persisted and new ones emerged, including the sassy, defiant, and aggressive Sapphire.
92. There are notable distinctions between northern and southern asylums. However, when it came to the care of the "colored insane," in both cases the policies and practices reflected proslavery psychiatric thought. Indeed, northern asylum superintendents largely left the question of how to treat the "colored insane" to southern psychiatrists' expertise and experience. Grob, *The Mad Among Us*, 88–89, and Grob, *Mental Institutions in America*, 248–56. Southern asylums, then, are ideal sites for examining how

notions of mental disability among formerly enslaved Black women continued to shape lives after emancipation.

93. Rana Hogarth, *Medicalizing Blackness: Making Racial Difference in the Atlantic World, 1780–1840* (University of North Carolina Press, 2017), 8.

94. Ellen Samuels, *Fantasies of Identification: Disability, Gender, Race* (New York University Press, 2014), 11, 13.

95. W. Camps, "Hysteria Considered as a Connecting Link between Mental and Bodily Diseases," *Southern Medical and Surgical Journal* 15 (October 1859): 701-3. As cited in Marli Frances Weiner and Mazie Hough, *Sex, Sickness, and Slavery: Illness in the Antebellum South* (University of Illinois Press, 2012), 143.

96. Green, "Cases of Inflammation and Ulceration of the Cervix Uteri," 54-55. As cited in Weiner and Hough, *Sex, Sickness, and Slavery*, 149.

97. Weiner and Hough, *Sex, Sickness, and Slavery*, 123. For historical accounts of the role of the medical field in studying the Black body and contributions to justifying existing social structures, see Haller, "The Negro and the Southern Physician," and Todd Savitt and James Harvey Young, eds., *Disease and Distinctiveness in the American South* (University of Tennessee Press, 1988).

98. A. P. Merrill, "An Essay on Some of the Distinctive Peculiarities of the Negro Race," *Southern Medical and Surgical Journal* 12, no. 1 (January 1856): 21–36; no. 2 (February 1856): 80–90; no. 3 (March 1856): 147–56, published in three parts. Although I focus here on Merrill, his conceptions were not uncommon among southern physicians. For more examples of his sentiments about insanity in the North, slave diet, and climate, see Gretchen Long, *Doctoring Freedom: The Politics of African American Medical Care in Slavery and Emancipation* (University of North Carolina Press, 2012), 32–39.

99. Merrill, "An Essay on Some of the Distinctive Peculiarities of the Negro Race," 21. Merrill directly relies on the most famous polygenist, Jean Louis Agassiz. He also references the notion that Blacks demonstrated "mental deterioration" that could only be corrected over thousands of years during which they could be influenced by whites' supposedly superior culture. Merrill, "An Essay on Some of the Distinctive Peculiarities of the Negro Race," 23. Debates with which he would have been familiar appeared in a host of scientific fields that by today's standards would be dismissed as pseudoscience but at the time were mainstream and consequential to debates about slavery, citizenship, and freedom from confinement in prisons and asylums. Various fields included naturalism, monogenesis, polygenesis, craniology, anthropometry, criminology, and phrenology. See Haller, *Outcasts from Evolution*; Stephen Tomlinson, *Head Masters: Phrenology, Secular Education, and Nineteenth-Century Social Thought* (University of Alabama Press, 2005); Nicole Hahn Rafter, *Creating Born Criminals* (University of Illinois Press, 1997); Gould, *The Mismeasure of Man*; George M. Fredrickson, *The Black Image in the White Mind: The Debate on Afro-American Character and Destiny, 1817–1914* (Harper & Row, 1971), 71–96.

100. Merrill, "An Essay on Some of the Distinctive Peculiarities of the Negro Race," 21. For more in-depth discussions of southern medical arguments about racial difference in disease in the South, particularity regarding health, see Savitt and Young, *Disease and*

228   1. ANTEBELLUM PSYCHIATRIC AND MEDICAL DISCOURSES

Distinctiveness; Long, *Doctoring Freedom*; Stephen Stowe, *Doctoring the South: Southern Physicians and Everyday Medicine in the Mid-Nineteenth Century* (University of North Carolina Press, 2004); and Margaret Humphreys, *Intensely Human: The Health of the Black Soldier in the American Civil War* (Johns Hopkins University Press, 2008), 11–43.

101. The fact that the interview took place reveals the fear, uneasiness, and incomprehensibility of Black resistance to slavery. Although the action was the result of a rational response to an illogical system of capitalistic human bondage on the part of Black people, it was pathologized as potentially irrational and "insane" in the eyes of their captors. This urge to pathologize Black resistance is carried on in the sentiments of Cartwright's formulation of drapetomania.

102. Amariah Brigham, "Exemption of the Cherokee Indians and Africans from Insanity," *American Journal of Insanity* 1 (1845): 287–88.

103. Amariah Brigham, *An Inquiry Concerning the Diseases and Functions of the Brain, the Spinal Cord, and the Nerves* (Elihu Geer, 1840), 22.

104. As I discuss elsewhere, race and gender impacted Black people's experiences with medical professionals and their lives in medical spaces, including asylums.

105. Merrill, "An Essay on Some of the Distinctive Peculiarities of the Negro Race," 21, 33.

106. Merrill, "An Essay on Some of the Distinctive Peculiarities of the Negro Race," 82.

107. For a discussion of alcohol abuse in the nineteenth century, see Matthew Warner Osborn, *Rum Maniacs: Alcoholic Insanity in the Early American Republic* (University of Chicago Press, 2014), 157–63.

108. Merrill, "An Essay on Some of the Distinctive Peculiarities of the Negro Race," 83.

109. Merrill, "An Essay on Some of the Distinctive Peculiarities of the Negro Race," 24.

110. Benjamin Rush, *Medical Inquiries and Observations Upon Diseases of the Mind* (Kimber & Richardson, 1812), 11.

111. Benjamin Rush, a Quaker and Presbyterian, was an ardent abolitionist. He used environmentalist arguments to prove that slavery was to blame for any inferiority, "immorality," or "ignorance" among Blacks. In 1773, he wrote, "Slavery is so foreign to the human mind, that the moral faculties, as well as those of the understanding are debased, and rendered torpid." Quoted in Jordan, *White Over Black*, 187. Still, Rush held fast to beliefs about the biological differences between Blacks and whites. For example, he concluded that African women were akin to "orang-outangs [sic]." Benjamin Rush, "Observations Intended to Favour a Supposition That the Black Color (as It Is Called) of the Negroes Is Derived from the Leprosy," *Transactions of the American Philosophical Society* 4, no. 1 (1799): 291.

2. MENTAL DISABILITY AND THE INTELLECTUAL THOUGHT OF JAMES McCUNE SMITH

1. At the Constitutional Convention of 1787, statesmen decided that congressional representation would depend on each state's population. Enumeration of the citizenry became the main focus of census data collection as a means of fulfilling the constitutional mandate. At the same convention, lawmakers devised the infamous three-fifths compromise.

The compromise—to count three out of every five slaves as people—in effect devalued Black Americans' humanity by considering their personhood solely in terms of legislative representation and taxation.

2. According to the findings, the total number of those reported to be "insane and feebleminded" in the United States was about 17,000, of whom nearly 3,000 were Black. The ratio of insanity among northern whites was 1:995. For southern whites, the ratio was 1:945. There were 2.7 million Blacks in the South, and of these, 1,734 were reported to be "insane or retarded," resulting in a ratio of 1:1,558. But in the free states, about 1,200 Blacks out of 171,894 were reported to be "insane or retarded," a ratio of 1:144. See Gerald N. Grob, *Edward Jarvis and the Medical World of Nineteenth-Century America* (University of Tennessee Press, 1978), 70–72.

3. For a discussion of how census data were used before and after emancipation to support research on the mental and physical health and mortality rates of Blacks, see John S. Haller, *Outcasts from Evolution: Scientific Attitudes of Racial Inferiority, 1859–1900* (University of Illinois Press, 1971), 40–68. For a discussion of the lasting discourses on Black mental inferiority and freedom, see Sander Gilman, *Difference and Pathology: Stereotypes of Sexuality, Race, and Madness* (Cornell University Press, 1985), 136–41.

4. The social statistician and physician Edward Jarvis first debunked the claims in an article in the *American Journal of the Medical Sciences*. Edward Jarvis, "Insanity Among the Coloured Population of the Free States," *American Journal of the Medical Sciences* 7, no. 14 (January 1844): 72–73.

5. John C. Calhoun, *The Works of John C. Calhoun*, ed. Richard Cralle, 6 vols. (D. Appleton 1863–1867), 5:337. Hayden was not alone in his assertions. Under the banner of medical science, other physicians made similar claims. See Samuel Forry, "Vital Statistics Furnished by the Sixth Census of the United States, Bearing Upon the Question of the Unity of the Human Race," *New York Journal of Medicine and the Collateral Sciences* 1 (1843): 151–67; and Samuel Forry, "On the Relative Proportion of Centenarians, of Deaf and Dumb, of Blind, and of Insane, in the Races of European and African Origin, as Shown by the Censuses of the United States," *New York Journal of Medicine and the Collateral Sciences* 2 (1844): 310–20.

6. James McCune Smith, "Freedom and Slavery for Afric-Americans," *The Liberator*, February 23, 1844.

7. Other notable achievements were made by Black women in the medical field in the nineteenth century. In 1864, Rebecca Davis Lee Crumpler was the first Black woman to earn a medical degree. She wrote *A Book of Medical Discourses* in 1883. In 1867, Rebecca J. Cole became the second Black woman in the United States to earn a medical degree.

8. On studies of Black intellectuals in antebellum America, see David W. Blight, "In Search of Learning, Liberty, and Self Definition: James McCune Smith and the Ordeal of the Antebellum Black Intellectual," *Afro-Americans in New York Life and History* 9, no. 2 (1985): 7–26; John Stauffer, *The Black Hearts of Men: Radical Abolitionists and the Transformation of Race* (Harvard University Press, 2002); Leslie M. Harris, *In the Shadow of Slavery: African Americans in New York City, 1626–1863* (University of Chicago Press, 2023); Kelly Harris, "Foreshadowing Du Bois: James McCune Smith and the Shaping of Nineteenth

Century Black Social Scientists," *Du Bois Review: Social Science Research on Race* (2024): 1–17. On studies of James McCune Smith in the history of medicine, see Heidi L. Lujan and Stephen E. DiCarlo, "First African American to Hold a Medical Degree: Brief History of James McCune Smith, Abolitionist, Educator, and Physician," *Advances in Physiological Education* 43, no. 2 (2019): 134–39; Thomas M. Morgan, "The Education and Medical Practice of Dr. James McCune Smith (1813–1865), First Black American to Hold a Medical Degree," *Journal of the National Medical Association* 95, no. 7 (2003): 603–14; Neil Krishan Aggarwal, "The Legacy of James McCune Smith, MD—the First US Black Physician," *Journal of the American Medical Association* 326, no. 22 (2021): 2245–46.

9. Judith Mulcahy is wary of scholars such as John Stauffer who position Smith as a representative figure. She contends that Smith would not see himself in such a light and that there were other venerable public intellectuals such as Martin Delany and Alexander Crummel. In a story about mental disability, Smith stands out as one of the most important figures for his breadth and depth of thinking about race and health and his deliberate attempts to generate a counterdiscourse to medical, scientific, and psychiatric discourses on the Black bodymind in every arena of his public and professional life. Judith Mulcahy, "James McCune Smith: The Communipaw Connection," *Nineteenth Century Prose* 34, nos. 1–2 (2007): 359–67.
10. Rusert explores the work of other Black scientists and physicians, including Benjamin Banneker and Martin Delany. Britt Rusert, *Fugitive Science: Empiricism and Freedom in Early African American Culture* (New York University Press, 2017), 7.
11. In 1799, New York State passed a Gradual Emancipation Act that freed enslaved children who were born after July 4, 1799, with the caveat that they were to be indentured servants until young adulthood. Before the official Emancipation Act that freed all enslaved people on July 4, 1827, Smith was "free" under the terms of the Gradual Emancipation Act because he was the child of an enslaved mother. Smith was the son of a white merchant named Samuel. Lujan and DiCarlo, "First African American to Hold a Medical Degree"; Graham Russell Hodges, *Root and Branch: African Americans in New York and New Jersey, 1613–1863* (University of North Carolina Press, 1999).
12. The most expansive study is John Stauffer, ed., *The Works of James McCune Smith: Black Intellectual and Abolitionist* (Oxford University Press, 2006). Also see Harris, "Foreshadowing Du Bois"; Morgan, "The Education and Medical Practice of Dr. James McCune Smith (1813–1865)"; Stauffer, *The Black Hearts of Men*; Aggarwal, "The Legacy of James McCune Smith, MD"; Lujan and DiCarlo, "First African-American to Hold a Medical Degree."
13. Foreword in Stauffer, *The Works of James McCune Smith*, xi.
14. Mulcahy, "James McCune Smith," 364.
15. Frederick Douglass, "Dr. James McCune Smith," *Douglass' Monthly*, March 1859.
16. He used these essays to make strong cases against racist currents of ethnology. Stauffer, *The Works of James McCune Smith*, 245.
17. Many well-known abolitionist figures contributed to these publications, including Martin Delany, Francis Watkins Harper, Frederick Douglass, J. W. C. Pennington, and William Cooper Nell.

18. John Stauffer uses this phrase to describe the ways religious beliefs undergirded their commitment to racial equality and abolition. Stauffer, *The Black Hearts of Men*, 2.
19. "Colored Orphan's Asylum: Physician's Report [with Reply]," *Colored American*, January 26, 1839.
20. James McCune Smith, "Hon. John C Calhoun and The Free Colored People," *New York Daily Tribune*, May 8, 1844.
21. James McCune Smith, "The Influence of Climate on Longevity: With Special Reference to Life Insurance," *Hunt's Merchant Magazine* 14, no. 5 (1846): 403–18.
22. Smith, "The Influence of Climate on Longevity," 415.
23. Smith, "The Influence of Climate on Longevity," 418. On discourses on climate and the idea of "racial seasoning," see Christopher Willoughby, *Masters of Health: Racial Science and Slavery in U.S. Medical Schools* (University of North Carolina Press, 2022).
24. Smith, "The Influence of Climate on Longevity," 416. Jefferson speculates that Blacks are "inferior to the whites in the endowments both of body and mind." Thomas Jefferson, *Notes on the State of Virginia* (Prichard and Hall, 1788), 153. Located in Documenting the American South, University Library, the University of North Carolina at Chapel Hill, 2006. Smith takes on Jefferson's ideas in a two-part 1859 essay entitled, "On the Fourteenth Query of Thomas Jefferson's *Notes on the State of Virginia*" in the *Anglo-African Magazine* 1, no. 8 (1859): 225–38. For a discussion of phrenology, see Roger Cooter, *The Cultural Meaning of Popular Science: Phrenology and the Organization of Consent in Nineteenth-Century Britain* (Cambridge University Press, 1984); and John D. Davis, *Phrenology, Fad and Science: A Nineteenth-Century American Crusade* (Yale University Press, 1955).
25. Morgan, "The Education and Medical Practice of Dr. James McCune Smith (1813–1865)," 610.
26. Smith advertised his practices in the newspaper. He offered bleeding, tooth-drawing, cupping, and shaker herbs from his pharmacy. "Multiple Classified Advertisements," *Colored American*, November 18, 1837, *Slavery and Anti-Slavery: A Transnational Archive*; "Multiple Classified Advertisements," *Colored American*, March 2, 1839, *Slavery and Anti-Slavery: A Transnational Archive*.
27. James McCune Smith, "On the Influence of Opium Upon the Catamenial Functions," *New York Journal of Medicine and Collateral Sciences* 2, no. 1 (1844): 56.
28. The psychiatrist Amariah Brigham contended that the health of the woman was critical to the health of the nation. He wrote, "It is a truth which cannot be too often repeated, that nothing is more essential to the welfare of any country, than the preservation of the health of its females, and I am pleased to see by an increased attention to their physical education, that many have become convinced of the fact." Amariah Brigham, *An Inquiry Concerning the Diseases and Functions of the Brain, the Spinal Cord, and the Nerves* (Elihu Geer, 1840), 205de.
29. Women's reproductive systems were broadly objects of study for psychiatrists, and as Elaine Showalter argues, regulating their bodies was a means of regulating their minds. Elaine Showalter, *The Female Malady: Women, Madness, and English Culture, 1830–1980* (Pantheon, 1985).

30. Patient Notebook, 1842–1843, Lucy Fankersby entry, ESH, as cited in Wendy Gonaver, *The Peculiar Institution and the Making of Modern Psychiatry 1840–1880* (University of North Carolina Press, 2018), 115.
31. Smith, "On the Influence of Opium," 57. The designation of her temperament is connected to humor theory, which identified four temperaments. The sanguine temperament was seen as a social personality and usually associated with impulsiveness, pleasure seeking, and talkativeness.
32. Smith, "On the Influence of Opium," 57.
33. Magdalen Asylum was a charitable institution that took in women and girls aged fifteen to forty years old from prisons and the streets, many of whom were sex workers, which at the time was seen as a social vice. Much like asylums and other socializing institutions, it emphasized daily routines and religious instruction, but it also focused much more on educational and vocational training and instilling "respectable habits" with the goal of reintegrating its residents into society. "Our Charitable Institutions: The New-York Magdalen Asylum-Incentives Offered the Penitent-Daily Routine ofFogel Life Led by the Inmates, &c., &c," *New York Times*, January 14, 1862. For more on institutions to reform women and girls, see Lu Ann De Cunzo, "Reform, Respite, Ritual: An Archaeology of Institutions: The Magdalen Society of Philadelphia, 1800–1850," *Historical Archaeology* 29, no. 3 (1995): 1–168; Miriam Haughton, Mary McAuliffe, and Emilie Pine, *Legacies of the Magdalen Laundries: Commemoration, Gender, and the Postcolonial Carceral State* (Manchester University Press, 2021); Steven Ruggles, "Fallen Women: The Inmates of the Magdalen Society Asylum of Philadelphia, 1836–1908," *Journal of Social History* 16, no. 4 (Summer 1983): 65–82; "Inwood's Old Magdalen Asylum," *My Inwood*, July 13, 2013; Saidiya V. Hartman, *Wayward Lives, Beautiful Experiments: Intimate Histories of Riotous Black Girls, Troublesome Women, and Queer Radicals* (Norton, 2019).
34. Smith also took issue with homeopathy, which he saw as illegitimate and harmful. He called homeopathy "the most deadly quackery that curses the nineteenth century." James McCune Smith, "Lay Puffery of Homeopathy, Letter from Dr. James McC. Smith," *The Annalist, a Record of Practical Medicine in the City of New-York* 2, no. 18 (June 15, 1848): 351. Also cited in Lujan and DiCarlo, "First African-American to Hold a Medical Degree."
35. Phrenology had adherents into the end of the nineteenth century even after it fell out of vogue.
36. Susan Branson, "Phrenology and the Science of Race in Antebellum America," *Early American Studies* 15, no. 1 (2017): 164–93.
37. On the influence of criminology in education, see Stephen Tomlinson, *Head Masters: Phrenology, Secular Education, and Nineteenth-Century Social Thought* (University of Alabama Press, 2005). On the links between criminology and phrenology, see Nicole Hahn Rafter, *Creating Born Criminals* (University of Illinois Press, 1997), 76–77. Phrenology also found widespread use in the burgeoning field of criminology, especially through the proliferation of the notion of "moral insanity." Although the person who coined the term, James Cowles Prichard, was not a phrenologist, particularly because he did not see moral insanity as an affliction that was not connected to the brain, phrenologists favored the concept as exemplary of their scientific schema. Prichard did not see moral insanity

as a subcategory of insanity. Both he and phrenologists saw moral insanity as a parallel ailment that shared with insanity the fact that an individual's actions and behavior were out of their control. Phrenologists believed that moral insanity was rooted in problems in the brain and that, as such, it came under the purview of medicine and science. Unlike insanity, which phrenologists believed affected the reason, intellect, and understanding of a person, when one fell victim to moral insanity, phrenologists believed their feelings, emotions, and empathy were defective.

38. Alan Gribben, "Mark Twain, Phrenology and the 'Temperaments': A Study of Pseudoscientific Influence," *American Quarterly* 24, no. 1 (1972): 45–68; Edward Hungerford, "Walt Whitman and His Chart of Bumps," *American Literature* 2, no. 4 (1931): 350–84; Nathaniel Mackey, "Phrenological Whitman," *Conjunctions* 29 (1997): 231–51; Robert E. Riegel, "The Introduction of Phrenology to the United States," *American Historical Review* 39, no. 1 (October 1933): 73–78; Madeleine B. Stern, "Mark Twain Had His Head Examined," *American Literature* 41, no. 2 (1969): 207–18.

39. Johann Gaspar Spurzheim, *Observations on the Deranged Manifestations of the Mind: Or Insanity*, 3rd American ed. (Marsh, Capen, and Lyon, 1836), 109. Also cited in Lawrence B. Goodheart, *Mad Yankees: The Hartford Retreat for the Insane and Nineteenth-Century Psychiatry* (University of Massachusetts Press, 2003), 93.

40. Tomlinson, *Head Masters*. On the links between criminology and phrenology, see Rafter, *Creating Born Criminals*, 221.

41. Many believed there were four to five species or racial types: Caucasian, Ethiopian, Mongolian, American, and Malay.

42. Charles Caldwell, *Elements of Phrenology*, 2nd ed. (A. G. Meriwether, 1827), 244, 245, 253–54.

43. Branson, "Phrenology and the Science of Race in Antebellum America."

44. Tomlinson, *Head Masters*, 232. Thomas Jefferson also alludes to the damaging effects slavery had on the psyches of white children in *Notes on the State of Virginia*. In Query XVIII, "Manners" of *Notes on the State of Virginia*, he writes: "The parent storms, the child looks on, catches the lineaments of wrath, puts on the same airs in the circle of smaller slaves, gives a loose to his worst of passions, and thus nursed, educated, and daily exercised in tyranny, cannot but be stamped by it with odious peculiarities. The man must be a prodigy who can retain his manners and morals undepraved by such circumstances." Jefferson, *Notes on the State of Virginia*, 173. Proslavery advocates such as John Taylor did not take kindly to his claim. For a discussion of Jefferson's comments and the political response to them, see Elizabeth Duquette, *American Tyrannies in the Long Age of Napoleon* (Oxford University Press, 2023). On Combe's antislavery perspective, see Branson, "Phrenology and the Science of Race in Antebellum America."

45. George Combe, *Notes on the United States of North America, During a Phrenological Visit in 1838-9-40* (Carey & Hart, 1841), 260. Also cited in Tomlinson, *Head Masters*, 233.

46. George Combe, *A System of Phrenology*, 3rd Edinburgh ed. (Benjamin B. Mussey, 1851), 562.

47. Frederick Douglass, *Life and Times of Frederick Douglass, Written by Himself*, new revised ed. (De Wolfe & Fiske, 1892), 299–300. Located in Documenting the American

South, University Library, the University of North Carolina at Chapel Hill, 2001. Other middle-class Blacks had similar respect for Combe but, like Douglass, found phrenology illegitimate science. "Mr. George Combe's Lectures," *Colored American*, May 18, 1839.

48. Douglass, *Life and Times of Frederick Douglass*, 299.
49. Frederick Douglass, *The Claims of the Negro, Ethnologically Considered: An Address Before the Literary Societies of Western Reserve College, at Commencement, July 12, 1854* (Lee, Mann, 1854), 1, 21.
50. Douglass, *The Claims of the Negro, Ethnologically Considered*, 8.
51. Douglass, *The Claims of the Negro, Ethnologically Considered*, 20–21, 8.
52. George Combe to Lucretia Mott, Edinburgh, June 7, 1846, MS 7390, F 16 Letter Book (copies of letter in reply), December 1844–February 1847, George Combe Papers, National Library of Scotland. Cited in Carla Bittel, "Testing the Truth of Phrenology: Knowledge Experiments in Antebellum American Cultures of Science and Health," *Medical History* 63, no. 3 (2019): 352–74.
53. "Frederick Douglas [sic]: Portrait, Character, and Biography," in *The American Phrenological Journal and Life Illustrated* (Fowler and Wells, 1866), 148.
54. "Dr. Smith," *Colored American*, September 30, 1837. Morgan, "The Education and Medical Practice of Dr. James McCune Smith (1813–1865)," 609. On October 14th, a newspaper editor wrote that in the wake of his two lectures on phrenology in September of 1837, there was "earnest solicitation" by learned men, "several scientific gentlemen," along with like-minded "friends who could not then gain admission" to hear Smith's astute denouncement of phrenology. I found no articles suggesting that he delivered another lecture. "Anti Phrenology," *Colored American*, October 14, 1837.
55. *The Colored American* was edited by several prominent members of the Black middle class: Samuel Cornish, Phillip Alexander Bell, and Charles Bennett Ray. James McCune Smith joined as a coeditor when Cornish retired.
56. "Phrenology," *Colored American*, September 23, 1837.
57. "Phrenology."
58. "Phrenology."
59. "Dr. Smith."
60. "Dr. Smith."
61. For a discussion of the origins of the asylum and its sometimes-contentious relationship with Black middle-class and working-class communities, see Harris, *In the Shadow of Slavery*, 145–69.
62. For a discussion of the daily routines of the children, see Harris, *In the Shadow of Slavery*, 163.
63. Morgan, "The Education and Medical Practice of Dr. James McCune Smith (1813–1865)," 609.
64. "Colored Orphan's Asylum: Physician's Report [with Reply]," *The Colored American*, January 26, 1839.
65. "Colored Orphan's Asylum: Physician's Report [with Reply]."
66. "Colored Orphan's Asylum: Physician's Report [with Reply]."
67. See chapter 1 for a discussion of Merrill.

68. "Colored Orphan's Asylum: Physician's Report [with Reply]."
69. "Colored Orphan's Asylum: Physician's Report [with Reply]."
70. "Colored Orphan's Asylum: Physician's Report [with Reply]."
71. "Colored Orphan's Asylum: Physician's Report [with Reply]."
72. James McCune Smith, "The Black News-Vender," in Stauffer, *The Works of James McCune Smith*, 190.
73. Apart from "The Heads of the Colored People," Smith had one other sketch that challenged the credibility of phrenology. He wrote an article in the *New York Correspondent* about Louis Kossuth, who led the Hungarian Revolution of 1848 for independence. He insisted that Kossuth, who was highly regarded internationally and toured in America, was a man of color and had the features such as a "low and slanted brow" that phrenologists would associate with smaller brains and lower intelligence. He addressed phrenologists directly and sarcastically, saying that according to their faulty metrics, they would misread Kossuth, who the world would agree was exceptional: "The greatest height of skull is just before the ear: he has not what Phrenologists call concentration or self-esteem." James McCune Smith, "Outside Barbarians," in Smith and Stauffer, *The Works of James McCune Smith*, 80, 82.
74. John Stauffer uses this phrase to describe the sketches, which he also contends are impressionistic, at times abstract, and experimental. Smith and Stauffer, *The Works of James McCune Smith*, 187.
75. Robert William Fogel, *Without Consent or Contract: The Rise and Fall of American Antislavery* (Norton, 1989), 356. Also quoted in Smith and Stauffer, *The Works of James McCune Smith*, 187. For other works on the state of Blacks in the North in light of gradual freedom, white riots, carceral systems, and religious cultures, see Harris, *In the Shadow of Slavery*; Joanne Pope Melish, *Disowning Slavery: Gradual Emancipation and "Race" in New England, 1780–1860* (Cornell University Press, 1998); Robin Bernstein, *Freeman's Challenge: The Murder That Shook America's Original Prison for Profit* (University of Chicago Press, 2024); Graham Russell Hodges, *Root and Branch: African Americans in New York and East Jersey, 1613–1863* (University of North Carolina Press, 1999).
76. James McCune Smith, "Report on the Social Condition of the People of Color Around New York City, and on the Best Means of Ameliorating the Same," *The North Star*, April 10, 1851.
77. Smith, "Report on the Social Condition of the People of Color Around New York City."
78. Smith, "Report on the Social Condition of the People of Color Around New York City."
79. Frederick Douglass, "Letter from the Editor (Frederick Douglass)," in Smith and Stauffer, *The Works of James McCune Smith*, 234.
80. Patrick Rael, *Black Identity and Black Protest in the Antebellum North* (University of North Carolina Press, 2002).
81. Jacob Crane, "'Razed to the Knees': The Anti-Heroic Body in James McCune Smith's 'The Heads of Colored People,'" *African American Review* 51, no. 1 (2018): 8. For a discussion of the ways ableism can become reproduced in discourses of freedom and emancipation, see Andrea Stone, "The Black Atlantic Revisited, the Body Reconsidered: On Lingering, Liminality, Lies, and Disability," *American Literary History* 24, no. 4 (2012): 814–26.

82. Tobin Siebers, *Disability Aesthetics* (University of Michigan Press, 2010), 27.
83. Smith, "The Black News-Vender" in Smith and Stauffer, *The Works of James McCune Smith*, 192–93, 191. All references to the sketches will be made with respect to the reprints in Stauffer's anthology.
84. Dea Boster, *African American Slavery and Disability: Bodies, Property, and Power in the Antebellum South, 1800–1860* (Routledge, 2013), 19.
85. Smith, "The Black News-Vender," 193.
86. Jenifer Barclay, *The Mark of Slavery: Disability, Race, and Gender in Antebellum America* (University of Illinois Press, 2021), 9.
87. For a discussion of disability and race in the nineteenth century, see Ellen Samuels, *Fantasies of Identification: Disability, Gender, Race* (New York University Press, 2014); Cassandra Jackson, "Visualizing Slavery: Photography and the Disabled Subject in the Art of Carrie Mae Weems," in *Blackness and Disability: Critical Examinations and Cultural Interventions*, ed. Christopher Bell (Michigan State University Press, 2011); Kim Nielsen, *A Disability History of the United States* (Beacon, 2012).
88. Stauffer, *The Works of James McCune Smith*, 193.
89. Classic studies on the concept of bearing witness in Black literature in the antebellum period include Robert Septo, "Storytelling in Early Afro-American Fiction: Frederick Douglass's 'The Heroic Slave,'" in *Black Literature and Literary Theory*, ed. Henry Louis Gates (Methuen, 1984); James Onley, "'I Was Born': Slave Narratives, Their Status as Autobiography and as Literature," *Callaloo*, no. 20 (Winter 1984): 46–73; Frances Foster, *Witnessing Slavery: The Development of Antebellum Slave Narratives* (Greenwood, 1979); William Andrews, *To Tell a Free Story: The First Century of Afro-American Autobiography, 1760–1865* (University of Illinois Press, 1986); Saidiya V. Hartman, *Scenes of Subjection: Terror, Slavery, and Self-Making in Nineteenth-Century America* (Oxford University Press, 1997). Also see Allissa V. Richardson, "The Origins of Bearing Witness While Black," in *Bearing Witness While Black: African Americans, Smartphones, and the New Protest #Journalism* (Oxford University Press, 2020).
90. For a discussion on Smith's references to Thomas Jefferson's bloodline and the nineteenth-century concept of character, see Hannah Spahn, "Blood and Character in Early African American Literature," in *The Cultural Politics of Blood, 1500–1900*, ed. Kimberly Anne Coles, Ralph Bauer, Zita Nunes, and Carla L. Peterson (Palgrave Macmillan, 2015), 146–67.
91. James McCune Smith, "The Black News-Vender," in Smith and Stauffer, *The Works of James McCune Smith*, 191.
92. Jefferson, *Notes on the State of Virginia*, 148.
93. Smith, "The Black News-Vender," 191.
94. Jefferson, *Notes on the State of Virginia*, 148, 149.
95. Smith, "The Black News-Vender," 193.
96. Smith, "Report on the Social Condition of the People of Color Around New York City."
97. Stauffer, *The Works of James McCune Smith*, 224.
98. Smith, "The Black News-Vender," 193.
99. John Haydn Baker, *Browning and Wordsworth* (Associated University Presses, 2004), 10.

100. T. S. Eliot, *Selected Prose of T. S. Eliot*, ed. Frank Kermode (Harcourt Brace Jovanovich, 1975), 246.
101. Stephen Greenblatt, Carol T. Christ, and Catherine Robson, eds., *The Norton Anthology of English Literature, Vol. E: The Victorian Age* (Norton, 2005), 1111.
102. Alfred Tennyson, *In Memoriam* (Edward Moxon, 1850), 37.
103. Smith, "The Black News-Vender," 194.
104. Smith, "The Washerwoman," in Stauffer, *The Works of James McCune Smith*, 201.
105. Smith, "The Washerwoman," 201.
106. Smith, "The Washerwoman," 201–2.
107. Stauffer, *The Works of James McCune Smith*, 233.
108. James McCune Smith, "The Whitewasher," in Stauffer, *The Works of James McCune Smith*, 222.
109. Boster, *African American Slavery and Disability*, 19.
110. Smith, "The Whitewasher," 223.
111. James McCune Smith, "The Black Boot-Black," in Smith and Stauffer, *The Works of James McCune Smith*, 198–99.
112. Smith, "The Black Boot-Black," 196, 198, 199.
113. James McCune Smith, "The Sexton," in Stauffer, *The Works of James McCune Smith*, 204.
114. James McCune Smith, "The Editor," in Stauffer *The Works of James McCune Smith*, 215, 212.
115. James McCune Smith, "The Inventor," in Smith and Stauffer, *The Works of James McCune Smith*, 217–18.
116. James McCune Smith, "The Schoolmaster (Continued)," in Smith and Stauffer, *The Works of James McCune Smith*, 230–32.

3. PSYCHOLOGICAL COSTS OF BLACK WOMEN'S ENSLAVEMENT IN HARRIET JACOBS'S *INCIDENTS IN THE LIFE OF A SLAVE GIRL* (1861)

1. To avoid rape by Norcom, Jacobs chose to have children with a neighboring white lawyer and slaveholder named Samuel Sawyer. Jacobs believed that if Norcom thought she had run away he would sell her children out of disgust. Using a middleman, she arranged for Sawyer to buy the children in the hope that he would eventually free them.
2. Harriet Ann Jacobs, *Incidents in the Life of a Slave Girl, Written by Herself*, ed. L Maria Child, 2nd ed. (Published for the Author, 1861), 241. Located in Documenting the American South, University Library, the University of North Carolina at Chapel Hill, 2003.
3. Historical studies that give considerable attention to the effects of slavery on the mind include Tyler D. Parry, "'How Much More Must I Suffer?': Post-Traumatic Stress and the Lingering Impact of Violence Upon Enslaved People," *Slavery and Abolition* 42, no. 2 (2021): 184–200; Kidada E. Williams, "The Wounds That Cried Out: Reckoning with African Americans' Testimonies of Trauma and Suffering from Night Riding," in *The World the Civil War Made*, ed. Gregory P. Downs and Kate Masur (University of

North Carolina Press, 2015); Diane Miller Sommerville, *Aberration of Mind: Suicide and Suffering in the Civil War-Era South* (University of North Carolina Press, 2018), 85–119; David Silkenat, *Moments of Despair: Suicide, Divorce and Debt in Civil War Era North Carolina* (University of North Carolina Press, 2011); Nell Irvin Painter, *Soul Murder and Slavery* (Markham Press Fund, 1995); Terri L. Snyder, *The Power to Die: Slavery and Suicide in British North America* (University of Chicago Press, 2015), 150–51. Disability studies scholars have written about the disabling features of slavery; see Jenifer Barclay, *The Mark of Slavery: Disability, Race, and Gender in Antebellum America* (University of Illinois Press, 2021); Dea H. Boster, *African American Slavery and Disability: Bodies, Property, and Power in the Antebellum South, 1800–1860* (Routledge, 2013); Stefanie Hunt-Kennedy, *Between Fitness and Death: Disability and Slavery in the Caribbean* (University of Illinois Press, 2020). Scholars who have called for more research on psychological trauma during slavery include Nell Irvin Painter, "Soul Murder and Slavery: Toward a Fully Loaded Cost Accounting," in *U.S. History as Women's History: New Feminist Essays*, ed. Linda K. Kerber, Alice Kessler-Harris, and Kathryn Kish Sklar (University of North Carolina Press, 1995), 125–46; Darlene Clark Hine, "Rape and the Inner Lives of Black Women in the Middle West," *Signs: Journal of Women in Culture and Society* 14, no. 4 (Summer, 1989): 912–20; Brenda E. Stevenson, *Life in Black and White: Family and Community in the Slave South* (Oxford University Press, 1997), 138.

4. Katherine McKittrick argues that Jacobs "recast[s] the meanings of slavery's geographic terrain . . . [and thereby presents] a black sense of space," setting new terms for her confinement and changing a seemingly captive space into one of instability and paradox. Katherine McKittrick, *Demonic Grounds: Black Women and the Cartographies of Struggle* (University of Minnesota Press, 2006), xxviii, xxvii. Saidiya Hartman demonstrates that Jacobs recasts the meaning of seduction by "recontextualiz[ing] virtue within the economy of slavery and [thereby] trouble[s] distinctions between the virtuous and the fallen." Saidiya V. Hartman, *Scenes of Subjection: Terror, Slavery, and Self-Making in Nineteenth-Century America* (Oxford University Press, 1997), 105. Both affirm Jacobs's ability to shape meaning in ways that conflict with and/or complicate conceptions upheld by slaveholders and the system of slavery. I contend that Jacobs's meaning-making enterprise includes complicated conceptions of health, in particular mental health.

5. Theri Alyce Pickens, *Black Madness :: Mad Blackness* (Duke University Press, 2019), x.

6. Several studies in the history of psychiatry have addressed race and mental health in a sustained fashion and do some work to discover the voices and perspectives of Black mentally disabled people and their families. See Wendy Gonaver, *The Peculiar Institution and the Making of Modern Psychiatry, 1840–1880* (University of North Carolina Press, 2018); Mab Segrest, *Administrations of Lunacy: Racism and the Haunting of American Psychiatry at the Milledgeville Asylum* (New Press, 2020); Martin Summers, *Madness in the City of Magnificent Intentions: A History of Race and Mental Illness in the Nation's Capital* (Oxford University Press, 2019); Elodie Edwards-Grossi, *Mad with Freedom: The Political Economy of Blackness, Insanity, and Civil Rights in the U.S. South, 1840–1940* (Louisiana State University Press, 2022). These studies are foundational to our understanding of the conditions of institutionalized Black psychiatric treatment, the racist

3. PSYCHOLOGICAL COSTS OF BLACK WOMEN'S ENSLAVEMENT 239

underpinnings of American psychiatric administration and care, and significantly, the role of slavery in the development of American psychiatry. They leave much room, however, for deeper explorations of Black people's intellectual traditions of theorizing about mental health and its connection to the system of slavery.

7. See chapter 2 for a discussion of Jefferson's commentary about the transiency of Black feeling.
8. For a full discussion of medical and psychiatric theories of mental disability, see chapters 1 and 2.
9. Sharla M. Fett, *Working Cures: Healing, Health, and Power on Southern Slave Plantations* (University of North Carolina Press, 2002), 59.
10. See chapter 1 for a discussion of medical and psychiatric perspectives on mental disability during slavery.
11. Todd L. Savitt, *Medicine and Slavery: The Diseases and Health Care of Blacks in Antebellum Virginia* (University of Illinois Press, 1978); Steven M. Stowe, *Doctoring the South: Southern Physicians and Everyday Medicine in the Mid-Nineteenth Century* (University of North Carolina Press, 2004); Marli Frances Weiner and Mazie Hough, *Sex, Sickness, and Slavery: Illness in the Antebellum South* (University of Illinois Press, 2012).
12. Jeffrey Geller and Maxine Harris, *Women of the Asylum: Voices from Behind the Walls, 1840–1945* (Anchor, 1994); Mary Elene Wood, *The Writing on the Wall: Women's Autobiography and the Asylum* (University of Illinois Press, 1994).
13. Barbara Christian, "The Race for Theory," in *The Black Feminist Reader*, ed. Joy James and Denean Sharpley-Whiting (Blackwell, 2000), 52.
14. Jacobs, *Incidents*, 119.
15. Jean Fagan Yellin, "Texts and Contexts of Harriet Jacobs' Incidents in the Life of a Slave Girl: Written by Herself," in *The Slave's Narrative*, ed. Charles T. Davis and Henry Louis Gates (Oxford University Press, 1985), 262–82.
16. Jacobs, *Incidents*, 6.
17. Painter, "Soul Murder and Slavery," 125–46.
18. Foundational histories of slavery, such as John Blassingame, *The Slave Community: Plantation Life in the Antebellum South*, rev. ed. (Oxford University Press, 1979), 298–302, and Ira Berlin, *Many Thousands Gone: The First Two Centuries of Slavery in North America* (Belknap, 1998), 106, have downplayed the incidence of mental disability. Studies that emphasize slave agency, rebellion, and resistance, especially in discussions of suicide, are plentiful. At the root of these claims is a master/slave tension in which slaves had an awareness of the economic consequences of their deaths. Key texts include Kenneth Stampp, *The Peculiar Institution: Slavery in the Ante-Bellum South* (Vintage, 1956), 101–5; Michael A. Gomez, *Exchanging Our Country Marks: The Transformation of African Identities in the Colonial and Antebellum South* (University of North Carolina Press, 1998), 120; Mark Schantz, *Awaiting the Heavenly Country: The Civil War and America's Culture of Death* (Cornell University Press, 2008), 126–62.
19. Her view contrasts with the Western philosophical tendency toward viewing the body as separate from the mind (with no utility for the spirit) commonly known as the "Cartesian split."

240   3. PSYCHOLOGICAL COSTS OF BLACK WOMEN'S ENSLAVEMENT

20. Black doctoring practices reflected a relational vision of health that refigured the spirit, mind, and body to support healing. See Fett, *Working Cures.*
21. George Gordon Byron, *The Lament of Tasso* (John Murray, Albemarle-Street, 1817). Jacobs chooses to sample from "The Lament of Tasso" instead of Byron's more famous poem, "The Prisoner of Chillon" (1816), which focuses on the plight of an imprisoned person. This might seem curious because of her substantial use of imprisonment imagery in *Incidents.* "Chillon," however, features a protagonist who is more concerned about being persecuted because of religious beliefs. The poem emphasizes the speaker's persecution, appreciation of nature, and acquired insight. In contrast, Jacobs is concerned with exposing the evils of slavery, not detailing introspection in confinement. Jacobs finds the "Lament" speaker's description of his confinement in a "madhouse" more fitting for depicting the institution of slavery.
22. Jacobs, *Incidents,* 58.
23. William Andrews, *To Tell a Free Story: The First Century of Afro-American Autobiography,* 1760–1865 (University of Illinois Press, 1986), 10, 11.
24. Mary Titus, "This Poisonous System: Social Ills, Bodily Ills, and Incidents in the Life of a Slave Girl," in *Harriet Jacobs and Incidents in the Life of a Slave Girl: New Critical Essays,* ed. Deborah M. Garfield and Rafia Zafar (Cambridge University Press, 1996), 199–200.
25. Dorothea Lynde Dix and U.S. Congress, House, and Senate, *Memorial of D.L. Dix: Praying a Grant of Land for the Relief and Support of the Indigent Curable and Incurable Insane in the United States,* 30th Cong., 1st sess., Misc. No. 150 (Tippin & Streeper, 1848), 2.
26. Jacobs, *Incidents,* 44.
27. Jennifer R. Greeson, "The 'Mysteries and Miseries' of North Carolina: New York City, Urban Gothic Fiction, and Incidents in the Life of a Slave Girl," *American Literature* 73, no. 2 (2001): 295.
28. Jacobs, *Incidents,* 44, 45.
29. Hartman, *Scenes of Subjection,* 55.
30. Jacobs, *Incidents,* 78, 79.
31. Dea H. Boster, "An 'Epeleptick' Bondswoman: Fits, Slavery, and Power in the Antebellum South," *Bulletin of the History of Medicine* 83, no. 2 (2009): 271–301; and *African American Slavery and Disability*; Savitt, *Medicine and Slavery*; Deborah Gray White, *Ar'n't I a Woman?: Female Slaves in the Plantation South* (Norton, 1999).
32. Diane Sommerville and Terri Snyder also make this point. Previous scholarship tended to interpret acts of self-murder as resistance. See Sommerville, *Aberration of Mind,* and Snyder, *The Power to Die.*
33. Byron, *The Lament of Tasso,* 12.
34. Jacobs, *Incidents,* 45.
35. Jean Fagan Yellin, *Harriet Jacobs: A Life* (Basic Civitas, 2004), xliii.
36. Elaine Showalter, *The Female Malady: Women, Madness and English Culture, 1830–1980* (Pantheon, 1985), 66–69.
37. Akasha Gloria Hull, Patricia Bell-Scott, and Barbara Smith, eds., *All the Women Are White, All the Blacks Are Men, but Some of Us Are Brave: Black Women's Studies* (Feminist, 1982).
38. Yellin, *Harriet Jacobs.*

39. Jacobs, *Incidents*, 224.
40. Painter, "Soul Murder and Slavery," 127. Also see Painter, *Soul Murder and Slavery*.
41. Jacobs, *Incidents*, 185.
42. Sarah L. Berry, "'[No] Doctor but My Master': Health Reform and Antislavery Rhetoric in Harriet Jacobs's Incidents in the Life of a Slave Girl," *Journal of Medical Humanities* 35, no. 1 (2014): 1–18.
43. Jacobs, *Incidents*, 94.
44. Benjamin Rush, *Medical Inquiries and Observations upon the Diseases of the Mind* (Kimber & Richardson, 1812), 11.
45. Thomas Parramore, "Harriet Jacobs, James Norcom, and the Defense of Hierarchy," *Carolina Comments* 38, no. 3 (1990): 82–87.
46. Jacobs, *Incidents*, 186.
47. Terri L. Snyder, "Suicide, Slavery, and Memory in North America," *Journal of American History* 97, no. 1 (2010): 39–62.
48. Frederick Douglass, *Narrative of the Life of Frederick Douglass, an American Slave, Written by Himself* (Anti-Slavery Office, 1845), 41, 65. Located in Documenting the American South, University Library, the University of North Carolina at Chapel Hill, 1999.
49. Jacobs, *Incidents*, 224.
50. Jacobs, *Incidents*, 150, 153, 237.
51. Samuel A. Cartwright, "Report on the Diseases and Physical Peculiarities of the Negro Race," *New Orleans Medical and Surgical Journal* 7 (1851): 707.
52. Stephanie Li, *Something Akin to Freedom: The Choice of Bondage in Narratives by African American Women* (State University of New York Press, 2010).
53. Jacobs, *Incidents*, 202.
54. John Brown, *Slave Life in Georgia: A Narrative of the Life, Sufferings, and Escape of John Brown, A Fugitive Slave, Now in England*, ed. L. A. Chamerovzow (1855), 17. Located in Documenting the American South, University Library, the University of North Carolina at Chapel Hill, 2001.
55. Galt believed that slaves' "mode of living" (labor) reinforced their already supposed stronger bodily constitutions. John Minson Galt, "Asylums for Colored Persons," *American Psychological Journal* 1, no. 3 (1853): 82–83.
56. Galt, "Asylums for Colored Persons," 83.
57. David Rothman, *The Discovery of the Asylum: Social Order and Disorder in the New Republic*, rev. ed. (Aldine de Gruyter, 2002).
58. Parry, "'How Much More Must I Suffer?,'" 191, 192.
59. Xiomara Santamarina, "Black Womanhood in North American Women's Slave Narratives," in *The Cambridge Companion to the African American Slave Narrative*, ed. Audrey Fisch (Cambridge University Press, 2007), 234.
60. Orlando Patterson, *Slavery and Social Death: A Comparative Study* (Harvard University Press, 1982), 5–6.
61. Blassingame, *The Slave Community*, 298.
62. Solomon Northup, *Twelve Years a Slave: Narrative of Solomon Northup, a Citizen of New-York, Kidnapped in Washington City in 1841, and Rescued in 1853 from a Cotton Plantation*

Near the Red River, in Louisiana (Derby and Miller, 1853), 53, 81, 82. Located in Documenting the American South, University Library, the University of North Carolina at Chapel Hill, 1997.
63. Northup, *Twelve Years a Slave*, 85.
64. Northup, *Twelve Years a Slave*, 85, 88.
65. Northup, *Twelve Years a Slave*, 53, 159, 160.
66. Jacobs, *Incidents*, 131, 132.
67. Parry, "'How Much More Must I Suffer?,'" 190.
68. Jacqueline Jones, *Labor of Love, Labor of Sorrow: Black Women, Work, and the Family from Slavery to the Present* (Basic, 1985), 36.
69. Patterson, *Slavery and Social Death*, 6.
70. Henry Bibb, *Narrative of the Life and Adventures of Henry Bibb, an American Slave, Written by Himself* (Published by the Author, 1849), 120, 122. Located in Documenting the American South, University Library, the University of North Carolina at Chapel Hill, 2000.
71. Jacobs, *Incidents*, 87.
72. Jacobs, *Incidents*, 26, 27.
73. Chapter 6 discusses the violence of post–Civil War America. Jacobs helped the contraband during the war. She wrote a report in which she detailed horrific scenes of mental suffering and neglect among formerly enslaved people. Harriet Jacobs, "Life Among the Contrabands," *The Liberator*, September 5, 1862. In 1864, she and her daughter opened a school for Black children in Alexandria, Virginia. In 1866, they continued their relief work in Savannah but were forced to leave on account of the violence toward Blacks after the war. By 1877, she had moved to Washington, DC, with her daughter, where they ran a boarding house until she died in 1897. She lost contact with her son and never saw him again after he went on a trip to Australia. Yellin, *Harriet Jacobs*, 175–89, 200–202.

4. HARRIET TUBMAN AND NINETEENTH-CENTURY CONCEPTIONS OF MENTAL DISABILITY

1. Wilbur H. Siebert, a professor at Ohio State University, collected materials and conducted interviews regarding the Underground Railroad. He described Tubman's sleeping spells in a letter to Earl Conrad. Lois E. Horton, *Harriet Tubman and the Fight for Freedom: A Brief History with Documents* (Bedford/St. Martin's, 2013), 153.
2. Edna Dow Cheney, "Moses," *Freedmen's Record 1*, no. 3 (March 1865): 34–35.
3. Beverly Lowry, *Harriet Tubman: Imagining a Life* (Anchor, 2007), 91–92; Cheney, "Moses"; Kate Clifford Larson, *Bound for the Promised Land: Harriet Tubman, Portrait of an American Hero* (Ballantine, 2004), 262. On hearing voices and heavenly melodies, also see "Harriet Tubman Home Free from Debt," *The New York Age*, November 2, 1918.
4. Lowry, *Harriet Tubman*, 92.
5. Emma P. Telford, "Harriet, the Modern Moses of Heroism and Visions," 5, 1905, the Telford Manuscript, Cayuga Museum of History and Art, Auburn, New York.

6. For more on soundness, see Sharla Fett, *Working Cures: Healing, Health, and Power on Southern Slave Plantations* (University of North Carolina Press, 2002); and Walter Johnson, *Soul by Soul: Life Inside the Antebellum Slave Market* (Harvard University Press, 1999).
7. Juriah Harriss, "What Constitutes Unsoundness in the Negro?" *Savannah Journal of Medicine* 1, no. 3 (September 1858): 147.
8. "Wiley M. Pearce Slave Bill of Sale, 1859," MS 1562, Georgia Historical Society, Savannah, Georgia.
9. Harriss, "What Constitutes Unsoundness in the Negro?" 147.
10. There are no reliable figures about the number of enslaved people with disability during slavery. Statistical data collected during the time were unreliable, and discrepancies arose in definitions of "soundness," which were not uniformly applied throughout an enslaved person's lifetime. Historians in the mid-twentieth century, notably William Postell, tried to use succession records to quantify disabilities. He came up with the figure of 4.1 percent disabled enslaved people in Adams County, Mississippi, and 9.6 percent in Montgomery County, Alabama, but he relied on one type of source and only a small geographical area. William Postell, *The Health of Slaves on Southern Plantations* (Louisiana State University Press, 1951), 159–63. More recent scholars have taken a more discursive rather than quantitative approach by using plantation records, runaway advertisements, and slave narratives to give a more textured picture of disability in slavery. See Jenifer L. Barclay, *The Mark of Slavery: Disability, Race, and Gender in Antebellum America* (University of Illinois Press, 2021); and Dea H. Boster, *African American Slavery and Disability: Bodies, Property and Power in the Antebellum South, 1800–1860* (Routledge, 2013).
11. A. B. Crook, "A Case of Injury of the Head, with Inquiries and Reflections on Fungus Cerebri," *Southern Journal of Medicine and Pharmacy* 1, no. 5 (September 1846): 483–86.
12. J. E. Pearson, "Fracture of the Cranium, with Depression, Attended with an Escape of a Portion of the Brain; Relieved by the Trephine; Death Four Years Afterwards, from Suppuration Within the Cranium, and Encroachment Upon the Brain, by a Sharp Projecting Exostosis Springing from the Inner Surface of the Fractured Bone," *Southern Journal of Medicine and Pharmacy* 2, no. 2 (March 1847): 156, Center for Research Libraries.
13. William Wells Brown, *Narrative of William W. Brown, A Fugitive Slave. Written by Himself* (Anti-Slavery Office, 1847), 30. Located in Documenting the American South, University Library, the University of North Carolina at Chapel Hill, 2001.
14. John Brown, *Slave Life in Georgia: A Narrative of the Life, Sufferings, and Escape of John Brown, a Fugitive Slave, Now in England*, ed. L. A. Chamerovzow (1855), 87. Located in Documenting the American South, University Library, the University of North Carolina at Chapel Hill, 2001.
15. Earl Conrad, *Harriet Tubman: Negro Soldier and Abolitionist* (International, 1942), 7; Samuel Hopkins Adams, *Grandfather Stories* (Random House, 1955), 273.
16. Bradford published an updated version of the biography in 1886 entitled *Harriet, the Moses of Her People*.
17. On the politics of white figures bringing Black slave narratives to the public, see John Sekora, "Black Message/White Envelope: Genre, Authenticity, and Authority in the Antebellum Slave Narrative," *Callaloo* 32 (1987): 482–515.

18. Sarah H. Bradford, *Scenes in the Life of Harriet Tubman* (W. J. Moses, 1869), 54–56. Located in Documenting the American South, University Library, the University of North Carolina at Chapel Hill, 2000.
19. Bradford, *Scenes in the Life of Harriet Tubman*, 56.
20. Sarah H. Bradford, *Harriet, the Moses of Her People* (Geo. R. Lockwood & Son, 1886), 14. Located in Documenting the American South, University Library, the University of North Carolina at Chapel Hill, 1995.
21. Here "stupidity" is not associated with the present-day notion of intelligence. In the nineteenth century, it was a colloquial synonym for mental illness. Telford, "Harriet, the Modern Moses of Heroism and Visions," 5.
22. Bradford, *Scenes in the Life of Harriet Tubman*, 15–16.
23. Milton C. Sernett, *Harriet Tubman: Myth, Memory, and History* (Duke University Press, 2007), 196.
24. Sernett, *Harriet Tubman*, 140.
25. Conrad, *Harriet Tubman*, 6, 7.
26. Although there are no explicit expressions by contemporary scholars to sanitize her image to the public in the way Conrad does in the mid-twentieth century, the stakes of Tubman's image are higher than ever before. Tubman's story became more accessible to the general public in 2017 when her home became a National Historic Park, thereby making the twenty-five-acre site a viable tourist destination. Tubman's story got its biggest stage by way of the 2019 biographical film *Harriet*, directed by Kasi Lemmons, which received moderate global commercial success. Tubman stands to receive even broader and enduring cultural notoriety if plans to have her likeness appear on the US twenty-dollar bill materialize. The move to replace Andrew Jackson with Tubman was initiated by US president Barack Obama's administration and was slated to be unveiled in 2020. Plans were halted by Donald Trump's administration. The plans were resumed by the Biden administration with no specific details on a timeline for completion.
27. Catherine Clinton, *Harriet Tubman: The Road to Freedom* (Little, Brown, 2004), 185.
28. Erica Armstrong Dunbar, *She Came to Slay: The Life and Times of Harriet Tubman* (Simon & Schuster, 2019), 24.
29. Larson, *Bound for the Promised Land*, 381–83.
30. Larson, *Bound for the Promised Land*, 43. Historian Tiya Miles also associates Tubman with the temporal lobe epilepsy diagnosis. In addition, she refers to Tubman as neuroatypical. Tiya Miles, *Night Flyer: Harriet Tubman and the Faith Dreams of a Free People* (Penguin, 2024), 14.
31. "Harriet Tubman Is Dead," *The Auburn Citizen*, Tuesday, March 11, 1913.
32. Adams, *Grandfather Stories*, 277.
33. "A Considerable Amount of Excitement," *Auburn (N.Y) Daily Advertiser*, October 13, 1884.
34. For more on Horace Mann's educational reform, see Stephen Tomlinson, *Head Masters: Phrenology, Secular Education, and Nineteenth-Century Social Thought* (University of Alabama Press, 2005).
35. Norman Dain, *Concepts of Insanity in the United States, 1789–1865* (Rutgers University Press, 1964), 173.

36. Frederick Norton Manning, *Report on Lunatic Asylums* (Thomas Richards, Government Printer, 1868); F. Norton Manning, "The Epileptic: His Treatment and Care," *The Australasian Medical Gazette: The Journal of the Australasian Branches of the British Medical Association* 19 (1900): 219.
37. Cheney, "Moses," 35.
38. Nancy Tomes, *The Art of Asylum-Keeping: Thomas Story Kirkbride and the Origins of American Psychiatry* (University of Pennsylvania Press, 1994), 122–23.
39. Amariah Brigham, *An Inquiry Concerning the Diseases and Functions of the Brain, the Spinal Cord, and the Nerves* (Elihu Geer, 1840), 220.
40. Brigham, *An Inquiry*, 108; Amariah Brigham, *Remarks on the Influence of Mental Cultivation and Mental Excitement Upon Health* (Lea & Blanchard, 1845), 57; Amariah Brigham, "Definition of Insanity–Nature of the Disease," *American Journal of Psychiatry* 151, no. 6 (1994): 104.
41. Although it garnered great criticism from his peers, he advocated for nonsegregated treatment of Black free and enslaved people at his asylum and employed enslaved attendants at his hospital, notwithstanding the fact that he was proslavery. Box III, folder 0045, JMG to "Gentlemen," ESH. Also quoted in Wendy Gonaver, *The Peculiar Institution and the Making of Modern Psychiatry* (University of North Carolina Press, 2018), 94.
42. Prior to the nineteenth century, mental disability was seen in Western European countries as having supernatural causes, and therefore, priests were seen as the best-equipped members of the community to address the issue, primarily through prayer and exorcisms. With the rise of Enlightenment thinking, mental disability was seen to be a natural phenomenon and best addressed by physicians. However, the most common forms of treatment for mental illness did not differ from the treatment of other ailments. Physicians were beholden to the idea that disease was most influenced by the humors, which were blood, yellow bile, black bile, and phlegm. Physicians would balance the humors through means such as bleeding and purging, which were the cornerstone of heroic medicine. In addition to heroic methods for treating mental illness, many mentally ill people were treated rather harshly, often being beaten or restrained in homes and jails. Dain, *Concepts of Insanity*, 3–27. See also Gerald N. Grob, *Mental Illness and American Society, 1875–1940* (Princeton University Press, 2019).
43. Dain, *Concepts of Insanity*, 16.
44. It should be noted that American psychiatrists' preoccupation with religious insanity was unique. Historian Roy Porter argues that British psychiatrists were not particularly concerned with religious "madness" in part because spiritual traditions characterized by "mass ecstasies" and "demonomania" in the general population were in decline with the advent of Methodism. Roy Porter, *Mind-forg'd Manacles: A History of Madness in England from the Restoration to the Regency* (Harvard University Press, 1987), 72–73.
45. The undergirding principle of moral therapy was the notion that people could be restored to their natural, God-intended order—an order that had been upended by any number of social vices or habits, including intemperance in drugs and alcohol, masturbation, a quest for wealth, physical changes caused by serious illness such as blows to the head, changes in normal bodily functions (like constipation, diarrhea, or menstruation), or

poor diet. Treatment entailed providing people with a home-like environment in which they were treated kindly and restored back to health through a structured environment with regularity in diet, sleep, and purposeful religious activities, amusements, and labor. She chapter 1 for more on moral therapy.

46. Gonaver, *Peculiar Institutions*, 86.
47. Dain, *Concepts of Insanity*, 184–85. There were diverging views about the utility of religion among Black people. Some planters in Jamaica were wary of the role religion might play in encouraging freed slaves to strike for better wages. Gonaver, *Peculiar Institution*s, 86–87.
48. Fanaticism was also associated with some political and ideological traditions. For example, psychiatrists thought Millerism and Spiritualism were fanatical religious sects. They were also critical of transcendentalism and abolition as fanatical ideologies. Dain, *Concepts of Insanity*, 189–90; Gonaver, *Peculiar Institutions*, 36–37, 47, 90–91; Benjamin Reiss, *Theaters of Madness, Insane Asylums and Nineteenth-Century American Culture* (University of Chicago Press, 2008), 103–5, 124–30; Amariah Brigham, "Millerism," *American Journal of Insanity* 1 (1845): 249–53.
49. Pliny Earle, "On the Causes of Insanity," *American Journal of Insanity* 4 (1848): 207.
50. Amariah Brigham, *Observations on the Influence of Religion Upon the Health and Physical Welfare of Mankind* (Marsh, Capen & Lyon, 1835), 274, 304.
51. Brigham, *Observations*, 210.
52. John M. Galt, Box VI, Folder 0047, ESH; see also Galt Family Papers I, Manuscripts, Box 20, Case Histories of Asylum Patients, 1844–1845, Phoebe Epps and Mary Britt entries, SSC. Also quoted in Gonaver, *Peculiar Institutions*, 106.
53. Bradford, *Harriet, the Moses of Her People*, 4. For a discussion of Bradford's portrayal of Tubman's spirituality, see Jean Humez, "In Search of Harriet Tubman's Spiritual Autobiography," *National Women's Studies Association Journal* 5, no. 2 (1993): 162–82.
54. James A. McGowan, "The Psychic Life of Harriet Tubman, Part 1," *Visions* (March 1995): 1–3, as cited by Sernett, *Harriet Tubman*, 376.
55. Dianne M. Stewart, *Three Eyes for the Journey: African Dimensions of the Jamaican Religious Experience* (Oxford University Press, 2005), x.
56. Franklin Sanborn, "Harriet Tubman," *The Commonwealth*, July 17, 1863. Also see Bradford, *Scenes in the Life of Harriet Tubman*, 82–83; Telford, "Harriet, the Modern Moses of Heroism and Visions," 13–14.
57. Horton, *Harriet Tubman and the Fight for Freedom*.
58. Telford, "Harriet, the Modern Moses of Heroism and Visions," 10.
59. Quoted in Horton, *Harriet Tubman and the Fight for Freedom*, 48.
60. Telford, "Harriet, the Modern Moses of Heroism and Visions," 15. Also see Bradford, *Harriet, the Moses of Her People*, 92.
61. Telford, "Harriet, the Modern Moses of Heroism and Visions," 15.
62. Larson, *Bound for the Promised Land*, 262.
63. Telford, "Harriet, the Modern Moses of Heroism and Visions," 13.
64. Alexis Wells-Oghoghomeh, *The Souls of Womenfolk: The Religious Cultures of Enslaved Women in the Lower South* (University of North Carolina Press, 2021), 161.
65. Wells-Oghoghomeh, *The Souls of Womenfolk*, 162.

66. One of her friends, Maria Coffin Wright, believed Tubman might have been chloroformed. Larson, *Bound for the Promised Land*, 379n47.
67. Among the articles were "The Gold Swindle and Greenback Robbery," *Auburn Daily Bulletin*, October 3, 1873, and "The Mysterious Robbery," *Auburn Daily Advertiser*, Monday, October 6, 1873, as cited by Larson, *Bound for the Promised Land*, 379.
68. "The Gold Swindle and the Greenback Robbery," *Auburn Daily Bulletin*, October 3, 1873, as cited by Larson, *Bound for the Promised Land*, 258.
69. "Harriet Tubman Is Dead."
70. Jean Humez is the first scholar to make this argument. Jean Humez, *Harriet Tubman: The Life and the Life Stories* (University of Wisconsin Press, 2003), 90. It is reiterated by Larson, *Bound for the Promised Land*, 259; and Lowry, *Harriet Tubman*, 368.
71. Wells-Oghoghomeh, *The Souls of Womenfolk*, 161.
72. Georgia Writers' Project, *Drums and Shadows: Survival Studies Among the Georgia Coastal Negroes* (University of Georgia Press, 1986), 15–16.
73. Georgia Writers' Project, *Drums and Shadows*, 15–16.
74. Many Black Americans had a belief in ghosts that were connected to African-derived understandings of the supernatural. George P. Rawick, ed., *The American Slave: A Composite Autobiography*, vol. 1 (Greenwood, 1972), 49–50; Georgia Writers' Project, *Drums and Shadows*, 2, 7, 17–18.
75. Georgia Writers' Project, *Drums and Shadows*, 2.
76. Yvonne P. Chireau, "'Our Religion and Superstition Was All Mixed Up': Conjure, Christianity, and African American Supernatural Traditions," in *Black Magic: Religion and the African American Conjuring Tradition* (University of California Press, 2003), 12. For more on the complex overlap of Conjure and Black religious expression, see Theophus H. Smith, *Conjuring Culture: Biblical Formations of Black America* (Oxford University Press, 1994); and Albert J. Raboteau, *Slave Religion: The "Invisible Institution" in the Antebellum South* (Oxford University Press, 1978), 275–88; Wells-Oghoghomeh, *The Souls of Womenfolk*, 164.
77. On Black Americans' ability to accommodate multiple spiritual orientations, see Chireau, *Black Magic* 11–34. Tubman has been most often associated with Christian church-based Black religious traditions. Kate Clifford Larson suggests that she might have attended Bazzel's Methodist Church or Scott's Chapel, also a Methodist church. She could have encountered Methodist, Catholic, Episcopal, and/or Baptist sects. Larson, *Bound for the Promised Land*, 46. For more on Black religious traditions, see Raboteau, *Slave Religion*; Albert J. Raboteau, *A Fire in the Bones: Reflections on African-American Religious History* (Beacon, 1995); Lawrence W. Levine, *Black Culture and Black Consciousness: Afro-American Folk Thought from Slavery to Freedom* (Oxford University Press, 1977); Mechal Sobel, *The World They Made Together: Black and White Values in Eighteenth-Century Virginia* (Princeton University Press, 1987); Sylvia R. Frey, *Water from the Rock: Black Resistance in a Revolutionary Age* (Princeton University Press, 1992); Sylvia R. Frey and Betty Wood, *Come Shouting to Zion: African American Protestantism in the American South and British Caribbean to 1830* (University of North Carolina Press, 1998); Eugene D. Genovese, *Roll, Jordan, Roll: The World the Slaves Made* (Pantheon, 1974); Milton C.

Sernett, ed., *African American Religious History: A Documentary Witness* (Duke University Press, 1999); Charles Joyner, *Down by the Riverside: A South Carolina Slave Community* (University of Illinois Press, 1984).

78. For a more in-depth discussion on the role of religion in the lives of nineteenth-century Blacks, see Raboteau, *Slave Religion*; Raboteau, *A Fire in the Bones*; Levine, *Black Culture and Black Consciousness*; Sobel, *The World They Made Together*; Frey, *Water from the Rock*; Frey and Wood, *Come Shouting to Zion*; Genovese, *Roll, Jordan, Roll*; Sernett, ed., *African American Religious History*; Joyner, *Down by the Riverside*.

79. Although Tubman's narrative was developed from interviews with Bradford, it had the benefit of a subject who had immediate memories of slavery, unlike many of the Works Progress Administration (WPA) narratives that were taken of Black people in the early twentieth century who had been children during slavery. For a discussion of other challenges with WPA narratives, see Norman R. Yetman, "The Background of the Slave Narrative Collection," *American Quarterly* 19, no. 3 (1967): 534–53; Sharon Ann Musher, "Contesting 'The Way the Almighty Wants It': Crafting Memories of Ex-Slaves in the Slave Narrative Collection," *American Quarterly* 53, no. 1 (2001): 1–31; Scott E. Casper, "Catherine A. Stewart. 'Long Past Slavery: Representing Race in the Federal Writers' Project,'" *The American Historical Review* 122, no. 5 (2017): 1642–43; Marie Jenkins Schwartz, "The WPA Narratives as Historical Sources," in *The Oxford Handbook of the African American Slave Narrative*, ed. John Ernest (Oxford University Press, 2014), 89–100.

80. John Blassingame, "Using the Testimony of Ex-Slaves: Approaches and Problems," *Journal of Southern History* 41, no. 4 (1975): 483.

81. Scholars have been rightly critical of Bradford as a biographer for several reasons. There are historical inaccuracies around names of family members and figures within and between both versions of the biography. In her own books, she also did not prove to be a diligent researcher because in at least one of her books she conflated, created, and omitted information. James McGowan, "Harriet Tubman: According to Sarah Bradford," *Harriet Tubman Journal* 2 (1994): 1–10, as cited by Sernett, *Harriet Tubman*, 332n53. Bradford was an inexperienced interviewer and wrote the narrative hastily as she had an upcoming trip to Europe. Her hurried product was criticized after its publication. She also was a moderately successful children's literature writer, which may have shaped her moralistic and sentimental preferences regarding literary construction. Humez, *Harriet Tubman*, 146–51. She only chose material she could corroborate, which may have limited the knowledge we have about Tubman's life. She also was a white woman who harbored racial bias and had limited knowledge of the realities of Black slavery and life. Larson, *Bound for the Promised Land*.

82. On Bradford's mediation of Tubman, see Humez, *Harriet Tubman*, 146–51.

83. Humez, *Harriet Tubman*, 150.

84. This process of translation and transformation was not unique to Bradford. Other women including Edna Dow Cheney translated Tubman's oral interviews into texts. The changes to meaning are sometimes profound and always shape the lasting image of figures like Tubman. This process of translation also happened with Sojourner Truth, whose speeches were made into a written text by Frances Gage. For more on mediation

and Sojourner Truth, see Karlyn Kohrs Campbell, "Style and Content in the Rhetoric of Early Afro-American Feminists," *Quarterly Journal of Speech* 72, no. 4 (1986): 434–45; Suzanne Pullon Fitch and Roseann M. Mandziuk, *Sojourner Truth as Orator: Wit, Story, and Song* (Greenwood, 1997); Suzanne Pullon Fitch and Roseann M. Mandziuk, "The Rhetorical Construction of Sojourner Truth," *Southern Communication Journal* 66, no. 2 (2001): 120–38; Nell Irvin Painter, *Sojourner Truth: A Life, a Symbol* (Norton, 1996); Olive Gilbert, *Narrative of Sojourner Truth*, ed. Margaret Washington (Vintage, 1993).

85. Bradford's first biography is referenced most in popular and historical accounts and studies of Tubman's life.
86. Horton, *Harriet Tubman and the Fight for Freedom*.
87. Adams, *Grandfather Stories*, 5.
88. Carla Peterson, *"Doers of the Word" African-American Women Speakers and Writers in the North (1830–1880)* (Oxford University Press, 1995), 17–19. It is important to note that although these women found such spaces empowering, Black male leaders often took issue with their claims to spiritual authority. Some of these women, such as Jarena Lee, were called "mad" because their religious expressions or their claim to sacred power was seen as delusional. Self-proclaimed preaching women subverted clerical authority and posed a challenge to the entire social order. For more on Black women religious leaders, see William Andrews, *Sisters of the Spirit: Three Black Women's Autobiographies of the Nineteenth Century* (Indiana University Press, 1986).
89. Humez, *Harriet Tubman*, 135.
90. Sernet, *Harriet Tubman*, 53–54.
91. Tiya Miles, *Night Flyer*, 14. Humez makes a similar point. He contends that Tubman's stories are sites at which we find "the most authentic embodiments of her own values and political and religious perspectives." Humez, *Harriet Tubman*, 141.
92. Humez, *Harriet Tubman*, 397n25.
93. Bradford, *Scenes in the Life of Harriet Tubman*, 32.
94. Bradford, *Harriet, the Moses of Her People*, 49.
95. Sernett, *Harriet Tubman*, 53.
96. Bradford, *Scenes in the Life of Harriet Tubman*, 32, 33.
97. Bradford, *Scenes in the Life of Harriet Tubman*, 34, 35.
98. Humez, *Harriet Tubman*, 200.
99. Sernett, *Harriet Tubman*, 145, 142.
100. For more on Black traditions of herbalism, see Leah Penniman, *Farming While Black: Soul Fire Farm's Practical Guide to Liberation on the Land* (Chelsea Green, 2018).
101. Rawick, *The American Slave*, vol. 1, 49.
102. Sharla Fett discusses the process of teaching and passing down knowledge in chapter 5, "Doctoring Women," in *Working Cures*.
103. Adams, *Grandfather Stories*, 278.
104. Susie King Taylor, the first Black nurse to publish a memoir, also had a fearless attitude toward sickness and used herbal practices to protect herself against diseases such as smallpox. Ella Forbes, *African American Women During the Civil War* (Routledge, 1998), 48. Susie King Taylor, *Reminiscences of My Life in Camp with the 33rd United States Colored*

250   4. HARRIET TUBMAN AND CONCEPTIONS OF MENTAL DISABILITY

        Troops Late 1st S.C. Volunteers (published by the author, 1904). Bradford also describes Tubman's lack of fear concerning smallpox. Bradford, *Harriet, the Moses of Her People*, 98.
105. Bradford, *Harriet, the Moses of Her People*, 141.
106. Larson, *Bound for the Promised Land*, 208.
107. Bradford, *Harriet, the Moses of Her People*, 98.
108. "Harriet Tubman Is Dead."
109. Rosa Belle Holt, "A Heroine in Ebony," *Chautauquan* 23 (July 1886): 45–462, as cited in Humez, *Harriet Tubman*, 94.
110. Bradford, *Harriet, the Moses of Her People*, 138–39.
111. "Harriet Tubman's Hogs," *Evening Auburnian* I, July 11, 1884, as cited in Humez, *Harriet Tubman*, 94.
112. Lille Buffman Chace Wyman, "Harriet Tubman," *New England Magazine* 6 (1896, March): 110–18, as cited in Humez, *Harriet Tubman*, 94.
113. "Harriet Tubman Home for Aged and Indigent Negroes," National Park Service, last updated on January 19, 2024. Tubman bid on the land for the home on her own. For a discussion of the bidding episode, see Humez, *Harriet Tubman*, 94. She sought financial assistance from the African Methodist Episcopal Zion Church for a $350 down payment and received a bank mortgage loan of $1,000. She was barely able to fulfill the financial obligation, so she took up public speaking and asked Sarah Bradford to publish the 1886 edition of her biography to generate income. She went to Boston to publicize the book and took a photo that could be sold for profit. When she was unable to raise the necessary funds to open the actual facility, Tubman deeded the property to the African Methodist Episcopal Zion Church in exchange for their opening and operating the home. The facility operated from 1908 until the early 1920s. Tubman was upset that under the operation of the church, people were charged one hundred dollars for admission.
114. Telford, "Harriet, the Modern Moses of Heroism and Visions," 20.
115. Alicia Dietrich, "UT Scholar Tells Forgotten Story of African-American Psychiatric Patients," *Alcalde*, January 17, 2014.
116. Tiya Miles, *Night Flyer*, 218.

5. BLACK WOMEN'S PSYCHIATRIC INCARCERATION AT GEORGIA LUNATIC ASYLUM IN THE NINETEENTH CENTURY

1. T. O. Powell, "A Sketch of Psychiatry in the Southern States," *American Journal of Insanity* 54, no. 1 (1897): 21–36, 29.
2. I use the term "bodymind" in this chapter and elsewhere in the book not to suggest there is any split between the body and the mind but rather to draw attention to the ways that Black bodies consist of both mental and physical dimensions, although the former is often unrecognized or not thoroughly considered. Southern psychiatrists were deeply interested in why there was an increase in insanity among Blacks and postulated that slavery and the Civil War were at the heart of the matter. Edwards-Grossi argues that southern medical men believed that madness was caused by "large-scale political and

social dysfunction, for which Northerners were largely responsible." Élodie Edwards-Grossi, *Mad with Freedom: The Political Economy of Blackness, Insanity, and Civil Rights in the U.S. South, 1840–1940* (Louisiana State University Press, 2022), 68. Modern historians argue that there was an actual increase of insanity as a result of the spread of venereal disease, the availability and use of alcohol, and childbirth trauma–related schizophrenia. Segrest suggests that trauma from the Civil War was also a cause. Mab Segrest, *Administrations of Lunacy: Racism and the Haunting of American Psychiatry at the Milledgeville Asylum* (New Press, 2020), 165–69.

3. Charlotte Perkins Gilman, "A Suggestion on the Negro Problem," *American Journal of Sociology* 14, no. 1 (July 1908).

4. In a speech to the Georgia State Agricultural Society, Felton urged that Black men should be lynched to protect rural white women from being raped by Black men. In response to the speech, which had been reprinted in newspapers, Alex Manly wrote a rebuttal in the *Daily Record*, a Black newspaper, that argued that Black women were more likely to be the victims of rape by white men and that Black men's sexual relations with white women were usually consensual. Manly's response ignited the 1898 Wilmington race massacre and coup d'etat, which I will discuss more in chapter 6. James A. Holloman, "'Lynch,' Says Mrs. Felton," *Atlanta Journal*, August 12, 1897, 1; "Mrs. Felton's Letter," *Atlanta Constitution*, August 20, 1897, 4.

5. See John Haller, *Outcasts from Evolution: Scientific Attitudes of Racial Inferiority, 1859–1900* (McGraw-Hill, 1971).

6. For a discussion of Powell in the context of eugenic discourses, see Segrest, *Administrations of Lunacy*, 169–84. For a discussion of the white psychiatric project's distinguishing the white psyche and prioritizing white patients, see Martin Summers, *Madness in the City of Magnificent Intentions: A History of Race and Mental Illness in the Nation's Capital* (Oxford University Press, 2019); and Segrest, *Administrations of Lunacy*, 168. It is important to note that there was a widespread cultural project of eugenics that was occurring within civil society and among Blacks themselves, who also created better baby contests and argued for the purification of the race along with white nationalists. See Daylanne K. English, *Unnatural Selections: Eugenics in American Modernism and the Harlem Renaissance* (University of North Carolina Press, 2004).

7. Studies in the field of psychiatry are numerous. A few notable examples that offer commentary on Blacks and white superintendents' ideas about them include Gerald N. Grob, *The Mad Among Us: A History of the Care of America's Mentally Ill* (Maxwell Macmillan, 1994), 88–90, 151; David Rothman, *The Discovery of the Asylum: Social Order and Disorder in the New Republic*, rev. ed. (Aldine de Gruyter, 2002), 112, 135, 229; Norman Dain, *Disordered Minds: The First Century of Eastern State Hospital in Williamsburg, Virginia 1766–1866* (Colonial Williamsburg Foundation, 1971), 19, 37, 99, 108–13, 186. Studies offering a more robust analysis of race and Black people in asylums include Segrest, *Administrations of Lunacy*; Summers, *Madness in the City of Magnificent Intentions*; Wendy Gonaver, *The Peculiar Institution and the Making of Modern Psychiatry, 1840–1880* (University of North Carolina Press, 2018); Edwards-Grossi, *Mad with Freedom*. For a history of another marginalized group's experiences of institutionalization that also

8. Jeffrey Geller and Maxine Harris, *Women of the Asylum: Voices from Behind the Walls, 1840–1945* (Anchor, 1994); Jeffrey Geller, "Women's Accounts of Psychiatric Illness and Institutionalization," *Hospital and Community Psychiatry* 36, no. 10 (October 1985): 1056–62; Mary Elene Wood, *The Writing on the Wall: Women's Autobiography and the Asylum* (University of Illinois Press, 1994); Linda Carlisle, *Elizabeth Packard: A Noble Fight* (University of Illinois Press, 2010).
9. See Segrest, *Administrations of Lunacy*.
10. First names and last initials are used to protect the identities of the women. After first use, only first names are used. References to psychiatric records include first name and "intake ledger." Alice and Jane do not appear in the asylum ledgers.
11. Gonaver, *The Peculiar Institution*, 80–84. In his copious study, Martin Summers has done much to bring to light the perspectives of Black family members and patients at St. Elizabeth's asylum. See Summers, *Madness in the City of Magnificent Intentions*.
12. Minor discrepancies exist between the asylum ledgers and the newspaper articles, including name spellings, ages, and admission dates. For example, Olivia's name in the newspaper article is spelled with an added "s." However, in the asylum ledger, her name is spelled without an "s" at the end. In Olivia's case, a census record confirms that her name was actually spelled without an added "s." Viney is listed as thirty years of age in the intake records but reported as being forty years old in the newspaper. The most curious discrepancy is in regard to admission dates. For example, the newspaper records indicate that Olivia was sent to the asylum on July 17; however, the intake ledger notes that she entered the hospital on July 16. The newspaper record indicates that Amanda was sent to the asylum on July 13; the asylum intake ledger indicates that she arrived at the hospital on July 12.
13. "1880 United States Federal Census About Olivia W.," Ancestry.com, accessed June 23, 2014. Original source: 1880 U.S. Census (National Archives Microfilm Publication T9, roll 1454); Records of the Bureau of the Census, Record Group 29; National Archives Building, Washington, DC. Beginning in 1840, the US census enumerated instances of insanity.
14. "In the Local Field," *Atlanta Constitution*, July 14, 1894.
15. "In the Local Field," *Atlanta Constitution*, July 18, 1894.
16. Olivia W., intake ledger, July 16, 1894, Collection 350, Box 22, vol. 11, Central State Hospital Admissions Registers, 1842–1924, Georgia Archives.
17. Amanda C., intake ledger, July 14, 1894, Collection 350, Box 22, vol. 9, Central State Hospital Admissions Registers, 1842–1924, Georgia Archives.
18. "Sent to the Lunatic Asylum: Ordinary Calhoun and a Jury Hear Two Lunacy Cases," *Atlanta Constitution*, July 4, 1888.
19. Viney W., intake ledger, July 11, 1888, Collection 350, Box 21, vol. 9, Central State Hospital Admissions Registers, 1842–1924, Georgia Archives.
20. "Yesterday's Arrests: Johnson's 83-An Insane Woman—Jackson Goes to Jail—Smith, the Vagrant—Stolen Jewelry—The Result of a Drunk," *Daily Constitution*, July 2, 1881.

21. Saidiya V. Hartman, *Wayward Lives, Beautiful Experiments: Intimate Histories of Riotous Black Girls, Troublesome Women, and Queer Radicals* (Norton, 2019), 25.
22. Saidiya V. Hartman, *Wayward Lives, Beautiful Experiments*, 21.
23. Ula Taylor, "Women in the Documents: Thoughts on Uncovering the Personal, Political, and Professional," *Journal of Women's History* 20, no.1 (2008): 191.
24. Gonaver, *The Peculiar Institution*, 112–44; Elizabeth Lunbeck, *The Psychiatric Persuasion: Knowledge, Gender, and Power in Modern America* (Princeton University Press, 1994), 204–5; Elaine Showalter, *The Female Malady: Women, Madness, and English Culture, 1830–1980* (Pantheon, 1985), 74–100.
25. Jacqueline Jones, *Labor of Love, Labor of Sorrow: Black Women, Work and the Family, from Slavery to the Present* (Basic, 1985), 70–72; Deborah Gray White, *Ar'n't I a Woman?: Female Slaves in the Plantation South* (Norton, 1999), 185, 189. For a thorough discussion of these tropes, see Patricia Hill Collins, *Black Feminist Thought: Knowledge, Consciousness, and the Politics of Empowerment* (Routledge, 2008).
26. Asylum physicians believed asylums were best suited for the most severe cases of insanity. Individuals who were most disruptive and violent toward family members were a priority for admission.
27. Jones, *Labor of Love, Labor of Sorrow*, 70.
28. "A Queer Case of Suicide," *Savannah Morning News*, January 9, 1894.
29. "Yesterday's Arrests."
30. Tera W. Hunter, *To 'Joy My Freedom: Southern Black Women's Lives and Labors after the Civil War* (Harvard University Press, 1997), 34.
31. "Yesterday's Arrests."
32. "In the Local Field," July 14, 1894.
33. "In the Local Field," July 14, 1894; "In the Local Field," July 18, 1894.
34. "In the Local Field," July 14, 1894.
35. "Sent to the Lunatic Asylum."
36. Noralee Frankel, *Break Those Chains at Last: African Americans 1860–1880* (Oxford University Press, 1996), 103; Leslie Schwalm, *A Hard Fight for We: Women's Transition from Slavery to Freedom in South Carolina* (University of Illinois Press, 1997), 260–68.
37. "Sent to the Lunatic Asylum."
38. Gonaver, *The Peculiar Institution*, 122.
39. For studies on the myriad forms of state, institutional, and sexualized violence against Black women in the postemancipation South, see Hannah Rosen, *Terror in the Heart of Freedom: Citizenship, Sexual Violence, and the Meaning of Race in the Postemancipation South* (University of North Carolina Press, 2009); and Sarah Haley, *No Mercy Here: Gender, Punishment, and the Making of Jim Crow Modernity* (University of North Carolina Press, 2016).
40. Medicalized views of insanity came from a range of actors, including both Black and white doctors, psychiatrists, and public health officials. Medical practitioners generally believed that emancipation brought about an increase in several diseases among Black people, including tuberculosis, syphilis, and insanity. Historians of medicine have considered how social discourses about race were interwoven with medical theories of

health. See Hunter, *To 'Joy My Freedom*, 188–89. Also see Charles E. Rosenburg, *Explaining Epidemics and Other Studies in the History of Medicine* (Cambridge University Press, 1992), 278–79, 301; Dorothy Roberts, *Fatal Invention: How Science, Politics, and Big Business Re-Create Race in the Twenty-First Century* (New Press, 2011).

41. These areas of inquiry were not mutually exclusive; in fact, many of the arguments were overlapping and used to support theories in another area. For example, debates about whether there were distinct types of man were a part of debates about the outcome of mixing supposedly different types, which was a chief concern for social evolutionists who used arguments about innate hereditary conditions to talk about the possibilities for a racial group's ability to develop and progress over time.

42. F. Tipton, "The Negro Problem from a Medical Standpoint," *New York Medical Journal* XLIII (May 1886): 569–72.

43. Frederick Hoffman argued that education did not do away with moral deficiencies in Blacks or mulattos. He argued further that any sort of philanthropic aid to Blacks impeded their ability to rise as a race, something that could only happen through virtues derived from struggle and self-help. See Frederick Hoffman, *Race Traits and Tendencies of the American Negro* (Published for the American Economic Association by the Macmillan Company, 1896).

44. Sanford B. Hunt, "The Negro as a Soldier," *Quarterly Journal of Psychological Medicine and Medical Jurisprudence* 1, no. 2 (October 1867): 185.

45. On Blacks' supposed undeveloped nervous system, see Summers, *Madness in the City of Magnificent Intentions*.

46. T. O. Powell, "The Increase of Insanity and Tuberculosis in the Southern Negro Since 1860, and Its Alliance, and Some of the Supposed Causes," *Journal of American Medical Association* 27, no. 23 (December 1896): 1185–88; Thomas McKie, "A Brief History of Insanity and Tuberculosis in the Southern Negro," *Journal of American Medical Association* 28, no. 12 (March 1897): 537–38; Thomas J. Mays, "Human Slavery as a Prevention of Pulmonary Consumption" (1904), in *Germs Have No Color Lines: Blacks and American Medicine, 1900–1940*, ed. Vanessa Northington Gamble (Garland, 1989), 6–11; William Frances Drewry, "History of the Central State Hospital of Virginia," *Annual Reports of Officers, Boards, and Institutions of the Commonwealth of Virginia* (1904): 105–28.

47. The census continued to label people as "insane" or "idiotic" through 1880 and, in 1890, dropped those words for "defective of mind." "The 1840 U.S. Census Was Overly Interested in Americans' Mental Health," History, May 15, 2019, https://www.history.com/news/census-change-mental-illness-controversy. Also see James Trent, *Inventing the Feeble Mind: A History of Intellectual Disability in the United States* (Oxford University Press, 2016).

48. J. F. Miller, "The Effects of Emancipation upon the Mental and Physical Health of the Negro in the South," *North Carolina Medical Journal* 38, no. 10 (November 1896): 286.

49. See chapter 1.

50. Miller, "The Effects of Emancipation," 289. For more on the Goldsboro hospital see Edwards-Grossi, *Mad with Freedom*. There were increases in both Black insanity rates and Blacks' admissions to asylums. This was in part because admission to asylums was in large part denied to Blacks before emancipation. Also, Blacks were seeking out care in the most

affordable forms; most asylums were funded by the state (although funding was meager and outpaced by high demand). Prior to admission to asylums after the Civil War and the establishment of the freedmen's bureau hospitals, most Blacks received care from family members and in some cases from physicians brought in by plantation owners and in other cases from Black healthcare providers, some of whom were Conjure women and men. For a discussion on preemancipation care of Blacks with mental disabilities, see chapters 1–3. Black doctors conceded that there were rising rates of insanity, but they were more likely to locate the source of disease in the social, political, and economic realities of Black life. John E. Hunter borrowed almost word for word the leading psychiatrists' formulations on disease, including the hygienic benefits of slavery, but even he placed most of the emphasis on socioeconomic disparities as the driving cause of disease. John E. Hunter, "Tuberculosis in the Negro: Causes and Treatment," in Gamble, ed., *Germs Have No Color Line*, 12–19.

51. See chapter 2.
52. J. F. Miller, "The Effects of Emancipation," 290.
53. Paul Topinard, "Chapter VIII: Influence of Milieux," in *Anthropology* (Chapman and Hall, 1878), 413. Also quoted in Haller, *Outcasts from Evolution*, 46.
54. J. Allison Hodges, "The Effect of Freedom Upon the Physical and Psychological Development of the Negro," *Richmond Journal of Practice* 14 (June 1900): 170–71. Seale Harris, "The Future of the Negro from the Standpoint of the Southern Physician," *Alabama Medical Journal* 14, no. 2 (January 1902): 58.
55. "Deterioration of the American Negro," *Atlanta Journal-Record of Medicine* V (July 1903): 287; H. M. Bannister and Ludwig Hektoen, "Race and Insanity," *American Journal of Insanity* 44, no. 4 (April 1888): 63. Black doctors were at odds with these claims on some accounts. E. Mayfield Boyle pointed to statistics that indicated lower Black suicide rates to argue that the low numbers of suicide among Blacks were indicative of the fact that whites had "inferior brain structures" and "mental endurance." E. Mayfield Boyle, "The Negro and Tuberculosis" (1912), in Gamble, ed., *Germs Have No Color Line*, 45; E. T. Easley, "The Sanitary Condition of the Negro," *American Weekly* 3 (July 31, 1875): 49–50.
56. Hoffman, *Race Traits and Tendencies of the American Negro*, 140–42. See D. M. Sommerville, *Aberration of Mind: Suicide and Suffering in the Civil War-Era South* (University of North Carolina Press, 2018) for a thorough discussion of suicide among Blacks and whites before and after slavery.
57. Hoffman, *Race Traits and Tendencies*, 143.
58. This sentiment resonated with Black social scientists and leaders of Black uplift movements such as Booker T. Washington, who compelled Blacks to rely on themselves to create economic, educational, and moral progress from within. For Black perspectives, See J. M. Keating, "Twenty Years of Negro Education," *Popular Science Monthly* 28 (November 1885): 25; D. Kerfoot Shute, "Racial Anatomical Peculiarities," *American Anthropologist* 9, no. 4 (April 1896): 131–32; M. Alfred Fouille, "Scientific Philanthropy," *Popular Science Monthly* XXII (February 1883): 521–35; Franklin Smith, "The Real Problems of Democracy," *Popular Science Monthly* LVI (November 1899): 1–3.
59. For a discussion of all-Black asylums in light of the many race massacres that occurred during Reconstruction, see Edwards-Grossi, *Mad with Freedom*, 69–70.

256   5. BLACK WOMEN'S PSYCHIATRIC INCARCERATION

60. Powell's sentiments about the "colored insane" appear in two local newspaper articles: "The Lunatic Asylum," *Union Recorder* 60, no. 20, November 19, 1889, 6; and "Superintendent Powell Talks About the State's Lunatics," *Union Recorder* 60, no. 29, January 21, 1890, 6.
61. The most extensive analysis of Powell can be found in Segrest, *Administrations of Lunacy*.
62. T. O. Powell, "Increase of Insanity and Its Supposed Causes, Etc.," in *Reports of the Trustees and Officers of the Lunatic Asylum, of the State of Georgia, from October 1st, 1885, to 1st October, 1886* (Union & Recorder—Barnes & Moore, 1886), 15. His emphasis on heredity was common among psychiatrists of his time. See Ian Dowbiggin, *Keeping America Sane: Psychiatry and Eugenics in the United States and Canada, 1880–1940* (Cornell University Press, 1997), 70–132.
63. For a discussion of the transition in the field of psychiatry from emphasizing environment to emphasizing genetics, see Gerald N. Grob, *The State and the Mentally Ill: A History of Worcester State Hospital in Massachusetts, 1830–1920* (University of North Carolina Press, 1966), 198–228. Powell, "Increase of Insanity and Its Supposed Causes, Etc.," 15–16.
64. Powell, "Increase of Insanity and Its Supposed Causes, Etc.," 17.
65. T. O. Powell, "Heredity and Invironment [sic]," *Union Recorder*, May 3, 1887, 2.
66. Powell, "Sketch," 32.
67. Powell, "Increase of Insanity and Its Supposed Causes, Etc.," 22.
68. T. O. Powell, "The Increase of Insanity and Tuberculosis in the Southern Negro Since 1860, and Its Alliance, and Some of the Supposed Causes," *Journal of the American Medical Association* 27, no. 23 (1896): 1185–88. For accounts of the actual proliferation of these diseases during slavery, see Hunter, *To 'Joy My Freedom*, 191–98.
69. Powell, "The Increase of Insanity and Tuberculosis in the Southern Negro," 1188.
70. See chapters 1 and 2.
71. Roberts, *Fatal Invention*, 5.
72. Summers, *Madness in the City of Magnificent Intentions*, 3.
73. Amanda, intake ledger.
74. Olivia, intake ledger.
75. Olivia, intake ledger; Ancestry.com, "1880 Census." According to the census of 1880, Olivia would be thirty-five not twenty-eight. John and Anna were three and one, respectively, in 1880.
76. Black mothers composed 48.33 percent of the population. "Annual Report of the Trustees of the Georgia Lunatic Asylum, for the Fiscal Year from October 1, 1893, to September 1, 1894," 1–21, in "Bi-ennial Report of the Trustees of the Georgia Lunatic Asylum for the Fiscal Year from October 1, 1890, to September 1, 1894 [1890–94]," (Richards & Shaver, Printers and Binders, 1894). Hereafter AR 1894.
77. Frankel, *Break Those Chains*, 7–8, 42–43, 89, 90, 97–98, 113.
78. Powell, "Increase of Insanity," 13; Rothman, *The Discovery of the Asylum*, 137.
79. Black wives composed 45 percent of the population and widows 20 percent. AR 1894.
80. Many slaves had long-standing marriages that lasted after emancipation. For more on marriage in Black communities before and after slavery, see Herbert Gutman, *The Black Family in Slavery and Freedom, 1750–1925* (Vintage, 1976), 50; Schwalm, *A Hard Fight for We*, 239–48.

81. Frankel, *Break Those Chains*, 100.
82. Tera W. Hunter, *Bound in Wedlock: Slave and Free Black Marriage in the Nineteenth Century* (Belknap, 2017), 15–16.
83. Frankel, *Break Those Chains*, 103.
84. Olivia, intake ledger; Amanda, intake ledger; Frankel, *Break Those Chains*, 102.
85. The restoration rate of all Black women at the hospital was about 23 percent. The rate for married Black women was 21 percent; for Black men, it was 29 percent. AR 1894.
86. Amanda, intake ledger; Olivia, intake ledger; Viney, intake ledger.
87. "The Lunatic Asylum: Dr. Powell, the Superintendent, Is in Atlanta with His Annual Statement," *Atlanta Constitution*, November 16, 1889.
88. Powell, "Sketch," 30.
89. "Reports of the Trustees and Officers of the Lunatic Asylum of the State of Georgia, from December 1st, 1878, to September 30th, 1879," 11–12, in "Reports of the Trustees and Superintendent, Resident Physician and Other Officers, of the Lunatic Asylum of the State of Georgia from December 1st, 1877, to September 30th, 1879 [1877–79]," (J. W. Burke, 1879).
90. Segrest, *Administrations of Lunacy*, 155.
91. Sharon Harley, "When Your Work is Not Who You Are: The Development of a Working-Class Consciousness Among Afro-American Women," in *"We Specialize in the Wholly Impossible": A Reader in Black Women's History*, ed. Darlene Clark Hine, Wilma King, and Linda Reed (Carlson, 1995), 25–38.
92. Peter McCandless, *Moonlight, Magnolias, and Madness: Insanity in South Carolina from the Colonial Period to the Progressive Era* (University of North Carolina Press, 1996), 10.
93. Frankel, *Break Those Chains*, 42.
94. Frankel, *Break Those Chains*, 7–8; Hunter, *To 'Joy My Freedom*, 27–28.
95. Powell, "Sketch," 32.
96. Summers, *Madness in the City of Magnificent Intentions*, 103, 29.
97. Testimony of Alfred Richardson, Washington, DC, July 7, 1871, in *Report of the Joint Select Committee to Inquire into the Condition of Affairs in the Late Insurrectionary States, Made to the Two Houses of Congress February 19, 1872* (Government Printing Office, 1872), https://hdl.handle.net/2027/miun.aca4911.0006.001.
98. See Rosen, *Terror in the Heart of Freedom*.
99. Grob, *The Mad Among Us*, 89–90.
100. Sallie M., intake ledger, June 28, 1879, Collection 350, Box 19, vol. 5, Central State Hospital Admissions Registers, 1878–1881, Georgia Archives.
101. Sallie, intake ledger.
102. Noel Ignatiev, *How the Irish Became White* (Routledge, 2009); Theodore W. Allen, *The Invention of the White Race, Volume 2: The Origin of Racial Oppression in Anglo-America* (Verso, 1997); Mary B., intake ledger, June 19, 1879, Collection 350, Box 19, vol. 5, Central State Hospital Admissions Registers, 1878–1881, Georgia Archives. For a comparative study of Irish and Black women's medical exploitation, see Deirdre Cooper Owens, *Medical Bondage: Race, Gender, and the Origins of American Gynecology* (University of Georgia Press, 2017), 89–107.

258   5. BLACK WOMEN'S PSYCHIATRIC INCARCERATION

103. Peter G. Cranford and Lois W. Lane, *Damnation Hospital* (Old Capital, 2009), 44.
104. Henry Mills Hurd et al., *The Institutional Care of the Insane in the United States and Canada*, ed. Henry Mills Hurd, reprint, vol. 4 (Johns Hopkins Press, 1917), 164.
105. Cranford and Lane, *Damnation*, 61. Over the course of the century, monies dedicated to colored buildings were modest compared to those for whites. For example, funding allocations for the expansion of facilities for the white population before 1860 were as follows: 1849, $10,500; 1851, $24,500; 1853, $56,500; 1855, $110,000; 1857, $63,500; and 1858, $30,000. Thus, before Blacks arrived, almost $300,000 had been appropriated for the construction of white buildings. After 1870, the appropriations for white facilities totaled $1,362,875: 1870–1871, $105,000; 1881, $165,000; 1883, $92,875; and 1893, $100,000. For Blacks, the allocations were as follows: 1866, $11,000; 1870, $18,000; 1879, $25,000; and 1881, $82,166. Over the course of a decade and a half, only $136,000 was spent on colored facilities. Thus, before 1881, white facilities received five times as much funding as Black facilities. Although the number of Blacks never exceeded the number of whites from 1866 to 1881, the Black-to-white ratio was certainly greater than 1:5. Figures from Hurd, *The Institutional Care*, vol. 4, 163–64.
106. As late as 1893, there were public discussions of overcrowding at the hospital and desperate appeals for more state funding to expand the facilities. "Lunatic Asylum," *Union Recorder* 64, no. 19, November 7, 1893. For discussions of Black people in segregated facilities or institutions, see Summers, *Madness in the City of Magnificent Intentions*, and Edwards-Grossi, *Mad with Freedom*.
107. North Carolina and Virginia had separate wards for Blacks starting in 1880 and 1885, respectively. McCandless, *Moonlight, Magnolias, and Madness*, 284. Alabama had a separate hospital for the "colored insane" under the same management as the original hospital for whites. Hurd, *The Institutional Care*, 377–78.
108. Segrest, *Administrations of Lunacy*, 189–90.
109. Cranford, *Damnation*, 65.
110. McCandless, *Moonlight, Magnolias, and Madness*, 283–84.
111. White women were dying at a rate of 6 percent and Black women at 10 percent. AR 1894.
112. Olivia, intake ledger.
113. "Exhaustion," a nineteenth-century term for what we now know as chronic fatigue syndrome, is characterized by extreme fatigue, memory or concentration difficulties, headaches, and sore muscles and joints.
114. "Dropsy" is the nineteenth-century term for what we now know as edema, a disease in which there is excess fluid in the tissues and cavities of the body.
115. Black people were dying at three times the rate of whites from tuberculosis. David McBride, *From TB to AIDS: Epidemics Among Urban Blacks since 1900* (State University of New York Press, 1991), 11; Marion M. Torchia, "The Tuberculosis Movement and the Race Question, 1890–1950," *Bulletin History of Medicine* 49, no. 2 (1975): 152–68. For a thorough examination of race and tuberculosis among Blacks in the twentieth century, see Samuel K. Roberts Jr., *Infectious Fear: Politics, Disease, and the Health Effects of Segregation* (University of North Carolina Press, 2009).
116. AR 1894.

117. White and Black female people died of marasmus at rates of 0.05 percent and 2 percent, respectively. AR 1894.
118. AR 1894.
119. Powell, "Sketch," 30.
120. Segrest, *Administrations of Lunacy*, 161–62.
121. Ayah Nuriddin, "Psychiatric Jim Crow: Desegregation at the Crownsville State Hospital, 1948–1970," *Journal of the History of Medicine and Allied Sciences* 74, no. 1 (2019): 85–106; Kylie Smith, *Talking Therapy: Knowledge and Power in American Psychiatric Nursing* (Rutgers University Press, 2020), 116.

6. CHARLES CHESNUTT AND MENTAL DISABILITY IN THE AGE OF BLACK FREEDOM

1. In 1931, Chesnutt called this period "Post-Bellum–Pre-Harlem," which refers to the period roughly following the Civil War and ending at the start of World War 1 (1877 to 1919). Charles W. Chesnutt, "Post-Bellum–Pre-Harlem," in *Charles W. Chesnutt: Essays and Speeches*, ed. Joseph R. McElrath Jr., Robert C. Leitz, and Jesse S. Crisler (Stanford University Press, 1999), 543–49. See also Barbara McCaskill and Caroline Gebhard, eds., *Post-Bellum-Pre-Harlem: African American Literature and Culture, 1877–1919* (New York University Press, 2006). Chesnutt shared the literary stage during this period with a preeminent group of Black writers, including the poet Paul Laurence Dunbar; novelist Sutton Griggs; poet, essayist, orator, and novelist Frances Harper; and dramatist, novelist, and editor Pauline Hopkins. The other writers' publication venues tended to be Black newspapers, journals, and magazines, including most notably the African Methodist Episcopal (AME) Church's *Christian Recorder* and the *Colored American Magazine*. See Andreá Williams, "Postbellum, Pre-Harlem: Black Writing Before the Renaissance," in *A Companion to the Harlem Renaissance*, ed. Cherene Sherrard-Johnson (Wiley, 2015), 37–38. For a discussion of early Black publishing outlets, see Frances Smith Foster, "A Narrative of the Interesting Origins and (Somewhat) Surprising Developments of African-American Print Culture," *American Literary History* 17, no. 4 (2005): 714–40.
2. For a comprehensive biography on Chesnutt and his works, see Tess Chakkalakal, *A Matter of Complexion: The Life and Fictions of Charles W. Chesnutt* (St. Martin's Press, 2025).
3. See Susanna Ashton and Bill Hardwig, eds., *Approaches to Teaching the Works of Charles W. Chesnutt* (Modern Language Association, 2017).
4. Dunbar was not as approving of Howells as Chesnutt because Dunbar eventually resented Howells's advice that he should produce Black dialect poetry, which he felt was harmful. Benjamin Brawley, *Paul Laurence Dunbar: Poet of His People* (University of North Carolina Press, 1936), 60. On white patrons of Black literature, see Francesca Sawaya, "'That Friendship of the Whites': Patronage, Philanthropy, and Charles Chesnutt's *The Colonel's Dream*," *American Literature* 83, no. 4 (December 2011): 775–801. On Howells's view on American imperialism, see Edwin H. Cady, *The Realist at War: The Mature Years,*

1885–1920, of William Dean Howells (Syracuse University Press, 1958). For a discussion of the support Chesnutt received from the white publishing establishment, see Kenneth M. Price, "Charles Chesnutt, the *Atlantic Monthly*, and the intersection of African-American Fiction and Elite Culture," in *Periodical Literature in Nineteenth-Century America*, ed. Kenneth M. Price and Susan Belasco Smith (University Press of Virginia, 1995).

5. W. D. Howells, "Mr. Charles W. Chesnutt's Stories," *Atlantic Monthly* 85 (May 1900): 699–701.
6. William D. Howells, "An Exemplary Citizen," *North American Review* 173, no. 537 (August 1901): 280–88.
7. William D. Howells, "A Psychological Counter-Current in Recent Fiction," *North American Review* 173, no. 541 (December 1901): 882. On it ending their relationship, see William L. Andrews, "William Dean Howells and Charles W. Chesnutt: Criticism and Race Fiction in the Age of Booker T. Washington," *American Literature* 48, no. 3 (November 1976): 329.
8. Howells, "An Exemplary Citizen," 280. Scholars have associated Howells's disdain with the representation of violence in the novel. However, *The Marrow of Tradition* does not end with violence, as this chapter shows. The Black characters exhibit forgiveness and help white Wellingtonians, something modern readers find too passive. I suggest here that in the context of the ideas circulating at the time, Howells might have been offended by the representation of Blacks not only as equal mentally and physically but also as moral authorities whom the white characters needed for survival. Charles W. Chesnutt, *The Marrow of Tradition* (Houghton, Mifflin, 1901).
9. Chesnutt, "The Future American: A Complete Race-Amalgamation Likely to Occur," in *Charles W. Chesnutt*, ed. McElrath et al., 134.
10. Vann Woodward, *The Strange Career of Jim Crow* (Oxford University Press, 1974), 70.
11. Black people were subject to widespread lynchings and racial terror in the wake of emancipation. For a description of mass lynchings by state, see "Reconstruction in America: Racial Violence After the Civil War, 1865–1876," Equal Justice Initiative, 2020, https://eji.org/report/reconstruction-in-america. For research on specific massacres and the general climate of racial and gendered terror, see Carolyn E. DeLatte, "The St. Landry Riot: A Forgotten Incident of Reconstruction Violence," *Louisiana History: The Journal of the Louisiana Historical Association* 17, no. 1 (1976): 41–49; Art Carden and Christoper J. Coyne, "The Political Economy of the Reconstruction Era's Race Riots," *Public Choice* 157, no. 1–2 (2013): 57–71; David T. Ballantyne, "Remembering the Colfax Massacre: Race, Sex, and the Meanings of Reconstruction Violence," *Journal of Southern History* 87, no. 3 (2021): 427–66; LeeAnna Keith, *The Colfax Massacre: The Untold Story of Black Power, White Terror, and the Death of Reconstruction* (Oxford University Press, 2009); Melinda Meek Hennessey, "Race and Violence in Reconstruction New Orleans: The 1868 Riot," *Louisiana History* 20, no. 1 (1979): 77–91; Sarah Haley, *No Mercy Here: Gender, Punishment, and the Making of Jim Crow Modernity* (University of North Carolina Press, 2016); Hannah Rosen, *Terror in the Heart of Freedom: Citizenship, Sexual Violence, and the Meaning of Race in the Postemancipation South* (University of North Carolina Press, 2009).
12. Chesnutt confirmed the sentiment in his acceptance speech for the Spingarn Medal in 1928. He noted that he was an "omnivorous reader" and that his maternal grandmother

remarked that "had she not been present at [his] delivery she could have believed that [he] was born with a book in [his] hand." Charles W. Chesnutt, "Remarks of Charles Waddell Chesnutt, of Cleveland, in Accepting the Spingarn Medal at Los Angeles," in *Charles W. Chesnutt*, ed. McElrath et al., 513.

13. When Chesnutt moved to the North, he successfully worked as a stenographer to support his family financially while also serving as a member of the NAACP, where he worked for equality in education and antidiscrimination laws.

14. William L. Andrews, *The Literary Career of Charles W. Chesnutt* (Louisiana State University Press, 1980), 181. Little scholarly attention has yet been given to the ways his commitment to intellectual debates about solving social ills of society manifested in his creative productions. William Andrews does provide some analysis of the ways Chesnutt's ideas in "The Future American" show up in the novel he published in the same month, *The House Behind the Cedars*. Andrews, *The Literary Career of Charles W. Chesnutt*, 137–74. Both the *Boston Transcript* articles and the novel were published in the same month, but the articles appeared first.

15. Chesnutt, "The Future American: A Stream of Dark Blood in the Veins of the Southern Whites," in *Charles W. Chesnutt*, ed. McElrath et al., 126.

16. Listing the barriers to racial amalgamation, Chesnutt writes: "Another obstacle to race fusion lies in the drastic and increasing proscriptive legislation by which the South attempts to keep the white and colored races apart in every place where their joint presence might be taken to imply equality; or, to put it more directly, the persistent effort to degrade the Negro to a distinctly and permanently inferior caste. This is undertaken by means of separate schools, separate railroad and street cars, political disfranchisement [sic], debasing and abhorrent prison systems, and an unflagging campaign of calumny, by which the vices and shortcomings of the Negroes are grossly magnified and their virtues practically lost sight of." Chesnutt, "The Future American: A Complete Race-Amalgamation Likely to Occur," 133. He writes that there are social forces in favor of amalgamation such as skin lightening in the Black community and slavery. He glosses over the violence of rape in slavery, the dominant process by which racial mixing occurred; he says slavery was "favorable to the mixing of races." Chesnutt, "The Future American: A Complete Race-Amalgamation Likely to Occur," 133. The premier Black intellectual W. E. B. Du Bois was more critical of racial mixing. Du Bois shared Chesnutt's view that antimiscegenation laws were unjust, but Du Bois was not eager to see racial mixing because of the American track record of violence. In a debate with a white supremacist eugenicist Lothrop Stoddard, Du Bois proclaimed that Blacks were not interested in marrying white people's daughters. These pro-Black communal, and what would become pan-African, leanings were troubling to Chesnutt because he believed that the erasure of contemporary racial strife depended on eliminating divisions based on arbitrary racial affinities. Ian Frazier, "When W. E. B. Du Bois Made a Laughingstock of a White Supremacist," *The New Yorker*, August 19, 2019.

17. Chesnutt, "The Future American: What the Race Is Likely to Become in the Process of Time," in *Charles W. Chesnutt*, ed. McElrath et al., 122.

18. Other works asserting the heredity argument, that is that no amount of philanthropic assistance could pull Blacks out of their inferior mental and moral defunctness, include

Charles F. Withington, "The Perils of Rapid Civilization," *Popular Science Monthly* 26 (1885): 233; Philip A. Bruce, *The Plantation Negro as a Freeman: Observations on His Character, Condition, and Prospects in Virginia* (G. P. Putnam's Sons, Knickerbocker Press, 1889), 260. For a discussion of amalgamation across various global social contexts and historical periods, see Jared Sexton, *Amalgamation Schemes: Antiblackness and the Critique of Multiracialism* (University of Minnesota Press, 2008); and Tavia Nyong'o, *The Amalgamation Waltz: Race, Performance, and the Ruses of Memory* (University of Minnesota Press, 2009). Black women activists such as Anna Julia Cooper, Frances Watkins Harper, and Victoria Earle Matthews offered commentary in their works in which they sided with the environmentalist arguments.

19. W. S. McCurley, "Impossibility of Racial Amalgamation," *Arena* 21 (1899): 449, 454.
20. Joseph Alexander Tillinghast, "The Negro in Africa and America," *Publications of the American Economic Association* 3, no. 2 (1902): 148.
21. Tillinghast, "The Negro in Africa and America," 136.
22. In the introduction to *Races of Europe*, Ripley writes, "Race, properly speaking, is responsible only for those peculiarities, mental or bodily, which are transmitted with constancy along the lines of direct physical descent from father to son. Many mental traits, aptitudes, or proclivities, on the other hand, which reappear persistently in successive populations may be derived from an entirely different source. They may have descended collaterally, along the lines of purely mental suggestion by virtue of mere social contact with preceding generations." William Zebina Ripley, *The Races of Europe: A Sociological Study* (Kegan Paul, Trench, Trubner, & Co., 1899), 1.
23. Ripley, *The Races of Europe*, 457.
24. Chesnutt, "The Future American: A Stream of Dark Blood in the Veins of the Southern Whites," in *Charles W. Chesnutt: Essays and Speeches*, ed. McElrath et al., 126. Eugenicists took up Ripley's research to prevent racial mixing first through antimiscegenation laws and eventually through sterilization. For more on how eugenicists used Ripley's work, see Richard B. Sherman, "'The Last Stand': The Fight for Racial Integrity in Virginia in the 1920s," *Journal of Southern History* 54, no. 1 (1988): 69–92; Thomas C. Leonard, *Illiberal Reformers: Race, Eugenics, and American Economics in the Progressive Era* (Princeton University Press, 2016); Jonathan Peter Spiro, *Defending the Master Race: Conservation, Eugenics, and the Legacy of Madison Grant* (University Press of New England, 2009).
25. Chesnutt, "The Future American: What the Race Is Likely to Become in the Process of Time," 123. Chesnutt is likely finding his scientific support from the work of Paul Broca, Charles Lyell, and John Bachman, who argued that mixed-race people were fertile. John S. Haller, *Outcasts from Evolution: Scientific Attitudes of Racial Inferiority, 1859–1900* (McGraw-Hill, 1971), 86. Willis Boughton, a professor at Ohio State University, argued that racial mixing occurred in ancient civilizations such as those of the Greeks and Romans and that their civilizations were better off for it. He believed racial fusion or amalgamation would result in a better racial type, which he believed would take place slowly over time rather than within a generation or two. Willis Boughton, "The Negro's Place in History," *Arena*, no. LXXXII (September 1896): 612–21.

26. Chesnutt was referring to the outbreak of the Spanish–American War in 1898, which he assumed would result in expanded national reach and ethnic diversity.
27. Also see Cherise A. Pollard, "Are We the 'Future Americans'?: Charles Chesnutt Anticipates a Postracial American Society," in *Postracial America?: An Interdisciplinary Study*, ed. Vincent L. Stephens and Anthony Stewart (Bucknell University Press, 2017), 112. Contemporary critic SallyAnn H. Ferguson is critical of the fact that in Chesnutt's view of a color-blind future, America would be white. SallyAnn H. Ferguson, "Chesnutt's Genuine Blacks and Future Americans," *Melus* 15, no. 3 (1988): 116.
28. Chesnutt believed that race was biological and socially constructed. "I use the word 'race' . . . in its popular sense—that of a people who look substantially alike, and are moulded by the same culture and dominated by the same ideals." Chesnutt, "The Future American: What the Race Is Likely to Become in the Process of Time," 123.
29. Chesnutt, "The Future American: What the Race Is Likely to Become in the Process of Time," 125.
30. Chesnutt, "The Future American: What the Race Is Likely to Become in the Process of Time," 122. Although he did not outline the undesirable traits of Black people in the articles, he did illuminate some desirable traits of Black people. From the narrator's omniscient point of view, Chesnutt proclaims in *The Marrow of Tradition* that the virtues of Blacks are their resiliency in the face of great wrongs, their ability to continue to outlast other races, and their "cheerfulness of spirit": "Was it not, after all, a wise provision of nature that had given to a race, destined to a long servitude and a slow emergence therefrom, a cheerfulness of spirit which enabled them to catch pleasure on the wing, and endure with equanimity the ills that seemed inevitable? The ability to live and thrive under adverse circumstances is the surest guaranty of the future. The race which at the last shall inherit the earth—the residuary legatee of civilization—will be the race which remains longest upon it. The negro was here before the Anglo-Saxon was evolved, and his thick lips and heavy-lidded eyes looked out from the inscrutable face of the Sphinx across the sands of Egypt while yet the ancestors of those who now oppress him were living in caves, practicing human sacrifice, and painting themselves with woad—and the negro is here yet." Chesnutt, *The Marrow of Tradition*, 61–62.
31. Chesnutt, "The Future American: A Complete Race-Amalgamation Likely to Occur," 135.
32. Although much has been written about Chesnutt's white audience, Tyrie Smith argues that Chesnutt's message to Black people in works such as *The Conjure Woman* is to "abandon their old folkways and, instead, work towards joining the ranks of the educated class." Tyrie Smith, " 'Your People Will Never Rise in the World': Chesnutt's Message to a Black Readership," in *Charles Chesnutt Reappraised: Essays on the First Major African American Fiction Writer*, ed. David Garrett Izzo and Maria Orban (McFarland, 2009), 113.
33. Chesnutt, "The Future American: A Complete Race-Amalgamation Likely to Occur," 133.
34. Dean McWilliams, *Charles W. Chesnutt and the Fictions of Race* (University of Georgia Press, 2002), 56.
35. Charles W. Chesnutt, "The Goophered Grapevine," in *The Conjure Woman* (Houghton, Mifflin, 1900), 9.

36. Charles W. Chesnutt, *Stories, Novels, and Essays* (Library of America, 2002), 722.
37. Several "mad" characters exist in Chesnutt's fiction. Tenie in "Po' Sandy" went "mad" as a result of her lover being killed. Dave in "Dave's Neckliss" went "mad" and committed suicide after harsh and degrading punishment by a slave master. Tom in "The Sheriff's Children" appeared to be "mad" as a result of being estranged from his father and former slave master. Rena in *The House Behind the Cedars* went "mad" because she could not reconcile her biracial identity. Slaveholder Malcolm in "The Colonel's Dream" went "mad" because he could not access his family wealth. Viney in "The Colonel's Dream" went "mad" and "mute" after she was beaten by an overseer. Viney in "The Dumb Witness" feigned madness until her treacherous master died. Josh's mother, "Silly Milly," in *The Marrow of Tradition*, went "mad" as a result of witnessing her husband's lynching, which I discuss in this chapter. More than merely including "mad" characters, *The Conjure Woman* forces readers to consider how Conjure was a mechanism for mental, physical, and social well-being for individuals and communities. More research needs to be done on mental disability in both Chesnutt's works broadly and the fiction of his contemporaries, including Paul Lawrence Dunbar, Sutton Griggs, Frances Watkins Harper, and Booker T. Washington, in which issues of mental disability, medical authority, and medical exploitation are prominent themes.
38. Chesnutt, *The Conjure Woman*, 59.
39. Chesnutt, *The Conjure Woman*, 72.
40. Chesnutt, *The Conjure Woman*, 17, 72, 82.
41. Chesnutt, *The Conjure Woman*, 100.
42. For another nineteenth-century fictional account of the race massacre, see Jack Thorne [David Bryant Fulton], *Hanover; or, the Persecution of the Lowly: A Story of the Wilmington Massacre* (M. C. L. Hill, 1901). For a discussion of the differences in Thorne and Chesnutt's account, see Linda Belau and Ed Cameron, "Charles W. Chesnutt, Jack Thorne and the African American Literary Response to the 1898 Wilmington Race Riot," in *Charles Chesnutt Reappraised: Essays on the First Major African American Fiction Writer*, ed. David Garrett Izzo and Maria Orban (McFarland, 2009).
43. Timothy B. Tyson and David S. Cecelski, eds., *Democracy Betrayed: The Wilmington Race Riot of 1898 and Its Legacy* (University of North Carolina Press, 1998).
44. During and after Reconstruction, Blacks made a concerted effort to create free and universal modern schools comparable to those in the North for Blacks throughout the South. Although the lion's share of their success depended on their sheer willpower and efforts, they did get support from white allies, including the Freedmen's Bureau, northern philanthropic organizations, and other white groups. Blacks were pushed out of the current Republican party gradually. See Boris Heersink and Jeffery A. Jenkins, *Republican Party Politics and the American South, 1865–1968* (Cambridge University Press, 2020).
45. "White Supremacy: Col. A. M. Waddell Addressed a Large Audience at the Opera House on Issues of the Campaign," *Morning Star* 63, no. 26, October 25, 1898. Waddell carried out his campaign; he, along with others, killed over three hundred Blacks, destroyed their property and businesses, and conducted the only successful coup d'état in US history. For more on him, see Edward McCrady, Jr. and Samuel A. Ashe, *Cyclopedia of*

Eminent and Representative Men of the Carolinas of the Nineteenth Century, Vol. 2 (Brant & Fuller, 1892); Cecelski and Tyson, eds., *Democracy Betrayed;* James M. Clifton, "Alfred Moore Waddell," in *Dictionary of North Carolina Biography*, Vol. 6, T–Z, ed. William S. Powell (University of North Carolina Press, 1996), 102–3; Jerome Dowd, *Sketches of Prominent Living North Carolinians* (Edwards & Broughton, 1888); H. Leon Prather Sr., *We Have Taken a City: Wilmington Racial Massacre and Coup of 1898* (Farleigh Dickinson University Press, 1984); Alfred Moore Waddell, *Some Memories of My Life* (Edwards & Broughton, 1908).

46. In addition to depicting the Wilmington massacre and coup, Chesnutt depicted aspects of "real life." Black doctors and by extension Black people made extraordinary efforts to care for their health, which they saw as a means of controlling their own bodies, a right they lacked as enslaved people.
47. Matthew Wilson, *Whiteness in the Novels of Charles W. Chesnutt* (University Press of Mississippi, 2004), 99.
48. Mary Eliza Church Terrell, *A Colored Woman in a White World* (Ransdell, 1940), 245. Black club woman Victoria Earle Matthews argued that creating "race literature" was key for developing ideas derived from the Black experience about timeless concepts such as heroism, womanhood, and religion. She, like leaders such as W. E. B. Du Bois, believed their ability to add to the story of civilization proved their own humanity and put them on par with all other nationalities and racial groups. They also believed that a race literature could correct American views on Blacks as a racial group and bring about a change in white thinking about Blacks.
49. Victoria Earle Matthews, "The Value of Race Literature: An Address Delivered at the First Congress of Colored Women of the United States, at Boston, Mass.," July 30, 1895, 9.
50. White newspapers at the time called it a "riot," terminology that stood for decades.
51. Daniel R. Biddle, "The Wilmington Massacre of 1898," *Equal Justice Initiative*, November 10, 2023.
52. Chesnutt, *The Marrow of Tradition*, 274–75.
53. Chesnutt, *The Marrow of Tradition*, 275–76.
54. For historical descriptions of Black responses to white vigilante violence in the post–Civil War period, see Kidada E. Williams, "The Wounds That Cried Out: Reckoning with African Americans' Testimonies of Trauma and Suffering from Night Riding," in *The World the Civil War Made*, ed. Kate Masur and Gregory P. Downs (University of North Carolina Press, 2015).
55. Chesnutt, *The Marrow of Tradition*, 111, 112, 294.
56. Chesnutt, *The Marrow of Tradition*, 25. Major Carteret's assertion that Black people as a group are deficient and made for servitude echoes similar early nineteenth-century medical and psychiatric proclamations. See chapters 1 and 2.
57. Chesnutt, *The Marrow of Tradition*, 79. (They were mutually informative. We see psychiatric ideas being reproduced in Black and white newspapers and then popular racist ideas being recapitulated by psychiatrists.)
58. Characterization is the representation of characters (persons, creatures, or other beings) in narrative and dramatic works. This representation may include direct methods, such as the attribution of qualities in description or commentary, and indirect (or "dramatic")

methods, which invite readers to infer qualities from characters' actions, dialogue, or appearance. Such a personage is called a "character."

59. Chesnutt, *The Marrow of Tradition*, 13, 25. Delamere's attitude toward Black Americans has an air of paternalism; still, he is a benevolent employer and sympathetic toward his Black workers. Delamere defends his servant Sandy's honor when he is in danger of being lynched for a crime he did not commit. Mr. Delamere's devious and morally bankrupt grandson Tom Delamere frames Sandy for the robbery and murder of Olivia Carteret's aunt, Polly Ochiltree. After investigating the matter, Delamere discovers that Tom disguised himself as the servant and planted evidence, gold, and an Ochiltree purse on the unaware Sandy. Mr. Delamere succeeds in establishing Sandy's innocence by offering himself as Sandy's alibi. Although he finds the false allegation dishonorable, he agrees to this course of action as a pact with Major Carteret to exonerate Sandy without implicating the true killer, his own grandson. He agrees to this to appease Major Carteret, who is intent on preserving the reputation of a respected white Wellington family.

60. Chesnutt, *The Marrow of Tradition*, 25.
61. Chesnutt, *The Marrow of Tradition*, 52.
62. For historical discussions on the relationships between white and Black doctors, see Thomas J. Ward Jr., *Black Physicians in the Jim Crow South* (University of Arkansas Press, 2003).
63. Chesnutt, *The Marrow of Tradition*, 65.
64. Psychiatry and medicine shared an emphasis on observing medical cases and publishing about them.
65. Dr. Burns is the first white man who comes under Black authority in the novel.
66. Several historical newspapers such as *Raleigh News* and *Observer* and Wilmington's *Morning Star* blamed the Black community for the horrific events and justified white violence against Blacks as necessary for political change and the restoration of white dominance. In addition to biased newspaper accounts, white nationalists also penned creative interpretations of the events, most notably Thomas Dixon Jr.'s *The Leopard's Spots: A Romance of the White Man's Burden—1865–1900*. Dixon was a widely popular speaker, preacher, lawyer, legislator, and writer. *The Leopard's Spots* presents a portrait of the South in which whites were the victims of injustice at the hands of northern whites and socially mobile Blacks. It promulgated the view that if Blacks gained political rights, it would lead to racial mixing, which Dixon saw as catastrophic. *The Leopard's Spots*, along with his novels *The Clansman* and *The Traitor*, was part of a trilogy. *The Clansman* was later adapted into the infamous film *The Birth of a Nation*, directed by David Wark Griffith, which romanticized slavery as a benevolent institution in which enslaved people were happy and which crystalized a sympathetic take on the rise of the Ku Klux Klan. In addition to Chesnutt, other Black citizens published corrective accounts of the events of November 10, 1898, including J. Allen Kirk, *A Statement of Facts Concerning the Bloody Riot in Wilmington, N.C. of Interest to Every Citizen of the United States* (Wilmington, NC, 1898).
67. A foil is a character who contrasts with another character, typically the protagonist, to better highlight or differentiate certain qualities of the protagonist. A foil to the protagonist may also be the antagonist of the plot. Peter Auger, *The Anthem Dictionary of Literary*

Terms and Theory (Anthem, 2010), 114. Thomas F. Gieryn places use of literary foils into three categories, which Tamara A. P. Metze explains as those that emphasize the *heightened contrast* (this is different because . . .), those that operate by *exclusion* (this is not X because . . .), and those that assign *blame* ("due to the slow decision-making procedures of government . . ."). Tamara Antoine Pauline Metze, *Innovation Ltd.: Boundary Work in Deliberative Governance in Land Use Planning* (Eburon Uitgeverij B.V., 2010), 62. Feminist scholarship has considered the sisters Janet and Olivia as foils for each other. Samina Najmi, "Janet, Polly, and Olivia: Constructs of Blackness and White Femininity in Charles Chesnutt's *The Marrow of Tradition*," *Southern Literary Journal* 32, no. 1 (1999): 1–19.

68. Chesnutt, *The Marrow of Tradition*, 37.
69. The modern concept of inheritance as in large part a product of genetic makeup and biological processes of transmission did not emerge until the early twentieth century. In the mid-nineteenth century, Gregor Mendel's experiments on cross-pollination of plants gave him a sense that genetic traits might comprise distinct units, but he was unaware of the chemical makeup of genes. This experimental model of discovering genetic inheritance was not replicated in the field of psychiatry. Starting in the late eighteenth century, psychiatrists across Europe and North America relied on observation and logical speculation about massive data on family histories to ascertain that certain mental health conditions, criminality, and mental traits seemed to reoccur. Heavily relying on their statistical evidence, psychiatrists were steadfast in the idea that people had hereditary predispositions to mental illness. Theodore M. Porter, *Genetics in the Madhouse: The Unknown History of Human Heredity* (Princeton University Press, 2018).
70. Koritha Mitchell, *Living with Lynching: African American Lynching Plays, Performance, and Citizenship, 1890–1930* (University of Illinois Press, 2011). Mitchell argues that Black plays looked more at the ways in which lynch mobs "mutilated black households, not just black bodies" and that Black-authored stories of lynching were not places in which the violent acts themselves were the featured content, but rather the plays honed in on how the familial and communal bonds of ordinary individuals were torn apart. Mitchell, *Living with Lynching*, 3. She argues that lynching plays offered a source of communal solace and a mechanism for survival in the midst of tragedy.
71. Chesnutt, *The Marrow of Tradition*, 324.
72. The women shared a white father, Samuel Merkell. Mrs. Carteret's mother, Elizabeth Merkell, was the white woman he married, whereas Janet's mother, Julia, was the servant he took up with after Elizabeth died. Samuel Merkell married Julia and, on his deathbed, left his fortune to his formerly enslaved wife. Elizabeth Merkell's sister, Polly Ochiltree, who was aware of the marriage, stole the license and expelled Julia from the estate, asserting that no one would believe the marriage between a wealthy southern gentleman and Black servant was legitimate. Polly Ochiltree successfully concealed the marriage and robbed Julia and Janet of their share of Merkell's estate.
73. Chesnutt, *The Marrow of Tradition*, 323, 324.
74. Chesnutt, *The Marrow of Tradition*, 325–6.
75. Chesnutt, *The Marrow of Tradition*, 10. To ward against misfortune, Mammy Jane put her faith in a conjure woman who gave her a charm that she then buried in the backyard.

76. Chesnutt, *The Marrow of Tradition*, 40.
77. Chesnutt, *The Marrow of Tradition*, 276.
78. Chesnutt, *The Marrow of Tradition*, 234.
79. Chesnutt, *The Marrow of Tradition*, 329.

CODA

1. My question is tied to the idea in Black feminist criticism that Black women are read according to longstanding archetypes of Black femininity, most notably the figures of the Mammy, Jezebel, Sapphire, Welfare Queen, and Crazy Bitch. See Patricia Hill Collins, *Black Feminist Thought: Knowledge, Consciousness, and the Politics of Empowerment* (Routledge, 2008); Kimberly Wallace-Sanders, *Mammy: A Century of Race, Gender, and Southern Memory* (University of Michigan Press, 2008); Joan Morgan, *When Chicken-Heads Come Home to Roost: My Life as a Hip-Hop Feminist* (Simon & Schuster, 1999); Diana Martha Louis, "Bitch You Must Be Crazy: Representations of Mental Illness in Ntozake Shange's *For Colored Girls Who Have Considered Suicide / When the Rainbow Is Enuf* (1976)," *Western Journal of Black Studies* 37, no. 3 (2013): 197–211.

2. For historical studies of Black healing ways, see Zora Neale Hurston, *Mules and Men* (Perennial Library, 1990); Sharla Fett, *Working Cures: Healing, Health, and Power on Southern Slave Plantations* (University of North Carolina Press, 2002); Londa Schiebinger, *Secret Cures of Slaves: People, Plants, and Medicine in the Eighteenth-Century Atlantic World* (Stanford University Press, 2017); Alexis Wells-Oghoghomeh, *The Souls of Womenfolk: The Religious Cultures of Enslaved Women in the Lower South* (University of North Carolina Press, 2021).

3. Research in the history of race and medicine that outlines histories of harm and precarity of Black health in America is vast. A few sources include Daina Ramey Berry, *The Price for Their Pound of Flesh: The Value of the Enslaved, from Womb to Grave, in the Building of a Nation* (Beacon, 2017); Deirdre Benia Cooper Owens, *Medical Bondage: Race, Gender, and the Origins of American Gynecology* (University of Georgia Press, 2017); Rana A. Hogarth, *Medicalizing Blackness: Making Racial Difference in the Atlantic World, 1780–1840* (University of North Carolina Press, 2017); Harriet A. Washington, *Medical Apartheid: The Dark History of Medical Experimentation on Black Americans from Colonial Times to the Present* (Doubleday, 2006); Susan L. Smith, *Sick and Tired of Being Sick and Tired: Black Women's Health Activism in America, 1890–1950* (University of Pennsylvania Press, 1995); Jim Downs, *Sick from Freedom: African-American Illness and Suffering During the Civil War and Reconstruction* (Oxford University Press, 2012).

4. Bettina Judd, "In 2006 I Had an Ordeal with Medicine," in *Patient* (Black Lawrence, 2014), 1.

5. Black feminist literature is vast and growing. A few key works include Akasha Gloria Hull, Patricia Bell-Scott, and Barbara Smith, eds., *All the Women Are White, All the Blacks Are Men, but Some of Us Are Brave: Black Women's Studies* (Feminist, 1982); bell hooks, *Ain't I a Woman: Black Women and Feminism* (Taylor and Francis, 2014); Deborah E. McDowell, "New Directions for Black Feminist Criticism," *Black American Literature*

Forum 14, no. 4 (1980): 153–59; Beverly Guy-Sheftall, ed., *Words of Fire: An Anthology of African-American Feminist Thought* (New Press, 1995); Audre Lorde, *Sister Outsider: Essays and Speeches* (Crossing Press, 2007); Tricia Hersey, *Rest Is Resistance: A Manifesto* (Little Brown, 2022); Bettina Judd, *Feelin: Creative Practice, Pleasure, and Black Feminist Thought* (Northwestern University Press, 2023); Candice Marie Benbow, *Red Lip Theology: For Church Girls Who've Considered Tithing to the Beauty Supply Store When Sunday Morning Isn't Enough* (Convergent, 2022); Alice Walker, *In Search of Our Mothers' Gardens: Womanist Prose* (Harcourt Brace Jovanovich, 1983); Ula Y. Taylor, "Making Waves: The Theory and Practice of Black Feminism," *Black Scholar* 28, no. 2 (Summer 1998): 18–28; Ula Y. Taylor, "The Historical Evolution of Black Feminist Theory and Praxis," *Journal of Black Studies* 29, no. 2 (November 1998): 234–53; Christina Sharpe, *In the Wake: On Blackness and Being* (Duke University Press, 2016); Kimberle Crenshaw, "Demarginalizing the Intersection of Race and Sex: A Black Feminist Critique of Antidiscrimination Doctrine, Feminist Theory and Antiracist Politics," *University of Chicago Legal Forum*, no. 1, article 8 (1989): 139–67; Katherine McKittrick, *Demonic Grounds: Black Women and Cartographies of Struggle* (University of Minnesota Press, 2006); Jennifer Nash, *The Black Body in Ecstasy: Reading Race, Reading Pornography* (Duke University Press, 2014).

6. Alexis Pauline Gumbs, *Spill: Scenes of Black Feminist Fugitivity* (Duke University Press, 2016); Ntozake Shange, *For Colored Girls Who Have Considered Suicide / When the Rainbow Is Enuf* (Scribner, 1976); Audre Lorde, *Zami: A New Spelling of My Name—A Biomythography* (Crossing, 1982).
7. Lorde, *Sister Outsider*, 112.
8. Brittney C. Cooper, *Beyond Respectability: The Intellectual Thought of Race Women* (University of Illinois Press, 2017), 9.
9. Michel Foucault, *Discipline and Punish: The Birth of the Prison*, trans. Alan Sheridan (Random House, 1977); Michel Foucault, *Madness and Civilization: A History of Insanity in the Age of Reason*, trans. Richard Howard (Random House, 1965).
10. Ellen Samuels, *Fantasies of Identification: Disability, Gender, Race* (New York University Press, 2014).
11. Recent works that exemplify this practice are Tiya Miles, *All That She Carried: The Journey of Ashley's Sack, a Black Family Keepsake* (Random House, 2021); and Saidiya V. Hartman, *Wayward Lives, Beautiful Experiments: Intimate Histories of Riotous Girls, Troublesome Women, and Queer Radicals* (Norton, 2019).
12. Saidiya Hartman's *Wayward Lives* is one of the best examples of speculative imagining of people who appear one-dimensionally in official documents. It is telling that at times it has the rigor of scholarship and the quality of creative fiction.
13. Some scholars have found particular genres of Black women's literature to be useful in their imaginings of new worlds, especially speculative fiction. I argue here that nineteenth-century genres are also ripe for new visions of Blackness, gender, and sexuality; this has been and should continue to be extended to include mental disability. Therí Pickens, *Black Madness :: Mad Blackness* (Duke University Press, 2019); Samantha Dawn Schalk, *Bodyminds Reimaged: (Dis)ability, Race, and Gender in Black Women's Speculative Fiction* (Duke University Press, 2018); Susana M. Morris, "Black Girls Are from the Future:

Afrofuturist Feminism in Octavia E. Butler's *Fledgling*," *Women's Studies Quarterly* 40, no. 3/4 (Fall/Winter 2012): 146–66.

14. Barbara Christian, "The Race for Theory," *Cultural Critique*, no. 6 (Spring 1987): 51–63.
15. Pickens, *Black Madness*, x.
16. Theophilus O. Powell, "The Increase of Insanity and Tuberculosis in the Southern Negro Since 1860, and Its Alliance, and Some of the Supposed Causes," *Journal of the American Medical Association* 27, no. 23 (December 1896): 1185–88; Thomas McKie, "A Brief History of Insanity and Tuberculosis in the Southern Negro," *Journal of the American Medical Association* 28, no. 12 (March 1897): 537–38; Thomas J. Mays, "Human Slavery as a Prevention of Pulmonary Consumption," in *Germs Have No Color Lines: Blacks and American Medicine, 1900-1940*, ed. Vanessa Northington Gamble (Garland, 1989), 6–11; William Frances Drewry, "History of the Central State Hospital of Virginia," in *Annual Reports of Officers, Boards, and Institutions of the Commonwealth of Virginia* (J. H. O'Bannon, 1904).
17. Other Black doctors pushed racist medical theories about insanity to their logical ends to subvert ideas about Black inferiority. John E. Hunter, "Tuberculosis in the Negro: Causes and Treatment," in *Germs Have No Color Line*, ed. Gamble, 12–19; E. Mayfield Boyle, "The Negro and Tuberculosis," in *Germs Have No Color Line*, ed. Gamble, 45; E. T. Easley, "The Sanitary Condition of the Negro," *American Weekly* 3 (July 31, 1875): 49–50.
18. Richard K. Scotch, "Medical Model of Disability," in *Encyclopedia of American Disability History*, ed. Susan Burch (Facts on File, 2009); Eli Clare, *Brilliant Imperfection: Grappling with Cure* (Duke University Press, 2017); Kim E. Nielsen, *A Disability History of the United States* (Beacon, 2012); Robert J. Menzies, Geoffrey Reaume, and Brenda A. LeFrançois, eds., *Mad Matters: A Critical Reader in Canadian Mad Studies* (Canadian Scholars' Press, 2013).

BIBLIOGRAPHY

Adams, Samuel Hopkins. *Grandfather Stories*. Random House, 1955.
Aggarwal, Neil Krishan. "The Legacy of James McCune Smith, MD—the First US Black Physician." *Journal of the American Medical Association* 326, no. 22 (2021): 2245–46.
Allen, Theodore W. *The Invention of the White Race*. Vol. 2: *The Origin of Racial Oppression in Anglo-America*. Verso, 1997.
Andrews, William L. *The Literary Career of Charles W. Chesnutt*. Louisiana State University Press, 1980.
Andrews, William L. *Sisters of the Spirit: Three Black Women's Autobiographies of the Nineteenth Century*. Indiana University Press, 1986.
Andrews, William L. *To Tell a Free Story: The First Century of Afro-American Autobiography, 1760–1865*. University of Illinois Press, 1986.
Andrews, William L. "William Dean Howells and Charles W. Chesnutt: Criticism and Race Fiction in the Age of Booker T. Washington." *American Literature* 48, no. 3 (1976): 327–39.
Asch, Adrienne. "Recognizing Death While Affirming Life: Can End of Life Reform Uphold a Disabled Person's Interest in Continued Life?" *Hastings Center Report* 35, no. 7 (2005): S31–36.
Ashton, Susanna, and Bill Hardwig, eds. *Approaches to Teaching the Works of Charles W. Chesnutt*. Modern Language Association, 2017.
Atlanta Constitution. "In the Local Field." July 14, 1894.
Atlanta Constitution. "In the Local Field." July 18, 1894.
Atlanta Constitution. "The Lunatic Asylum: Dr. Powell, the Superintendent, Is in Atlanta with His Annual Statement." November 16, 1889.
Atlanta Constitution. "Sent to the Lunatic Asylum: Ordinary Calhoun and a Jury Hear Two Lunacy Cases." July 4, 1888.
Auburn Citizen. "Harriet Tubman Is Dead." March 11, 1913.

Auger, Peter. *The Anthem Dictionary of Literary Terms and Theory*. Anthem, 2010.
Baker, John Haydn. *Browning and Wordsworth*. Associated University Presses, 2004.
Ballantyne, David T. "Remembering the Colfax Massacre: Race, Sex, and the Meanings of Reconstruction Violence." *Journal of Southern History* 87, no. 3 (2021): 427–66.
Bannister, H. M., and Ludwig Hektoen. "Race and Insanity." *American Journal of Insanity* 44, no. 4 (April 1888): 455–70. https://doi.org/10.1176/ajp.1888.44.4.455.
Barclay, Jenifer. *The Mark of Slavery: Disability, Race, and Gender in Antebellum America*. University of Illinois Press, 2021.
Bayer, Ronald. *Homosexuality and American Psychiatry*. Princeton University Press, 1987.
Baynton, Douglas. "Slaves, Immigrants, and Suffragists: The Uses of Disability in Citizenship Debates." *PMLA* 120, no. 2 (2005): 562–67.
Belau, Linda, and Ed Cameron. "Charles W. Chesnutt, Jack Throne and the African American Literary Response to the 1898 Wilmington Race Riot." In *Charles Chesnutt Reappraised: Essays on the First Major African American Fiction Writer*, ed. David Garrett Izzo and Maria Orban. McFarland, 2009.
Bell, Christopher. "Is Disability Studies Actually White Disability Studies?" In *The Disability Studies Reader*, ed. Lennard Davis. Routledge, 1997.
Bell, Leland. *Treating the Mentally Ill: From Colonial Times to the Present*. Praeger, 1980.
Benbow, Candice Marie. *Red Lip Theology: For Church Girls Who've Considered Tithing to the Beauty Supply Store When Sunday Morning Isn't Enough*. Convergent, 2022.
Berlin, Ira. *The Making of African America: The Four Great Migrations*. Viking Adult, 2010.
Berlin, Ira. *Many Thousands Gone: The First Two Centuries of Slavery in North America*. Belknap, 1998.
Bernstein, Robin. *Freeman's Challenge: The Murder That Shook America's Original Prison for Profit*. University of Chicago Press, 2024.
Berry, Daina Ramey. *The Price for Their Pound of Flesh: The Value of the Enslaved, from Womb to Grave, in the Building of a Nation*. Beacon, 2017.
Berry, Sarah L. "'[No] Doctor but My Master': Health Reform and Antislavery Rhetoric in Harriet Jacobs's Incidents in the Life of a Slave Girl." *Journal of Medical Humanities* 35, no. 1 (2014): 1–18.
Bibb, Henry. *Narrative of the Life and Adventures of Henry Bibb, an American Slave, Written by Himself*. Published by the Author, 1849. From Documenting the American South, University Library, the University of North Carolina at Chapel Hill, 2000. https://docsouth.unc.edu/neh/bibb/bibb.html.
Biddle, Daniel R. "The Wilmington Massacre of 1898." *Equal Justice Initiative* (blog), November 10, 2024. https://eji.org/news/wilmington-massacre-of-1898/.
Bittel, Carla. "Testing the Truth of Phrenology: Knowledge Experiments in Antebellum American Cultures of Science and Health." *Medical History* 63, no. 3 (2019): 352–74. https://doi.org/10.1017/mdh.2019.31.
Blassingame, John W. *The Slave Community: Plantation Life in the Antebellum South*. Revised ed. Oxford University Press, 1979.
Blassingame, John W. "Using the Testimony of Ex-Slaves: Approaches and Problems." *Journal of Southern History* 41, no. 4 (1975): 473–92. https://doi.org/10.2307/2205559.

Blight, David W. "In Search of Learning, Liberty, and Self Definition: James McCune Smith and the Ordeal of the Antebellum Black Intellectual." *Afro-Americans in New York Life and History* 9, no. 2 (1985): 7–26.
Bockoven, J. Sanbourne. *Moral Treatment in American Psychiatry*. Springer, 1963.
Boster, Dea H. *African American Slavery and Disability: Bodies, Property and Power in the Antebellum South, 1800–1860*. Routledge, 2013.
Boster, Dea H. "An 'Epeleptick' Bondswoman: Fits, Slavery, and Power in the Antebellum South." *Bulletin of the History of Medicine* 83, no. 2 (2009): 271–301. https://doi.org/10.1353/bhm.0.0206.
Boughton, Willis. "The Negro's Place in History." *The Arena (1889–1909)*, September 1896.
Boyle, E. Mayfield. "The Negro and Tuberculosis." In *Germs Have No Color Lines: Blacks and American Medicine, 1900–1940*, ed. Vanessa Northington Gamble. Garland, 1989.
Bradford, Sarah H. *Harriet, the Moses of Her People*. Geo. R. Lockwood & Son, 1886. From Documenting the American South, University Library, the University of North Carolina at Chapel Hill, 1995. https://docsouth.unc.edu/neh/harriet/harriet.html.
Bradford, Sarah H. *Scenes in the Life of Harriet Tubman*. W. J. Moses, Printer, 1869. From Documenting the American South, University Library, the University of North Carolina at Chapel Hill, 2000. https://docsouth.unc.edu/neh/bradford/bradford.html.
Branson, Susan. "Phrenology and the Science of Race in Antebellum America." *Early American Studies* 15, no. 1 (2017): 164–93. https://doi.org/10.1353/eam.2017.0005.
Brawley, Benjamin. *Paul Laurence Dunbar, Poet of His People*. University of North Carolina Press, 1936.
Brigham, Amariah. "Definition of Insanity—Nature of the Disease." *American Journal of Psychiatry* 151, no. 6 (1994): 97–102. https://doi.org/10.1176/ajp.151.6.97.
Brigham, Amariah. *An Inquiry Concerning the Diseases and Functions of the Brain, the Spinal Cord, and the Nerves*. Elihu Geer, 1840.
Brigham, Amariah. "Millerism." *American Journal of Insanity* 1 (1845): 249–53.
Brigham, Amariah. *Observations on the Influence of Religion Upon the Health and Physical Welfare of Mankind*. Marsh, Capen & Lyon, 1835.
Brigham, Amariah. *Remarks on the Influence of Mental Cultivation and Mental Excitement Upon Health*. Lea & Blanchard, 1845.
Brown, John. *Slave Life in Georgia: A Narrative of the Life, Sufferings, and Escape of John Brown, a Fugitive Slave, Now in England*, ed. L. A. Chamerovzow. London, 1855. From Documenting the American South, University Library, the University of North Carolina at Chapel Hill, 2001. https://docsouth.unc.edu/neh/jbrown/jbrown.html.
Brown, Thomas E. "Dance of the Dialectic? Some Reflections (Polemic and Otherwise) on the Present State of Nineteenth-Century Asylum Studies." *Canadian Bulletin of Medical History* 11, no. 2 (1994): 267–95.
Brown, William Wells. *Narrative of William W. Brown, A Fugitive Slave. Written by Himself*. Anti-Slavery Office, 1847. From Documenting the American South, University Library, the University of North Carolina at Chapel Hill, 2001. https://docsouth.unc.edu/neh/brown47/brown47.html.
Bruce, La Marr Jurelle. *How to Go Mad Without Losing Your Mind: Madness and Black Radical Creativity*. Duke University Press, 2021.

Bruce, Philip A. *The Plantation Negro as a Freeman: Observations on His Character, Condition, and Prospects in Virginia*. G. P. Putnam's Sons, the Knickerbocker Press, 1889.

Burch, Susan. *Committed: Remembering Native Kinship in and Beyond Institutions*. University of North Carolina Press, 2021.

Burnett, Williams. "On the Effects Produced by Poisonous Fish on the Human Frame." *Southern Medical and Surgical Journal* 2, no. 12 (December 1846): 730–31.

Byron, George Gordon. *The Lament of Tasso*. John Murray, Albemarle-Street, 1817.

Cady, Edwin. *The Realist at War: The Mature Years, 1885–1920, of William Dean Howells*. Syracuse University Press, 1958.

Caldwell, Charles. *Elements of Phrenology*. 2nd ed. A.G. Meriwether, 1827.

Calhoun, John C. *The Works of John C. Calhoun*, ed. Richard Cralle. 6 vols. New York, 1863.

Campbell, Karlyn Kohrs. "Style and Content in the Rhetoric of Early Afro-American Feminists." *Quarterly Journal of Speech* 72, no. 4 (1986): 434–45. https://doi.org/10.1080/00335638609383786.

Carden, Art, and Christopher J. Coyne. "The Political Economy of the Reconstruction Era's Race Riots." *Public Choice* 157, no. 1–2 (2013): 57–71. https://doi.org/10.1007/s11127-012-9955-7.

Carlisle, Linda V. *Elizabeth Packard: A Noble Fight*. University of Illinois Press, 2010.

Carlson, Eric, and Norman Dain. "The Psychotherapy That Was Moral Treatment." *American Journal of Psychiatry* 117, no. 6 (1960): 519–24. https://doi.org/10.1176/ajp.117.6.519.

Cartwright, Samuel A. "The Diseases of Negroes: Pulmonary Congestions, Pneumonia, & c." *De Bow's Review of the Southern and Western States* 11 (1851): 209–13.

Cartwright, Samuel A. "Dr. Cartwright on the Caucasians and the Africans." *De Bow's Review and Industrial Resources, Statistics, Etc.* 25 (1858): 45–56.

Cartwright, Samuel A. "Remarks on Dysentery Among Negroes." *New Orleans Medical and Surgical Journal* 11, no. 2 (September 1854): 145–63.

Cartwright, Samuel A. "Report on the Diseases and Physical Peculiarities of the Negro Race." *The New Orleans Medical and Surgical Journal* 7 (May 1851): 691–715.

Casey, H. R. "Contribution to the History of Typhoid Fever." *Southern Medical and Surgical Journal* 7, no. 12 (December 1851): 707–18.

Casper, Scott E. "Long Past Slavery: Representing Race in the Federal Writers' Project." *American Historical Review* 122, no. 5 (2017): 1642–43. https://doi.org/10.1093/ahr/122.5.1642.

Castel, Robert. "Moral Treatment: Mental Therapy and Social Control in the Nineteenth Century." In *Social Control and the State: Historical and Comparative Essays*, ed. Stanley Cohen and Andrew Scull, trans. Peter Miller. Robertson, 1983.

Cecelski, David S., and Timothy B. Tyson, eds. *Democracy Betrayed: The Wilmington Race Riot of 1898 and Its Legacy*. University of North Carolina Press, 1998.

Chakkalakal, Tess. *A Matter of Complexion: The Life and Fictions of Charles W. Chesnutt*. St. Martin's, 2025.

Chakrabarty, Dipesh. *Provincializing Europe: Postcolonial Thought and Historical Difference*. Princeton University Press, 2000.

Cheney, Edna Dow. "Moses." *Freedmen's Record* 1, no. 3 (March 1865): 34–38.

Chesler, Phyllis. *Women and Madness*. Doubleday, 1972.

Chesnutt, Charles W. *Charles W. Chesnutt: Essays and Speeches*, ed. Joseph R. McElrath, Robert C. Leitz, and Jesse S. Crisler. Stanford University Press, 1999.

Chesnutt, Charles W. *The Conjure Woman*. Houghton, Mifflin, 1900.

Chesnutt, Charles W. *An Exemplary Citizen: Letters of Charles W. Chesnutt, 1906–1932*, ed. Joseph R. McElrath Jr., Robert C. Leitz, and Jesse S. Crisler. Stanford University Press, 2002.

Chesnutt, Charles W. *The Marrow of Tradition*. Houghton, Mifflin, 1901.

Chireau, Yvonne P. *Black Magic: Religion and the African American Conjuring Tradition*. University of California Press, 2003. https://doi.org/10.1525/california/9780520209879.003.0002.

Chireau, Yvonne P. "Conjure and Christianity in the Nineteenth Century: Religious Elements in African American Magic." *Religion and American Culture: A Journal of Interpretation* 7, no. 2 (Summer 1997): 225–46.

Chireau, Yvonne P. "'Our Religion and Superstition Was All Mixed Up': Conjure, Christianity, and African American Supernatural Traditions." In *Black Magic: Religion and the African American Conjuring Tradition*. University of California Press, 2003. https://doi.org/10.1525 /california/9780520209879.003.0002.

Christian, Barbara. "The Race for Theory." *Cultural Critique*, no. 6 (1987): 51–63.

Christian, Barbara. "The Race for Theory." In *The Black Feminist Reader*, ed. Joy James and T. Denean Sharpley-Whiting. Blackwell, 2000.

Christian Recorder. "General Intelligence." June 9, 1866.

Clare, Eli. *Brilliant Imperfection: Grappling with Cure*. Duke University Press, 2017.

Clinton, Catherine. *Harriet Tubman: The Road to Freedom*. Little, Brown, 2004.

Collins, Patricia Hill. *Black Feminist Thought: Knowledge, Consciousness, and the Politics of Empowerment*. Routledge, 2008.

Colored American. "Anti Phrenology." October 14, 1837.

Colored American. "Colored Orphan's Asylum." January 26, 1839.

Colored American. "Dr. Smith." September 30, 1837.

Colored American. "Mr. George Combe's Lectures." May 18, 1839.

Colored American. "Multiple Classified Advertisements." November 18, 1837.

Colored American. "Multiple Classified Advertisements." March 2, 1839.

Colored American. "Phrenology." September 23, 1837.

Combe, George. *Notes on the United States of North America, During a Phrenological Visit in 1838-9-40*. Carey & Hart, 1841.

Combe, George. *A System of Phrenology*. 3rd Edinburgh ed. Benjamin B. Mussey, 1851.

Commonwealth. "Harriet Tubman." July 17, 1863.

Conrad, Earl. *Harriet Tubman: Negro Soldier and Abolitionist*. International, 1942.

Cooper, Brittney. *Beyond Respectability: The Intellectual Thought of Race Women*. University of Illinois Press, 2017.

Cooper Owens, Deirdre Benia. *Medical Bondage: Race, Gender, and the Origins of American Gynecology*. University of Georgia Press, 2017.

Cooter, Roger. *The Cultural Meaning of Popular Science: Phrenology and the Organization of Consent in Nineteenth-Century Britain*. Cambridge University Press, 1984.

Cox, David G. "Race, Reconstruction, and the Invention of 'Negro Superstition,' 1862–1877." *Journal of American Studies* 55, no. 5 (December 2021): 1125–52. https://doi.org/10.1017/S0021875820001723.

Coxe, John Redman. *The Philadelphia Medical Dictionary*. 2nd ed. Thomas Dobson and Son, 1817.

Crane, Jacob. "'Razed to the Knees': The Anti-Heroic Body in James McCune Smith's 'The Heads of Colored People.'" *African American Review* 51, no. 1 (2018): 7–21. https://doi.org/10.1353 /afa.2018.0001.

Cranford, Peter G., and Lois W. Lane. *Damnation Hospital*. Old Capital Press, 2009.

Creel, Margaret Washington. *A Peculiar People: Slave Religion and Community Culture Among the Gullahs*. New York University Press, 1988.

Crenshaw, Kimberle. "Demarginalizing the Intersection of Race and Sex: A Black Feminist Critique of Antidiscrimination Doctrine, Feminist Theory and Antiracist Politics." *University of Chicago Legal Forum*, no. 1, article 8 (1989): 139.

Crook, A. B. "A Case of Injury of the Head, with Inquiries and Reflections on Fungus Cerebri." *Southern Journal of Medicine and Pharmacy* 1, no. 5 (September 1846): 483–86. From Center for Research Libraries. https://dds.crl.edu/crldelivery/5570.

Crumpler, Rebecca Davis Lee. *A Book of Medical Discourses*. Cashman, Keating & Co., 1883.

Daily Constitution. "Yesterday's Arrests: Johnson's 83-An Insane Woman—Jackson Goes to Jail—Smith, the Vagrant—Stolen Jewelry—The Result of a Drunk." July 2, 1881.

Dain, Norman. *Concepts of Insanity in the United States, 1789–1865*. Rutgers University Press, 1964.

Dain, Norman. *Disordered Minds: The First Century of Eastern State Hospital in Williamsburg, Virginia 1766–1866*. Colonial Williamsburg Foundation, 1971.

Davis, Charles T., and Henry Louis Gates, Jr., eds. *The Slave's Narrative*. Oxford University Press, 1991.

Davis, John D. *Phrenology, Fad and Science: A Nineteenth-Century American Crusade*. Yale University Press, 1955.

Davis, Lennard J. "Constructing Normalcy." In *The Disability Studies Reader*, ed. Lennard J. Davis, 3rd ed. Routledge, 2010.

Davis, Lennard J. "Crips Strike Back: The Rise of Disability Studies." *American Literary History* 11, no. 3 (1999): 500–512.

Davis, Lennard J. *Enforcing Normalcy: Disability, Deafness, and the Body*. Verso, 1995.

De Cunzo, Lu Ann. "Reform, Respite, Ritual: An Archaeology of Institutions: The Magdalen Society of Philadelphia, 1800–1850." *Historical Archaeology* 29, no. 3 (1995): 1–168.

DeLatte, Carolyn E. "The St. Landry Riot: A Forgotten Incident of Reconstruction Violence." *Louisiana History: The Journal of the Louisiana Historical Association* 17, no. 1 (1976): 41–49.

"Deterioration of the American Negro." *Atlanta Journal-Record of Medicine* 5, no. 4 (1903): 287.

Dhejne, Cecilia, Roy Van Vlerken, Gunter Heylens, and Jon Arcelus. "Mental Health and Gender Dysphoria: A Review of the Literature." *International Review of Psychiatry* 28, no. 1 (2016): 44–57.

Dietrich, Alicia. "UT Scholar Tells Forgotten Story of African-American Psychiatric Patients." *Alcalde*, January 17, 2014.

Dix, Dorothea Lynde, and U.S. Congress, House, and Senate. *Memorial of D.L. Dix: Praying a Grant of Land for the Relief and Support of the Indigent Curable and Incurable Insane in the United States*. 30th Congress, 1st Session, Misc. No. 150. Tippin & Streeper, 1848.

Dixon, Jr., Thomas. *The Leopard's Spots; A Romance of the White Man's Burden–1865–1900*. A. Wessels, 1906.

Donaldson, Elizabeth J. "The Corpus of the Madwoman: Toward a Feminist Disability Studies Theory of Embodiment and Mental Illness." *NWSA* 14, no. 3 (2002): 99–119.

Donaldson, Elizabeth J. *Literatures of Madness: Disability Studies and Mental Health*. Springer, 2018.

Donaldson, Elizabeth J. "Revisiting the Corpus of the Madwoman: Further Notes Toward a Feminist Disability Studies Theory of Mental Illness." In *Feminist Disability Studies*, ed. Kim Hall. Indiana University Press, 2011.

Douglass, Frederick. *The Claims of the Negro, Ethnologically Considered: An Address Before the Literary Societies of Western Reserve College, At Commencement, July 12, 1854*. Lee, Mann & Co., 1854. https://www.loc.gov/resource/rbaapc.07900/.

Douglass, Frederick. "The Colored Insane." *Frederick Douglass' Paper*, April 1, 1852.

Douglass, Frederick. "Dr. James McCune Smith." *Douglass' Monthly*, March 1859.

Douglass, Frederick. *Life and Times of Frederick Douglass, Written by Himself*. New revised ed. De Wolfe & Fiske Co., 1892. From Documenting the American South, University Library, the University of North Carolina at Chapel Hill, 2001. https://docsouth.unc.edu/neh/dougl92/dougl92.html.

Douglass, Frederick. *Narrative of the Life of Frederick Douglass, an American Slave, Written by Himself*. Anti-Slavery Office, 1845. From Documenting the American South, University Library, the University of North Carolina at Chapel Hill, 1999. https://docsouth.unc.edu/fpn/jacobs/jacobs.html.

Dowbiggin, Ian Robert. *Keeping America Sane: Psychiatry and Eugenics in the United States and Canada, 1880–1940*. Cornell University Press, 1997.

Dowd, Jerome. *Sketches of Prominent Living North Carolinians*. Edwards & Broughton, 1888.

Downs, Jim. *Sick from Freedom: African-American Illness and Suffering During the Civil War and Reconstruction*. Oxford University Press, 2012.

Doyle, Dennis A. *Psychiatry and Racial Liberalism in Harlem, 1936–1968*. University of Rochester Press, 2016.

Drewry, William Frances. "History of the Central State Hospital of Virginia." *Annual Reports of Officers, Boards and Institutions of the Commonwealth of Virginia* (1904): 105–28.

Dunbar, Erica Armstrong. *She Came to Slay: The Life and Times of Harriet Tubman*. Simon & Schuster, Inc., 2019.

Duquette, Elizabeth. *American Tyrannies in the Long Age of Napoleon*. Oxford University Press, 2023.

Dwyer, Ellen. *Homes for the Mad: Life Inside Two Nineteenth-Century Asylums*. Rutgers University Press, 1987.

Earle, Pliny. "On the Causes of Insanity." *American Journal of Insanity* 4 (1848): 185–211.

Easley, E. T. "The Sanitary Condition of the Negro." *American Weekly* 3 (July 31, 1875): 49–50.

Edwards-Grossi, Élodie. *Mad with Freedom: The Political Economy of Blackness, Insanity, and Civil Rights in the U.S. South, 1840–1940*. Louisiana State University Press, 2022.

Eliot, T. S. *Selected Prose of T. S. Eliot*, ed. Frank Kermode. Harcourt Brace Jovanovich, 1975.

English, Daylanne K. *Unnatural Selections: Eugenics in American Modernism and the Harlem Renaissance*. University of North Carolina Press, 2004.

Equal Justice Initiative. "Reconstruction in America: Racial Violence After the Civil War, 1865–1976." 2020. https://eji.org/report/reconstruction-in-america/.

Erevelles, Nirmala. "Race." In *Keywords for Disability Studies*, ed. Rachel Adams, Benjamin Reiss, and David Serlin. New York University Press, 2015.

Ferguson, SallyAnn H. "Chesnutt's Genuine Blacks and Future Americans." *Melus* 15, no. 3 (1988): 109–19.

Fett, Sharla M. *Working Cures: Healing, Health, and Power on Southern Slave Plantations.* University of North Carolina Press, 2002.

Finkelman, Paul. *Defending Slavery: Proslavery Thought in the Old South: A Brief History with Documents.* Bedford/St. Martin's, 2003.

Fitch, Suzanne Pullon, and Roseann M. Mandziuk. "The Rhetorical Construction of Sojourner Truth." *Southern Communication Journal* 66, no. 2 (2001): 120–38. https://doi.org/10.1080/10417940109373192.

Fitch, Suzanne Pullon, and Roseann M. Mandziuk. *Sojourner Truth as Orator: Wit, Story, and Song.* Greenwood, 1997.

Fitzhugh, George. *Sociology for the South, or the Failure of Free Society.* A. Morris, 1854.

Fogel, Robert William. *Without Consent or Contract: The Rise and Fall of American Slavery.* Norton, 1989.

Foner, Eric. *The Fiery Trial: Abraham Lincoln and American Slavery.* Norton, 2011.

Forbes, Ella. *African American Women During the Civil War.* Routledge, 1998.

Forry, Samuel. "On the Relative Proportion of Centenarians, of Deaf and Dumb, of Blind, and of Insane, in the Races of European and African Origin, as Shown by the Censuses of the United States." *New York Journal of Medicine and the Collateral Sciences* 2, no. 6 (1844): 310–20.

Forry, Samuel. "Vital Statistics Furnished by the Sixth Census of the United States, Bearing Upon the Question of the Human Race." *New York Journal of Medicine and the Collateral Sciences* 1, no. 2 (1843): 151–67.

Forwood, W. S. "Serpent Worship Among the Negroes." *De Bow's Review: Agricultural, Commercial, Industrial Progress and Resources* 6, no. 1 (1861): 97–99.

Foster, Frances Smith. "A Narrative of the Interesting Origins and (Somewhat) Surprising Developments of African-American Print Culture." *American Literary History* 17, no. 4 (2005): 714–40.

Foster, Frances Smith. *Witnessing Slavery: The Development of Antebellum Slave Narratives.* Greenwood, 1979.

Foucault, Michel. *Discipline and Punish: The Birth of the Prison.* Trans. Alan Sheridan. Random House, 1977.

Foucault, Michel. *Madness and Civilization: A History of Insanity in the Age of Reason.* Trans. Richard Howard. Random House, 1965.

Foucault, Michel. *Psychiatric Power: Lectures at the Collège de France, 1973–1974*, ed. Jacques Lagrange. Palgrave Macmillan, 2006.

Fouille, M. Alfred. "Scientific Philanthropy." *Popular Science Monthly* 22 (February 1883): 521–35.

Frankel, Noralee. *Break Those Chains at Last: African Americans 1860–1880.* Oxford University Press, 1996.

Frazier, Ian. "When W. E. B. Du Bois Made a Laughingstock of a White Supremacist." *New Yorker*, August 19, 2019. https://www.newyorker.com/magazine/2019/08/26/when-w-e-b-du-bois-made-a-laughingstock-of-a-white-supremacist.

Fredrickson, George M., and American Council of Learned Societies. *The Black Image in the White Mind: The Debate on Afro-American Character and Destiny, 1817–1914.* Harper & Row, 1971.

Frey, Sylvia R. *Water from the Rock: Black Resistance in a Revolutionary Age.* Princeton University Press, 1991.

Frey, Sylvia R., and Betty Wood. *Come Shouting to Zion: African American Protestantism in the American South and British Caribbean to 1830.* University of North Carolina Press, 1998.

Galt, John Minson. "Asylums for Colored Persons." *American Psychological Journal* 1, no. 3 (1853): 78–88.

Garland-Thomson, Rosemarie. *Extraordinary Bodies: Figuring Physical Disability in American Culture and Literature.* Columbia University Press, 1997.

Garland-Thomson, Rosemarie. "Feminist Disability Studies." *Signs* 30, no. 2 (2005): 1557–87.

Geddings, E. "Case of Extraordinary Enlargement and Ossific Transformation of the Ovaria." *Southern Medical and Surgical Journal* 2, no. 10 (May 1838): 579–85.

Geller, Jeffrey. "Women's Accounts of Psychiatric Illness and Institutionalization." *Hospital and Community Psychiatry* 36, no. 10 (October 1985).

Geller, Jeffrey, and Maxine Harris. *Women of the Asylum: Voices from Behind the Walls, 1840–1945.* Anchor, 1994.

Genovese, Eugene D. *Roll, Jordan, Roll: The World the Slaves Made.* Vintage, 1976.

Georgia Lunatic Asylum. "Bi-Ennial Report of the Trustees of the Georgia Lunatic Asylum for the Fiscal Year from October 1, 1890, to September 1, 1894 [1890–94]." Richards & Shaver, 1894.

Georgia Lunatic Asylum. "Reports of the Trustees and Superintendent, Resident Physician and Other Officers, of the Lunatic Asylum of the State of Georgia from December 1st, 1877, to September 30th, 1879 [1877–79]." J W. Burke & Co., 1879.

Georgia Writers' Project. *Drums and Shadows: Survival Studies Among the Georgia Coastal Negroes.* University of Georgia Press, 1940.

Gilbert, Olive. *Narrative of Sojourner Truth*, ed. Margaret Washington. Vintage, 1993.

Gilman, Charlotte Perkins. "A Suggestion on the Negro Problem." *American Journal of Sociology* 14, no. 1 (July 1908).

Gilman, Sander. *Difference and Pathology: Stereotypes of Sexuality, Race, and Madness.* Cornell University Press, 1985.

Goldsby, Jacqueline. *A Spectacular Secret: Lynching in American Life and Literature.* University of Chicago Press, 2006.

Gollaher, David. *Voice for the Mad: The Life of Dorothea Dix.* Free Press, 1995.

Gomez, Michael. *Exchanging Our Country Marks: The Transformation of African Identities in the Colonial and Antebellum South.* University of North Carolina Press, 1998.

Gonaver, Wendy. *The Peculiar Institution and the Making of Modern Psychiatry, 1840–1880.* University of North Carolina Press, 2018.

Goodheart, Lawrence B. *Mad Yankees: The Hartford Retreat for the Insane and Nineteenth-Century Psychiatry.* University of Massachusetts Press, 2003.

Gould, Stephen Jay. *The Mismeasure of Man.* Norton, 1996.

Greenblatt, Stephen, Carol T. Christ, and Catherine Robson, eds. *The Norton Anthology of English Literature.* Vol. E: *The Victorian Age.* Norton, 2005.

Greeson, Jennifer Rae. "The 'Mysteries and Miseries' of North Carolina: New York City, Urban Gothic Fiction, and *Incidents in the Life of a Slave Girl.*" *American Literature* 73, no. 2 (2001): 277–309. https://doi.org/10.1215/00029831-73-2-277.

Gribben, Alan. "Mark Twain, Phrenology and the 'Temperaments': A Study of Pseudoscientific Influence." *American Quarterly* 24, no. 1 (1972): 45–68.

Griffith, David Wark, dir. *The Birth of a Nation*. Epoch Producing Co., 1915.

Grob, Gerald N. "Class, Ethnicity, and Race in American Mental Hospitals, 1830–75." *Journal of the History of Medicine and Allied Sciences* 28, no. 3 (July 1973): 207–29.

Grob, Gerald N. *Edward Jarvis and the Medical World of Nineteenth-Century America*. University of Tennessee Press, 1978.

Grob, Gerald N. *From Asylum to Community: Mental Health Policy in Modern America*. Princeton University Press, 1991.

Grob, Gerald N. *The Mad Among Us: A History of the Care of America's Mentally Ill*. Maxwell Macmillan, 1994.

Grob, Gerald N. *Mental Illness and American Society, 1875–1940*. Princeton University Press, 2019.

Grob, Gerald N. *Mental Institutions in America: Social Policy to 1875*. Free Press, 1972. Reprint, Transaction, 2009.

Grob, Gerald N. *The State and the Mentally Ill: A History of Worcester State Hospital in Massachusetts, 1830–1920*. University of North Carolina Press, 1966.

Gumbs, Alexis Pauline. *Spill: Scenes of Black Feminist Fugitivity*. Duke University Press, 2016.

Gutman, Herbert G. *The Black Family in Slavery and Freedom, 1750–1925*. Vintage, 1976.

Guy-Sheftall, Beverly, ed. *Words of Fire: An Anthology of African-American Feminist Thought*. New Press, 1995.

Haegele, Justin Anthony, and Samuel Hodge. "Disability Discourse: Overview and Critiques of the Medical and Social Models." *Quest* 68, no. 2 (2016). https://doi.org/10.1080/00336297.2016.1143849.

Haley, Sarah. *No Mercy Here: Gender, Punishment, and the Making of Jim Crow Modernity*. University of North Carolina Press, 2016.

Haller, John. "The Negro and the Southern Physician: A Study of Medical and Racial Attitudes, 1800–1860." *Medical History* 16, no. 3 (1972): 238–53.

Haller, John. *Outcasts from Evolution: Scientific Attitudes of Racial Inferiority, 1859–1900*. McGraw-Hill, 1971.

Harley, Sharon. "When Your Work Is Not Who You Are: The Development of a Working-Class Consciousness Among Afro-American Women." In *"We Specialize in the Wholly Impossible": A Reader in Black Women's History*, ed. Darlene Clark Hine, Wilma King, and Linda Reed. Carlson, 1995.

Harris, Kelly. "Foreshadowing Du Bois: James McCune Smith and the Shaping of Nineteenth Century Black Social Scientists." *Du Bois Review: Social Science Research on Race* 22 (2024): 1–17.

Harris, Leslie M. *In the Shadow of Slavery: African Americans in New York City, 1626–1863*. Historical Studies of Urban America. University of Chicago Press, 2003.

Harris, Seale. "The Future of the Negro from the Standpoint of the Southern Physician." *The Alabama Medical Journal* 14, no. 2 (1902): 57–68.

Harriss, Juriah. "What Constitutes Unsoundness in the Negro?" *The Savannah Journal of Medicine* 1, no. 3 (September 1858): 145–52.

Hartman, Saidiya V. *Scenes of Subjection: Terror, Slavery, and Self-Making in Nineteenth-Century America*. Oxford University Press, 1997.

Hartman, Saidiya V. *Wayward Lives, Beautiful Experiments: Intimate Histories of Riotous Black Girls, Troublesome Women, and Queer Radicals*. Norton, 2019.
Haughton, Miriam, Mary McAuliffe, and Emilie Pine. *Legacies of the Magdalen Laundries: Commemoration, Gender, and the Postcolonial Carceral State*. Manchester University Press, 2021.
Hayden, C. B. "On the Distribution of Insanity in the U. States." *Southern Literary Messenger* 10 (1844): 178–81.
Heersink, Boris, and Jeffery A. Jenkins. *Republican Party Politics and the American South, 1865–1968*. Cambridge University Press, 2020. https://doi.org/10.1017/9781316663950.
Hennessey, Melinda Meek. "Race and Violence in Reconstruction New Orleans: The 1868 Riot." *Louisiana History: The Journal of the Louisiana Historical Association* 20, no. 1 (1979): 77–91.
Hersey, Tricia. *Rest Is Resistance: A Manifesto*. Little Brown, 2022.
Hine, Darlene Clark. "Rape and the Inner Lives of Black Women in the Middle West." *Signs: Journal of Women in Culture and Society* 14, no. 4 (1989): 912–20.
Hinton, Anna. "On Fits, Starts, and Entry Points: The Rise of Black Disability Studies." *CLA* 64, no. 1 (2021): 11–29.
Hodges, Graham Russell. *Root and Branch: African Americans in New York and East Jersey, 1613–1863*. University of North Carolina Press, 1999.
Hodges, J. Allison. "The Effect of Freedom Upon the Physical and Psychological Development of the Negro." *Richmond Journal of Practice* 14 (June 1900).
Hoffman, Frederick L. *Race Traits and Tendencies of the American Negro*. Published for the American Economic Association by the Macmillan Company, 1896.
Hofstadter, Richard. "From Calhoun to the Dixiecrats." *Social Research* 82, no. 1 (2015): 245–61.
Hogarth, Rana A. *Medicalizing Blackness: Making Racial Difference in the Atlantic World, 1780–1840*. University of North Carolina Press, 2017.
Holloman, James A. "'Lynch,' Says Mrs. Felton." *Atlanta Journal*, August 12, 1897.
Holloman, James A. "Mrs. Felton's Letter." *Atlanta Constitution*, August 20, 1897.
Holloway, K. G. "Remarkable Case of Fibro-Schirro Cartilaginous Enlargement of the Ovaria." *Southern Medical and Surgical Journal* 2, no. 12 (n.d.): 714–20.
Holt, W. Stull. *The Bureau of the Census: Its History, Activities, and Organization*. Brookings Institution, 1929.
hooks, bell. *Ain't I a Woman: Black Women and Feminism*. Taylor and Francis, 2014.
Horton, Lois E. *Harriet Tubman and the Fight for Freedom: A Brief History with Documents*. Bedford/St. Martin's, 2013.
Howells, William Dean. "An Exemplary Citizen." *North American Review* 173, no. 537 (August 1901): 280–88.
Howells, William Dean. "Mr. Charles W. Chesnutt's Stories." *Atlantic Monthly* 85 (May 1900): 699–701.
Howells, William Dean. "A Psychological Counter-Current in Recent Fiction." *North American Review* 173, no. 541 (December 1901): 872–88.
Hull, Akasha Gloria, Patricia Bell-Scott, and Barbara Smith, eds. *All the Women Are White, All the Blacks Are Men, but Some of Us Are Brave: Black Women's Studies*. Feminist Press, 1982.
Humez, Jean M. *Harriet Tubman: The Life and the Life Stories*. University of Wisconsin Press, 2003.

Humez, Jean M. "In Search of Harriet Tubman's Spiritual Autobiography." *National Women's Studies Association Journal* 5, no. 2 (1993): 162–82.

Humphreys, Margaret. *Intensely Human: The Health of the Black Soldier in the American Civil War.* Johns Hopkins University Press, 2008.

Hungerford, Edward. "Walt Whitman and His Chart of Bumps." *American Literature* 2, no. 4 (1931): 350–84.

Hunt, Sanford B. "The Negro as a Soldier." *Quarterly Journal of Psychological Medicine and Medical Jurisprudence* 1, no. 2 (October 1867): 161–86.

Hunt-Kennedy, Stefanie. *Between Fitness and Death: Disability and Slavery in the Caribbean.* University of Illinois Press, 2020.

Hunter, John E. "Tuberculosis in the Negro: Causes and Treatment." In *Germs Have No Color Lines: Blacks and American Medicine, 1900–1940*, ed. Vanessa Northington Gamble. Garland, 1989.

Hunter, Tera W. *Bound in Wedlock: Slave and Free Black Marriage in the Nineteenth Century.* Belknap Press, 2017.

Hunter, Tera W. *To 'Joy My Freedom: Southern Black Women's Lives and Labors After the Civil War.* Harvard University Press, 1997.

Hurd, Henry Mills, William F. Drewry, Richard Dewey, Charles W. Pilgrim, G. Alder Blumer, and T. J. W. Burgess. *The Institutional Care of the Insane in the United States and Canada*, ed. Henry Mills Hurd. Reprint. Vol. 4. Johns Hopkins Press, 1917.

Hurston, Zora Neale. *Mules and Men.* Perennial Library, 1990.

Ignatiev, Noel. *How the Irish Became White.* Routledge, 2009.

Imada, Adria L. "A Decolonial Disability Studies?" *Disability Studies Quarterly* 37, no. 3 (2017). https://doi.org/10.18061/dsq.v37i3.5984.

Jackson, Bruce, ed. *The Negro and His Folklore in Nineteenth-Century Periodicals.* University of Texas Press, 1967.

Jackson, Cassandra. "Visualizing Slavery: Photography and the Disabled Subject in the Art of Carrie Mae Weems." In *Blackness and Disability: Critical Examinations and Cultural Interventions*, ed. Christopher Bell. Michigan State University Press, 2011.

Jacobs, Harriet. *Incidents in the Life of a Slave Girl, Written by Herself*, ed. L. Maria Child. 2nd ed. Published for the Author, 1861. From Documenting the American South, University Library, the University of North Carolina at Chapel Hill, 2003. https://docsouth.unc.edu/fpn/jacobs/jacobs.html.

Jacobs, Harriet. "Life Among the Contrabands." *The Liberator*, September 5, 1862.

James, Jennifer C., and Cynthia Wu. "Editors' Introduction: Race, Ethnicity, Disability, and Literature: Intersections and Interventions." *Melus* 31, no. 3 (2006): 3–13.

Jarvis, Edward. "Insanity Among the Coloured Population of the Free States." *American Journal of the Medical Sciences* 7, no. 13 (1844): 71.

Jarvis, Edward. "Statistics of Insanity in the United States." *Boston Medical and Surgical Journal* 27, no. 7 (1842): 116–21. https://doi.org/10.1056/NEJM184209210270703.

Jefferson, Thomas. *Notes on the State of Virginia.* Prichard and Hall, 1788. From Documenting the American South, University Library, the University of North Carolina at Chapel Hill, 2006. https://docsouth.unc.edu/southlit/jefferson/jefferson.html.

Johnson, Walter. *Soul by Soul: Life Inside the Antebellum Slave Market.* Harvard University Press, 1999.

Jones, Jacqueline. *Labor of Love, Labor of Sorrow: Black Women, Work, and the Family, from Slavery to the Present*. Basic, 1985.
Jordan, Winthrop. *White Over Black: American Attitudes Toward the Negro 1550–1812*. University of North Carolina Press, 1968.
Joyner, Charles. *Down by the Riverside: A South Carolina Slave Community*. University of Illinois Press, 1984.
Judd, Bettina. *Feelin: Creative Practice, Pleasure, and Black Feminist Thought*. Northwestern University Press, 2023.
Judd, Bettina. "In 2006 I had an Ordeal with Medicine." In *Patient*. Black Lawrence, 2014.
Kafer, Alison. *Feminist, Queer, Crip*. Indiana University Press, 2013.
Keating, J. M. "Twenty Years of Negro Education." *Popular Science Monthly* 28 (1885): 24–37.
Keith, LeeAnna. *The Colfax Massacre: The Untold Story of Black Power, White Terror, and the Death of Reconstruction*. Oxford University Press, 2009.
Kett, Joseph F. *The Formation of the American Medical Profession: The Role of Institutions, 1780–1860*. Yale University Press, 1968.
Kirk, J. Allen. *A Statement of Facts Concerning the Bloody Riot in Wilmington, N.C. of Interest to Every Citizen of the United States*. Wilmington, NC, 1898.
Kudlick, Catherine. "Comment: On the Borderland of Medical and Disability History." *Bulletin of the History of Medicine* 87, no. 4 (2013). https://doi.org/10.1353/bhm.2013.0086.
Kudlick, Catherine. "Social History of Medicine and Disability History." In *The Oxford Handbook of Disability History*, ed. Michael Rembis, Catherine Kudlick, and Kim E. Nielsen. Oxford University Press, 2018. https://doi.org/10.1093/oxfordhb/9780190234959.013.1.
Larson, Kate Clifford. *Bound for the Promised Land: Harriet Tubman, Portrait of an American Hero*. Ballantine, 2004.
LeFrançois, Brenda A., Robert Menzies, and Geoffrey Reaume. *Mad Matters: A Critical Reader in Canadian Mad Studies*. Canadian Scholars' Press, 2013.
Lemmons, Kasi, dir. *Harriet*. Focus Features, Universal Pictures, 2019.
Leonard, Thomas C. *Illiberal Reformers: Race, Eugenics, and American Economics in the Progressive Era*. Princeton University Press, 2016.
Levine, Lawrence W. *Black Culture and Black Consciousness: Afro-American Folk Thought from Slavery to Freedom*. Oxford University Press, 1978.
Li, Stephanie. *Something Akin to Freedom: The Choice of Bondage in Narratives by African American Women*. State University of New York Press, 2010.
Little, Becky. "The 1840 U.S. Census Was Overly Interested in Americans' Mental Health." *History*, May 15, 2019. https://www.history.com/news/census-change-mental-illness-controversy.
Long, Gretchen. *Doctoring Freedom: The Politics of African American Medical Care in Slavery and Emancipation*. University of North Carolina Press, 2012.
Lorde, Audre. *Sister Outsider: Essays and Speeches*. Crossing, 2007.
Lorde, Audre. *Zami: A New Spelling of My Name—A Biomythography*. Crossing, 1982.
Louis, Diana Martha. "Bitch You Must Be Crazy: Representations of Mental Illness in Ntozake Shange's *For Colored Girls Who Have Considered Suicide / When the Rainbow Is Enuf* (1976)." *Western Journal of Black Studies* 37, no. 3 (2013): 197–211.
Lowry, Beverly. *Harriet Tubman: Imagining a Life*. Anchor, 2007.

Lujan, Heidi L., and Stephen E. DiCarlo. "First African American to Hold a Medical Degree: Brief History of James McCune Smith, Abolitionist, Educator, and Physician." *Advances in Physiological Education* 43, no. 2 (2019): 134–39.

Lunbeck, Elizabeth. *The Psychiatric Persuasion: Knowledge, Gender, and Power in Modern America*. Princeton University Press, 1994.

Mackey, Nathaniel. "Phrenological Whitman." *Conjunctions* 29 (Fall 1997). https://conjunctions.com/articles/nathaniel-mackey-c29/.

Manning, Frederick Norton. "The Epileptic: His Treatment and Care." *Australasian Medical Gazette: The Journal of the Australasian Branches of the British Medical Association* 19 (1900): 217–23.

Manning, Frederick Norton. *Report on Lunatic Asylums*. Thomas Richards, 1868.

Matthews, Victoria Earle. "The Value of Race Literature: An Address Delivered at the First Congress of Colored Women of the United States, at Boston, Mass." July 30, 1895.

Mays, Thomas J. "Human Slavery as a Prevention of Pulmonary Consumption." In *Germs Have No Color Lines: Blacks and American Medicine, 1900–1940*, ed. Vanessa Northington Gamble. Garland, 1989.

McBride, David. *From TB to AIDS: Epidemics Among Urban Blacks Since 1900*. State University of New York, 1991.

McCandless, Peter. *Moonlight, Magnolias, and Madness: Insanity in South Carolina from the Colonial Period to the Progressive Era*. University of North Carolina Press, 1996.

McCaskill, Barbara, and Caroline Gebhard, eds. *Post-Bellum-Pre-Harlem: African American Literature and Culture, 1877–1919*. New York University Press, 2006.

McCoy, Ambrose. "Voodooism in the South." *Louisville Medical News*, December 13, 1884.

McCrady, Jr., Edward, and Samuel A. Ashe. *Cyclopedia of Eminent and Representative Men of the Carolinas of the Nineteenth Century*. Vol. 2. Brant & Fuller, 1892.

McCurley, W. S. "Impossibility of Racial Amalgamation." *The Arena*, 1899.

McDowell, Deborah E. "New Directions for Black Feminist Criticism." *Black American Literature Forum* 14, no. 4 (1980): 153–59.

McGovern, Constance M. *Masters of Madness: Social Origins of the American Psychiatric Profession*. University of Vermont by University Press of New England, 1985.

McGovern, Constance M. "The Myths of Social Control and Custodial Oppression: Patterns of Psychiatric Medicine in Late Nineteenth-Century Institutions." *Journal of Social History* 20, no. 1 (Fall 1986): 3–23.

McKie, Thomas. "A Brief History of Insanity and Tuberculosis in the Southern Negro." *Journal of the American Medical Association* 28, no. 12 (March 1897): 537–38.

McKittrick, Katherine. *Demonic Grounds: Black Women and the Cartographies of Struggle*. University of Minnesota Press, 2006.

McRuer, Robert. "Crip Eye for the Normate Guy: Queer Theory and the Disciplining of Disability Studies." *PMLA* 120, no. 2 (2005): 586–92.

McWilliams, Dean. *Charles W. Chesnutt and the Fictions of Race*. University of Georgia Press, 2002.

Melish, Joanne Pope. *Disowning Slavery: Gradual Emancipation and "Race" in New England, 1780–1860*. Cornell University Press, 1998.

Mendes, Gabriel N. *Under the Strain of Color: Harlem's Lafargue Clinic and the Promise of an Antiracist Psychiatry.* Cornell University Press, 2015.

Merrill, A. P. "An Essay on Some of the Distinctive Peculiarities of the Negro Race." *Southern Medical and Surgical Journal* 12, no. 1–3 (January 1856): 21–36, 80–90, 147–56.

Metze, Tamara. *Innovation Ltd: Boundary Work in Deliberative Governance in Land Use Planning.* Eburon Uitgeverij B.V., 2010.

Metzl, Jonathan. *The Protest Psychosis: How Schizophrenia Became a Black Disease.* Beacon, 2009.

Miles, Tiya. *All That She Carried: The Journey of Ashley's Sack, a Black Family Keepsake.* Random House, 2021.

Miles, Tiya. *Night Flyer: Harriet Tubman and the Faith Dreams of a Free People. Significations.* Penguin, 2024.

Miller, John F. "The Effects of Emancipation Upon the Mental and Physical Health of the Negro of the South." *North Carolina Medical Journal* 38, no. 10 (November 1896): 285–94.

Miron, Janet. *Prisons, Asylums, and the Public: Institutional Visiting in the Nineteenth Century.* University of Toronto Press, 2011.

Mitchell, David T., and Sharon Snyder. *Narrative Prosthesis: Disability and the Dependencies of Discourse.* University of Michigan Press, 2000.

Mitchell, Koritha. *Living with Lynching: African American Lynching Plays, Performance, and Citizenship, 1890–1930.* University of Illinois Press, 2011.

Mollow, Anna. "'When Black Women Start Going on Prozac': Race, Gender, and Mental Illness in Meri Nana-Ama Danquah's 'Willow Weep for Me.'" *Melus* 31, no. 3 (2006): 67–99.

Morgan, Joan. *When ChickenHeads Come Home to Roost: My Life as a Hip-Hop Feminist.* Simon & Schuster, 1999.

Morgan, Thomas M. "The Education and Medical Practice of Dr. James McCune Smith (1813–1865), First Black American to Hold a Medical Degree." *Journal of the National Medical Association* 95, no. 7 (2003): 603–14.

Morning Star. "White Supremacy: Col. A. M. Waddell Addressed a Large Audience at the Opera House On Issues of the Campaign." October 25, 1898.

Morris, Susana M. "Black Girls Are from the Future: Afrofuturist Feminism in Octavia E. Butler's *Fledgling*." *Women's Studies Quarterly* 40, no. 3/4 (Fall/Winter 2012): 146–66.

Morrison, Linda J. *Talking Back to Psychiatry: The Psychiatric Consumer/Survivor/Ex-Patient Movement.* Routledge, 2005.

Mulcahy, Judith. "James McCune Smith: The Communipaw Connection." *Nineteenth Century Prose* 34, no. 1–2 (2007): 359+.

Musher, Sharon Ann. "Contesting 'The Way the Almighty Wants It': Crafting Memories of Ex-Slaves in the Slave Narrative Collection." *American Quarterly* 53, no. 1 (2001): 1–31. https://doi.org/10.1353/aq.2001.0009.

My Inwood. "Inwood's Old Magdalen Asylum." July 13, 2013. http://myinwood.net/inwoods-old-magdalen-asylum/.

Najmi, Samina. "Janet, Polly, and Olivia: Constructs of Blackness and White Femininity in Charles Chesnutt's The Marrow of Tradition." *Southern Literary Journal* 32, no. 1 (1999): 1–19.

Nash, Jennifer. *The Black Body in Ecstasy: Reading Race, Reading Pornography.* Duke University Press, 2014.

National Park Service. "Harriet Tubman Home for Aged and Indigent Negroes." Last updated on January 19, 2024. https://www.nps.gov/places/tubmanagedhome.htm.

New York Age. "Harriet Tubman Home Free from Debt." November 2, 1918.

New York Times. "Our Charitable Institutions." January 14, 1862.

Nicki, Andrea. "The Abused Mind: Feminist Theory, Psychiatric Disability, and Trauma." *Hypatia* 16, no. 4 (2001): 80–104. https://doi.org/10.1111/j.1527-2001.2001.tb00754.x.

Nielsen, Kim E. *A Disability History of the United States.* Beacon, 2012.

Noll, Steven. "Southern Strategies for Handling the Black Feeble-Minded: From Social Control to Profound Indifference." *Journal of Policy History* 3, no. 2 (1991): 130–51.

Northup, Solomon. *Twelve Years a Slave: Narrative of Solomon Northup, a Citizen of New-York, Kidnapped in Washington City in 1841, and Rescued in 1853, from a Cotton Plantation Near the Red River, in Louisiana.* Derby and Miller, 1853. From Documenting the American South, University Library, the University of North Carolina at Chapel Hill, 1997. https://docsouth.unc.edu/fpn/northup/northup.html.

Numbers, Ronald L., and Todd Savitt, eds. *Science and Medicine in the Old South.* Louisiana State University Press, 1989.

Nuriddin, Ayah. "Psychiatric Jim Crow: Desegregation at the Crownsville State Hospital, 1948–1970." *Journal of the History of Medicine and Allied Sciences* 74, no. 1 (2019): 85–106. https://doi.org/10.1093/jhmas/jry025.

Nyong'o, Tavia. *The Amalgamation Waltz: Race, Performance, and the Ruses of Memory.* University of Minnesota Press, 2009.

Onley, James. "'I Was Born': Slave Narratives, Their Status as Autobiography and as Literature." *Callaloo*, no. 20 (Winter 1984): 46–73.

Osborn, Matthew Warner. *Rum Maniacs: Alcoholic Insanity in the Early American Republic.* University of Chicago Press, 2014.

Owens, Deirdre Cooper. *Medical Bondage: Race, Gender, and the Origins of American Gynecology.* University of Georgia Press, 2017.

Painter, Nell Irvin. *Sojourner Truth: A Life, a Symbol.* Norton, 1996.

Painter, Nell Irvin. "Soul Murder and Slavery: Toward a Fully Loaded Cost Accounting." In *U.S. History as Women's History: New Feminist Essays*, ed. Linda K. Kerber, Alice Kessler-Harris, and Kathryn Kish Sklar. University of North Carolina Press, 1995.

Painter, Nell Irvin. *Soul Murder and Slavery.* Markham Press Fund, 1995.

Parramore, Thomas. "Harriet Jacobs, James Norcom, and the Defense of Hierarchy." *Carolina Comments* 38, no. 3 (1990): 82–87.

Parry, Tyler D. "'How Much More Must I Suffer?': Post-Traumatic Stress and the Lingering Impact of Violence Upon Enslaved People." *Slavery and Abolition* 42, no. 2 (2021): 184–200. https://doi.org/10.1080/0144039X.2021.1896187.

Pasamanick, Benjamin. "Myths Regarding Prevalence of Mental Disease in the American Negro: A Century of Misuse of Mental Hospital Data and Some New Findings." *Journal of National Medical Association* 56, no. 1 (1964): 6–17.

Patterson, Orlando. *Slavery and Social Death: A Comparative Study.* Harvard University Press, 1982.

Pearson, J. E. "Fracture of the Cranium, with Depression, Attended with an Escape of a Portion of the Brain; Relieved by the Trephine; Death Four Years Afterwards, from Suppuration Within the Cranium, and Encroachment Upon the Brain, by a Sharp Projecting Exostosis Springing from the Inner Surface of the Fractured Bone." *Southern Journal of Medicine and Pharmacy* 2, no. 2 (March 1847): 155–57. From Center for Research Libraries. https://dds.crl.edu/crldelivery/5570.

Penniman, Leah. *Farming While Black: Soul Fire Farm's Practical Guide to Liberation on the Land*. Chelsea Green, 2018.

Peterson, Carla. *"Doers of the Word": African-American Women Speakers and Writers in the North (1830–1880)*. Oxford University Press, 1995.

Pickens, Therí A. *Black Madness :: Mad Blackness*. Duke University Press, 2019.

Pickens, Therí A. "Blue Blackness, Black Blueness: Making Sense of Blackness and Disability." *African American Review* 50, no. 2 (2017): 93–103.

Pollard, Cherise A. "Are We the 'Future Americans'?: Charles Chesnutt Anticipates a Postracial American Society," in *Postracial America?: An Interdisciplinary Study*, ed. Vincent L. Stephens and Anthony Stewart. Bucknell University Press, 2017.

Porter, Roy. *The Cambridge Illustrated History of Medicine*. Cambridge University Press, 2001.

Porter, Theodore M. *Genetics in the Madhouse: The Unknown History of Human Heredity*. Princeton University Press, 2018.

Postell, William. *The Health of Slaves on Southern Plantations*. Louisiana State University Press, 1951.

Powell, T. O. "Heredity and Invironment [Sic]." *Union Recorder* LVII, no. 43, May 3, 1887.

Powell, T. O. "Increase of Insanity and Its Supposed Causes, Etc." In *Reports of the Trustees and Officers of the Lunatic Asylum, of the State Of Georgia, from October 1st, 1885, to 1st October, 1886*. Union & Recorder-Barnes & Moore, Printers, 1886.

Powell, T. O. "The Increase of Insanity and Tuberculosis in the Southern Negro Since 1860, and Its Alliance, and Some of the Supposed Causes." *Journal of the American Medical Association* 27, no. 23 (December 1896): 1185–88. https://doi.org/10.1001/jama.1896.02431010013002f.

Powell, T. O. "A Sketch of Psychiatry in the Southern States." *American Journal of Insanity* 54, no. 1 (1897): 21–36. https://doi.org/10.1176/ajp.54.1.21.

Powell, William S., ed. *Dictionary of North Carolina Biography*. Vol. 6, T–Z. University of North Carolina Press, 1996.

Prather, Sr., H. Leon. *We Have Taken a City: Wilmington Racial Massacre and Coup of 1898*. Fairleigh Dickinson University Press, 1984.

Price, Kenneth M. "Charles Chesnutt, the *Atlantic Monthly*, and the Intersection of African-American Fiction and Elite Culture." In *Periodical Literature in Nineteenth-Century America*, ed. Kenneth M Price and Susan Belasco Smith. University Press of Virginia, 1995.

Price, Margaret. "The Bodymind Problem and the Possibilities of Pain." *Hypatia* 30, no. 1 (2015): 268–84.

Price, Margaret. *Mad at School: Rhetorics of Mental Disability and Academic Life*. University of Michigan Press, 2011.

Raboteau, Albert J. *A Fire in the Bones: Reflections on African-American Religious History*. Beacon, 1995.

Raboteau, Albert J. *Slave Religion: The "Invisible Institution" in the Antebellum South*. Oxford University Press, 1978.
Rael, Patrick. *Black Identity and Black Protest in the Antebellum North*. University of North Carolina Press, 2002.
Rafter, Nicole Hahn. *Creating Born Criminals*. University of Illinois Press, 1997.
Ramas, Maria. "Freud's Dora, Dora's Hysteria: The Negation of a Woman's Rebellion." *Feminist Studies* 6, no. 3 (1980): 472.
Rawick, George P., ed. *The American Slave: A Composite Autobiography*. Vol. 1. Greenwood, 1972.
Raz, Mical. *What's Wrong with the Poor?: Psychiatry, Race, and the War on Poverty*. University of North Carolina Press, 2013.
Reaume, Geoffrey. "Mad People's History." *Radical History Review*, no. 94 (Winter 2006): 170–82.
Records of Eastern State Hospital, 1770–2009. Accession 44812. State Government Records Collection, the Library of Virginia, Richmond, Virginia.
Reiss, Benjamin. *Theaters of Madness: Insane Asylums and Nineteenth-Century American Culture*. University of Chicago Press, 2008.
Richardson, Allissa V. "The Origins of Bearing Witness While Black." In *Bearing Witness While Black: African Americans, Smartphones, and the New Protest #Journalism*. Oxford University Press, 2020. https://doi.org/10.1093/oso/9780190935528.003.0002.
Riegel, Robert E. "The Introduction of Phrenology to the United States." *American Historical Review* 39, no. 1 (1933): 73–78. https://doi.org/10.2307/1839225.
Ripley, William Zebina. *The Races of Europe: A Sociological Study*. Kegan Paul, Trench, Trubner, & Co., 1899.
Roberts, Dorothy. *Fatal Invention: How Science, Politics, and Big Business Re-Create Race in the Twenty-First Century*. New Press, 2011.
Roberts, Jr., Samuel K. *Infectious Fear: Politics, Disease, and the Health Effects of Segregation*. University of North Carolina Press, 2009.
Rosen, Hannah. *Terror in the Heart of Freedom: Citizenship, Sexual Violence, and the Meaning of Race in the Postemancipation South*. University of North Carolina Press, 2009.
Rosenberg, Charles E. "The American Medical Profession: Mid-Nineteenth Century." *Mid America* 44 (July 1962): 163–71.
Rosenberg, Charles E. *Explaining Epidemics and Other Studies in the History of Medicine*. Cambridge University Press, 1992.
Rosengarten, Theodore. *Tombee: Portrait of a Cotton Planter with the Plantation Journal of Thomas B. Chaplin (1822–1890)*, edited by Susan W. Walker. Morrow, 1986.
Rothman, David. *The Discovery of the Asylum: Social Order and Disorder in the New Republic*. Revised ed. Aldine de Gruyter, 2002.
Rothstein, William. *American Physicians in the Nineteenth Century: From Sects to Science*. Johns Hopkins University Press, 1972.
Ruggles, Steven. "Fallen Women: The Inmates of the Magdalen Society Asylum of Philadelphia, 1836–1908." *Journal of Social History* 16, no. 4 (Summer 1983): 65–82.
Rusert, Britt. *Fugitive Science: Empiricism and Freedom in Early African American Culture*. New York University Press, 2017.
Rush, Benjamin. *Medical Inquiries and Observations Upon the Diseases of the Mind*. Kimber & Richardson, 1812.

Rush, Benjamin. "Observations Intended to Favour a Supposition That the Black Color (as It Is Called) of the Negroes Is Derived from the Leprosy." *Transactions of the American Philosophical Society* 4, no. 1 (1799): 289–97. https://doi.org/10.2307/1005108.
Samuels, Ellen. *Fantasies of Identification: Disability, Gender, Race*. New York University Press, 2014.
Santamarina, Xiomara. "Black Womanhood in North American Women's Slave Narratives." In *The Cambridge Companion to the African American Slave Narrative*, ed. Audrey Fisch. Cambridge University Press, 2007. https://doi.org/10.1017/CCOL0521850193.015.
Savannah Morning News. "A Queer Case of Suicide." January 9, 1894.
Savitt, Todd L. *Medicine and Slavery: The Diseases and Health Care of Blacks in Antebellum Virginia*. University of Illinois Press, 1978.
Savitt, Todd L., and James Harvey Young. *Disease and Distinctiveness in the American South*. University of Tennessee Press, 1988.
Sawaya, Francesca. "'That Friendship of the Whites': Patronage, Philanthropy, and Charles Chesnutt's The Colonel's Dream." *American Literature* 83, no. 4 (2011): 775–801. https://doi.org/10.1215/00029831-1437216.
Schalk, Samantha Dawn. *Bodyminds Reimagined: (Dis)Ability, Race, and Gender in Black Women's Speculative Fiction*. Duke University Press, 2018.
Schantz, Mark. *Awaiting the Heavenly Country: The Civil War and America's Culture of Death*. Cornell University Press, 2008.
Schiebinger, Londa. *Secret Cures of Slaves: People, Plants, and Medicine in the Eighteenth-Century Atlantic World*. Stanford University Press, 2017.
Schwalm, Leslie A. *A Hard Fight for We: Women's Transition from Slavery to Freedom in South Carolina*. University of Illinois Press, 1997.
Schwartz, Marie Jenkins. "The WPA Narratives as Historical Sources." In *The Oxford Handbook of the African American Slave Narrative*, ed. John Ernest. Oxford University Press, 2014.
Scotch, Richard K. "Medical Model of Disability." In *Encyclopedia of American Disability History*, ed. Susan Burch. Facts on File, 2009.
Scull, Andrew T. "Madness and Segregative Control: The Rise of the Insane Asylum." *Social Problems* 24, no. 3 (1977): 337–51. https://doi.org/10.1525/sp.1977.24.3.03a00040.
Scull, Andrew T. "Psychiatry and Social Control in the Nineteenth and Twentieth Centuries." *History of Psychiatry* 2, no. 6 (1991): 149–69.
Segrest, Mab. *Administrations of Lunacy: Racism and the Haunting of American Psychiatry at the Milledgeville Asylum*. New Press, 2020.
Sekora, John. "Black Message/White Envelope: Genre, Authenticity, and Authority in the Antebellum Slave Narrative." *Callaloo*, no. 32 (1987): 482–515. https://doi.org/10.2307/2930465.
Septo, Robert. "Storytelling in Early Afro-American Fiction: Frederick Douglass's 'The Heroic Slave.'" In *Black Literature and Literary Theory*, ed. Henry Louis Gates. Methuen, 1984.
Sernett, Milton C. *African American Religious History: A Documentary Witness*. 2nd ed. Duke University Press, 1999.
Sernett, Milton C. *Harriet Tubman: Myth, Memory, and History*. Duke University Press, 2007.
Sexton, Jared. *Amalgamation Schemes*. University of Minnesota Press, 2008.
Shakespeare, Tom. "The Social Model of Disability." In *The Disability Studies Reader*, ed. Lennard J. Davis. 3rd ed. Routledge, 2010.

Shange, Ntozake. *For Colored Girls Who Have Considered Suicide / When the Rainbow Is Enuf.* Scribner, 1976.

Sharpe, Christina. *In the Wake: On Blackness and Being.* Duke University Press, 2016.

Sherman, Richard B. "'The Last Stand': The Fight for Racial Integrity in Virginia in the 1920s." *Journal of Southern History* 54, no. 1 (1988): 69–92. https://doi.org/10.2307/2208521.

Showalter, Elaine. *The Female Malady: Women, Madness, and English Culture, 1830–1980.* Pantheon, 1985.

Shryock, Richard H. *Medicine and Society in America, 1660–1860.* New York University Press, 1960.

Shute, D. K. "Racial Anatomical Peculiarities." *American Anthropologist* 9, no. 4 (April 1896): 123–32.

Siebers, Tobin. *Disability Aesthetics.* University of Michigan Press, 2010.

Silkenat, David. *Moments of Despair: Suicide, Divorce, and Debt in Civil War Era North Carolina.* University of North Carolina Press, 2011.

Sinha, Manisha. *The Slave's Cause: A History of Abolition.* Yale University Press, 2016.

Smith, Franklin. "The Real Problems of Democracy." *Popular Science Monthly* LVI (November 1899): 1–13.

Smith, James McCune. "Freedom and Slavery for Afric-Americans." *The Liberator (1831–1865),* February 23, 1844.

Smith, James McCune. "Hon. John C Calhoun and The Free Colored People." *New York Daily Tribune,* May 8, 1844.

Smith, James McCune. "The Influence of Climate on Longevity: With Special Reference to Life Insurance." *Hunt's Merchant Magazine,* 1846.

Smith, James McCune. "Lay Puffery of Homeopathy, Letter from Dr. James McC. Smith." *The Annalist, a Record of Practical Medicine in the City of New-York, 1847–1848* 2, no. 18 (June 15, 1848): 348–51.

Smith, James McCune. "On the Fourteenth Query of Thomas Jefferson's Notes on the State of Virginia." *Anglo-African Magazine* 1, no. 8 (1859): 225–38.

Smith, James McCune. "On the Influence of Opium Upon the Catamenial Functions." *New York Journal of Medicine and Collateral Sciences* 2 (1844): 56–58.

Smith, James McCune. "Report on the Social Condition of the People of Color Around New York City, and on the Best Means of Ameliorating the Same." *North Star,* April 10, 1851.

Smith, Kylie. *Talking Therapy: Knowledge and Power in American Psychiatric Nursing.* Rutgers University Press, 2020.

Smith, Susan L. *Sick and Tired of Being Sick and Tired: Black Women's Health Activism in America, 1890–1950.* University of Pennsylvania Press, 1995.

Smith, Theophus H. *Conjuring Culture: Biblical Formations of Black America.* Oxford University Press, 1994.

Smith, Tyrie J. "'Your People Will Never Rise in the World': Chesnutt's Message to a Black Readership." In *Charles Chesnutt Reappraised: Essays on the First Major African American Fiction Writer,* ed. David Garrett Izzo and Maria Orban. McFarland, 2009.

Snyder, Terri L. *The Power to Die: Slavery and Suicide in British North America.* University of Chicago Press, 2015.

Snyder, Terri L. "Suicide, Slavery, and Memory in North America." *Journal of American History* 97, no. 1 (2010): 39–62. https://doi.org/10.2307/jahist/97.1.39.

Sobel, Mechal. *The World They Made Together*. Princeton University Press, 1987.

Sommerville, Diane Miller. *Aberration of Mind: Suicide and Suffering in the Civil War-Era South*. University of North Carolina Press, 2018.

Spahn, Hannah. "Blood and Character in Early African American Literature." In *The Cultural Politics of Blood, 1500–1900*, ed. Kimberly Anne Coles, Ralph Bauer, Zita Nunes, and Carla L. Peterson. Palgrave Macmillan, 2015.

Spiro, Jonathan. *Defending the Master Race: Conservation, Eugenics, and the Legacy of Madison Grant*. University Press of New England, 2009.

Spurzheim, Johann Gaspar. *Observations on the Deranged Manifestations of the Mind: Or, Insanity*. 3rd American ed. Marsh, Capen & Lyon, 1836.

St-Amand, Nérée, and Eugène LeBlanc. "Women in 19th-Century Asylums: Three Exemplary Women; A New Brunswick Hero." In *Mad Matters: A Critical Reader in Canadian Mad Studies*, ed. Robert J. Menzies, Geoffrey Reaume, and Brenda A. LeFrançois. Canadian Scholars' Press, 2013.

Stampp, Kenneth. *The Peculiar Institution: Slavery in the Antebellum South*. Vintage, 1956.

Stanton, William. *The Leopard's Spots: Scientific Attitudes Toward Race in America, 1815–59*. University of Chicago Press, 1960.

Stauffer, John. *The Black Hearts of Men: Radical Abolitionists and the Transformation of Race*. Harvard University Press, 2002.

Stauffer, John, ed. *The Works of James McCune Smith: Black Intellectual and Abolitionist*. Oxford University Press, 2006.

Stern, Madeleine B. "Mark Twain Had His Head Examined." *American Literature* 41, no. 2 (1969): 207–18. https://doi.org/10.2307/2923950.

Stevenson, Brenda E. *Life in Black and White: Family and Community in the Slave South*. Oxford University Press, 1997.

Stewart, Dianne M., ed. *Three Eyes for the Journey: African Dimensions of the Jamaican Religious Experience*. Oxford University Press, 2005. https://doi.org/10.1093/0195154150.002.0001.

Stone, Andrea. "The Black Atlantic Revisited, the Body Reconsidered: On Lingering, Liminality, Lies, and Disability." *American Literary History* 24, no. 4 (2012): 814–26. https://doi.org/10.1093/alh/ajs044.

Stowe, Steven M. *Doctoring the South: Southern Physicians and Everyday Medicine in the Mid-Nineteenth Century*. University of North Carolina Press, 2004.

Summers, Martin. *Madness in the City of Magnificent Intentions: A History of Race and Mental Illness in the Nation's Capital*. Oxford University Press, 2019.

Szasz, Thomas S. "The Sane Slave: An Historical Note on the Use of Medical Diagnosis as Justificatory Rhetoric." *American Journal of Psychotherapy* 25, no. 2 (1971): 228–39.

Taylor, Susie King. *Reminiscences of My Life in Camp with the 33rd United States Colored Troops Late 1st S.C. Volunteers*. Published by the author, 1904.

Taylor, Ula. "The Historical Evolution of Black Feminist Theory and Praxis." *Journal of Black Studies* 29, no. 2 (November 1998): 234–53.

Taylor, Ula. "Making Waves: The Theory and Practice of Black Feminism." *Black Scholar* 28, no. 2 (Summer, 1998): 18–28.

Taylor, Ula. "Women in the Documents: Thoughts on Uncovering the Personal, Political, and Professional." *Journal of Women's History* 20, no. 1 (2008): 187–96. https://dx.doi.org/10.1353/jowh.2008.0010.

Telford, Emma P. "Harriet, The Modern Moses of Heroism and Visions," 1905. The Telford Manuscript, Cayuga Museum of History and Art, Auburn, NY.

Tennyson, Alfred. *In Memoriam*. Edward Moxon, 1850.

Terrell, Mary Eliza Church. *A Colored Woman in a White World*. Ransdell, 1940.

"Testimony of Alfred Richardson, Washington, D.C., July 7, 1871." In *Report of the Joint Select Committee to Inquire into the Condition of Affairs in the Late Insurrectionary States, Made to the Two Houses of Congress February 19, 1872*. Vol. 6. Government Printing Office, 1872.

Thorne, Jack. *Hanover; or, The Persecution of the Lowly: A Story of the Wilmington Massacre*. M.C.L. Hill, 1901.

Tillinghast, Joseph Alexander. "The Negro in Africa and America." *Publications of the American Economic Association* 3, no. 2 (1902).

Tipton, F. "The Negro Problem from a Medical Standpoint." *New York Medical Journal* 43 (1886): 569–72.

Titus, Mary. "This Poisonous System: Social Ills, Bodily Ills, and Incidents in the Life of a Slave Girl." In *Harriet Jacobs and Incidents in the Life of a Slave Girl: New Critical Essays*, ed. Rafia Zafar and Deborah M. Garfield. Cambridge University Press, 1996. https://doi.org/10.1017/CBO9780511570414.

Tomes, Nancy. *The Art of Asylum-Keeping: Thomas Story Kirkbride and the Origins of American Psychiatry*. University of Pennsylvania Press, 1994.

Tomes, Nancy. *A Generous Confidence: Thomas Story Kirkbride and the Art of Asylum-Keeping, 1840–1883*. Cambridge University Press, 1983.

Tomlinson, Stephen. *Head Masters: Phrenology, Secular Education, and Nineteenth-Century Social Thought*. University of Alabama Press, 2005.

Topinard, Paul. "Chapter VIII: Influence of Milieux." In *Anthropology*. Chapman and Hall, 1878.

Torchia, Marion M. "The Tuberculosis Movement and the Race Question, 1890–1950." *Bulletin of the History of Medicine* 49, no. 2 (1975): 152–68.

Trent, James, ed. *Inventing the Feeble Mind: A History of Intellectual Disability in the United States*. Oxford University Press, 2016. https://doi.org/10.1093/med/9780199396184.002.0003.

Tucker, George A. *Lunacy in Many Lands*. Charles Potter, Government Printer, 1887.

Union Recorder. "The Lunatic Asylum." November 19, 1889.

Union Recorder. "Lunatic Asylum." November 7, 1893.

Union Recorder. "Superintendent Powell Talks About the State's Lunatics." January 21, 1890.

US Census. *Sixth Census of the United States, 1840: Compendium of the Enumeration of the Inhabitants and Statistics of the United States, as Obtained at the Department of State, from the Returns of the Sixth Census*. Census of the United States; Sixth Decennial Census, 1841.

Virginia. *Acts of the General Assembly of Virginia, 1845–1846*. J.E. Goode, 1846.

Waddell, Alfred Moore. *Some Memories of My Life*. Edwards & Broughton, 1908.

Walker, Alice. *In Search of Our Mothers' Gardens: Womanist Prose*. Harcourt Brace Jovanovich, 1983.

Wallace-Sanders, Kimberly. *Mammy: A Century of Race, Gender, and Southern Memory.* University of Michigan Press, 2008.
Ward, Jr., Thomas J. *Black Physicians in the Jim Crow South.* University of Arkansas Press, 2003.
Washington, Harriet A. *Medical Apartheid: The Dark History of Medical Experimentation on Black Americans from Colonial Times to the Present.* Doubleday, 2006.
Weiner, Marli Frances, and Mazie Hough. *Sex, Sickness, and Slavery: Illness in the Antebellum South.* University of Illinois Press, 2012.
Weld, Theodore Dwight. *American Slavery as It Is: Testimony of a Thousand Witnesses.* American Anti-Slavery Society, 1839. From Documenting the American South, University Library, the University of North Carolina at Chapel Hill, 2000. https://docsouth.unc.edu/neh/weld/weld.html.
Wells, Samuel R., ed. "Frederick Douglas [Sic]: Portrait, Character, and Biography." *American Phrenological Journal and Life Illustrated* 43, no. 5 (May 1866): 148.
Wells-Oghoghomeh, Alexis. *The Souls of Womenfolk: The Religious Cultures of Enslaved Women in the Lower South.* University of North Carolina Press, 2021.
White, Deborah Gray. *Ar'n't I a Woman?: Female Slaves in the Plantation South.* Norton, 1999.
"Wiley M. Pearce Slave Bill of Sale, 1859." MS 1562. Georgia Historical Society, Savannah, Georgia.
Williams, Andreá. "Postbellum, Pre-Harlem: Black Writing before the Renaissance." In *A Companion to the Harlem Renaissance,* ed. Cherene Sherrard-Johnson. Wiley, 2015.
Williams, Kidada E. *They Left Great Marks on Me: African American Testimonies of Racial Violence from Emancipation to World War I.* New York University Press, 2012.
Williams, Kidada E. "The Wounds That Cried Out: Reckoning with African Americans' Testimonies of Trauma and Suffering from Night Riding." In *The World the Civil War Made,* ed. Gregory P. Downs and Kate Masur. University of North Carolina Press, 2015.
Willoughby, Christopher D. E. *Masters of Health: Racial Science and Slavery in U.S. Medical Schools.* University of North Carolina Press, 2022.
Wilson, Matthew. *Whiteness in the Novels of Charles W. Chesnutt.* University Press of Mississippi, 2004.
Withington, Charles F. "The Perils of Rapid Civilization." *Popular Science Monthly* 26 (1885): 224–39.
Wood, Mary Elene. *The Writing on the Wall: Women's Autobiography and the Asylum.* University of Illinois Press, 1994.
Woodward, C. Vann. *The Strange Career of Jim Crow.* 3rd rev. ed. Oxford University Press, 1974.
Wright, Carroll D., and William C. Hunt. *The History and Growth of the United States Census.* 56th Congress, 1st Session, No. 239. Government Printing Office, 1900.
Yellin, Jean Fagan. *Harriet Jacobs: A Life.* Basic Civitas, 2004.
Yellin, Jean Fagan. "Texts and Contexts of Harriet Jacobs' Incidents in the Life of a Slave Girl: Written by Herself." In *The Slave's Narrative,* ed. Charles T. Davis and Henry Louis Gates. Oxford University Press, 1985.
Yetman, Norman R. "The Background of the Slave Narrative Collection." *American Quarterly* 19, no. 3 (1967): 534–53.
Zaks, Zosia. "Changing the Medical Model of Disability to the Normalization Model of Disability: Clarifying the Past to Create a New Future Direction." *Disability and Society* 39, no. 12 (2024): 3233–60.

INDEX

abolition: slave narratives goal of, 97; J. Smith on, 48, 50–51, 52; Tubman organizing for, 111, 121
Adams, Samuel Hopkins, 136
African-derived healing traditions, of Tubman: Adams on, 136; Civil War treatment, 135–37; in Underground Railroad, 135, 136
alcohol abuse, 43–44, 160, 228n107, 250n107
Alice M. narrative, on GLA, 143, 146–51, 170
Amanda C. narrative, on GLA, 143, 146–47, 162–65, 168, 170
American Anti-Slavery Society, 47, 52
American future, Chesnutt vision of, 194–98
American Journal of Insanity, Brigham beginning of, 6, 22, 42, 125
American Medical Association, 22, 155
American Medico-Psychological Association, 140
American Slavery as It Is (Weld), 27–28, 221n33
AMSAII. *See* Association of Medical Superintendents of American Psychiatric Association
Andrews, William, 94, 175

antebellum psychiatric and medical discourses, on Black bodymind: Conjure culture and mental disability, 28–31; history of, 19–24; medical perspectives on mental disability, 40–45; regimes of care for colored insane before emancipation, 24–28, 221n33; scientific racism and proslavery psychiatry, 31–40
apes, Jefferson and Cartwright comparison of Black people to, 36–37
Association of Medical Superintendents of American Psychiatric Association (AMSAII), 22, 121, 125
Asylum of St. Anna's, Tasso confined to, 93
asylums, 218n1; Black people segregation in, 10, 23, 24, 26, 27, 122, 142, 165–66, 258n107; Black treatment of mental disabilities at, 2, 19, 23; Black women labor in, 10, 165; case narratives, 11–12; Dix and movement for, 121; Foucault on relations of power in, 12; Gonaver on domestic violence normalization, 152; medical organizations for, 22; moral therapy in, 20; multidirectional power in, 12; physical and sexual violence in, 10; poor cure

asylums (*continued*)
rates at, 122; Powell address on southern, 140–41; relationship with broader culture, 16, 19; religion practice in, 124; violent racially charged fights at, 27. *See also* Georgia Lunatic Asylum; *specific asylum*
Auden, W. H., 79

Ball, Charles, 103
Barclay, Jennifer, 77
Beardsley, Monroe, 94
Black-authored documents, 11, 12–14
Black bodymind, 20, 250n2; antebellum psychiatric and medical discourses on, 19–45; Chesnutt on, 4, 18; Jacobs on slavery harm to, 87; medical and psychiatric discourses on, 3, 9; Merrill on, 42, 70; Powell on South as experts in, 140–41; proslavery psychiatry, 19, 153, 202; psychiatrists on freedom from slavery harm to, 19, 153; Rush on, 21, 219n5; J. Smith on, 17, 48, 53, 77–78; Tubman on mental and physical toll of slavery, 112; Weiner and Hough on, 41
Black feminism, 4, 90, 144; Black women asylum confinement and, 152; literature, 201, 269n5
Black feminist theory, 10, 13, 215n17
Black maternal mental health in Michigan, on PMAD diagnoses rates, 199
Black mental disability, 2, 39; Black people as primitive and, 25; Cartwright on drapetomania and dysaesthesia aethiopis, 38–39, 102, 226n87; Chesnutt criticism of medicalized conceptualization of, 173–74; conceptions about Conjure and, 20; Conjure and, 20, 28–31, 125, 129, 182, 218n2, 222n34, 222n38, 222n49, 247n76; kinship networks and, 91; medicalized thought on, 152–61; physician belief in brain abnormalities for, 26; study of history of, 15–16; terminology of, 4–10

Black mental health: Jacobs on alternative ideas about, 90; renarration of nineteenth-century medical discourses, 202; J. Smith on multifactorial elements of, 50
"Black News-Vender, The" (Smith, J.), 73, 79, 80; Black bodymind and, 77–78; Boster on, 76; on fugitive slave being disabled, 76
Black people: articulation of slavery psychological impact, 2; Brigham on smaller brain of, 42; census of 1840 on mortality rates, 229n3; conceptualizations of individual and communal mental health, 2; enthusiasm about marriage after emancipation, 163–64, 257n80; Fitzhugh paternalist view on, 37–38; Fogel on hidden depression of Black people, 73; genetic makeup and transmission, 267n69; C. Gilman on detention center assignment of, 142; intellectuals, 47, 48, 229n8; Jefferson and Cartwright comparison to apes of, 36–37; Jefferson on capacity for feeling by, 90; physicians on constitution of, 41–42; Powell on hereditary mental disease of, 142, 156–57; as primitive, 25; psychiatrists on anatomical differences of, 42; segregation in asylums, 10, 23, 24, 26, 27, 122, 142, 165–66, 258n107; J. Smith on active participants of lives, 51; J. Smith on capacity to suffer emotionally, 78; Washington on, 141–42
Black women: belief in ghosts, 128–29; experience of being a patient, 201; Frankel on freedom and motherhood, 162; Hartman on classification of social deviance, 148; Jacobs attentive to experiences of, 92; Jefferson sexual relationships with, 77, 236n90; J. Jones on violent label of, 150; labor in asylums, 10, 165; literature, 203, 270n13; medical

degrees of, 229n7; mental disease tied to menstrual cycles, 25, 57–58, 98, 145, 157, 164, 232n29; after slavery conceptions, 226n91; slavery psychological cost to, 88–110; stereotypes, 149, 268n1; U. Taylor on, 148; White on sexual violence against, 16

Black women psychiatric incarceration, at GLA, 9, 11–12, 140–44; Black femininity societal views and, 144; Black women journey to, 149–52; Black women of, 145–49; medicalized thought on Black mental disability, 152–61; race, gender and Black women narratives, 161–67; segregation and standards of care, 167–70, *168*, 258nn105–6, 259n115. *See also* Georgia Lunatic Asylum

bodymind. *See* Black bodymind

"Boot-Black, The" (Smith, J.), 83

Boster, Dea, 76, 82

Bow's Review, De proslavery southern magazine, 31

Bradford, Sarah, 116–18, 130–34, 137, 248n79, 248n81

brain: Brigham on smaller Black, 42; mental illness term for health concerns of, 5, 213n4; physicians on Black mental disability and abnormalities of, 26; Tubman surgery on, 120

Brickler, Alice, 118

Brigham, Amariah, 32, 231n28; *American Journal of Insanity* beginning by, 6, 22, 42, 125; on phrenology and mental disease, 60–61; on religious expressions, 125; on smaller Black brain, 42

Bronte, Charlotte, 98

Brown, John, 53, 115, 116; Tubman vision of death of, 118, 126

Browning, Robert, 79

Bucktown General Store, Tubman head injury at, 112–13, *113*

Byron, Lord, 93–97, 240n21

Caldwell, Charles, 61–62

Calhoun, John, 32, 229n5; on Blacks slavery suitability, 35; J. Smith debunking statements of, 54, 55

Camp, W., 41

Carrtarr, Surrah, 82–83

Cartesian split, 240n19

Cartwright, Samuel, 31, 32, 226n80; on Black drapetomania and dysaesthesia aethiopis, 38–39, 102, 226n87; comparison of Blacks to apes, 36–37; S. Gilman on, 39; on physical and mental differences between races, 226n77; on slavery protection against mental disability, 37

census of 1840, 36, 254n47; Black mental disability concern from, 32; on Black mortality rates, 229n3; Calhoun on Blacks suitability to slavery and, 35; categories of, 46–47, 223n52; S. Gilman on, 33, 224n56; Hayden on freedom and mental disability correlation, 35; Jarvis on errors in, 32–34, 47, 229n4; mental disability data collection, 20, 32, 47, 229n2; J. Smith on errors of, 54–55; statistics from, 32, 223n54

Cheney, Edna Dow, 122

Chesnutt, Charles, 13–15, *172*, *175*, 200, 205, 254n43, 261nn12–13; as Black American fiction writer, 3, 9, 171; on Black bodymind, 4, 18; as Black intellectual, 48; on color line problem, 141; *The Conjure Woman*, 171, 174, 179–85, *180*, 263n32; *The Marrow of Tradition*, 16, 171, 172, 174, 185–94, *187*, 263n30, 266n59; mental disability in age of black freedom and, 171–98; theory of racial amalgamation, 174, 175–79, 261n16

Child, Lydia Maria, 88

children: in Colored Orphan Asylum courtyard, 69; Jacobs school for Black, 242n73; of Jacobs with Sawyer,

children (*continued*)
    237n1; Jefferson on slavery damage to white, 233n44; mental suffering from being severed from, 104; motherhood and slavery practice of selling, 104–7; proslavery psychiatry on Black comparison to, 37–38
Chireau, Yvonne, 129, 222n34
Christian, Barbara, 91, 205
Christian Recorder, on Blacks equal access to psychiatric facilities, 27
Cinqué, Joseph, 42
civilization state belief, 224n59, 224n61; Cartwright on Black halted development, 37, 226n80; mental disability link to, 34
Civil War, 16; African-derived healing traditions of Tubman, 135–37; Tubman as spy and nurse in, 111, 136; Tubman vision of commencement of, 118, 127
Clinton, Catherine, 119
Cole, Rebecca J., 229n7
Colored American, The (newspaper), 52; "Physician's Report" on Colored Orphan Asylum, 68, 70; J. Smith phrenology fallacy lectures in, 65, 234n54
colored insane: mental disability approach, 9–10; Powell on care in southern asylums, 140; psychiatric discourses on Tubman as, 111–12; regimes of care before emancipation of, 24–28, 221n33
Colored Orphan Asylum, 67–72, 68; children in courtyard of, 69; emphasis on good health, 67; McDonald and Proudfit as white physicians for, 68–70; J. Smith as chief physician at, 53, 67, 67–69
color line, Du Bois and Chesnutt on problem of, 141
Combe, George, 59, 60, 61–63, 234n45; belief in racial hierarchies, 61
Communipaw, as pen name of J. Smith, 72
Conjure and mental disability, 20, 125, 129, 182, 247n76; Cartwright on, 31; as cause and cure, 29–30; Chireau on enchanted universe, 222n34; direct and indirect treatments by, 30; dominant role in physical and mental ailments, 28; Fett on, 28; insanity treatment with interpersonal social conflict, 29; Pinckney on, 30; T. Smith on, 28–29; supernatural and magical explanations, 29, 218n2, 222n49; unexplained disease and, 222n38
Conjure Woman, The (Chesnutt), 171, 174, 180, 263n32; "Mars Jeem's Nightmare" chapter on mental disability, 181–85; mental disability in, 179–85
Conrad, Earl, 118–19
Constitution of Man (Combe), 62
Cornish, Samuel, 80
Crane, Jacob, 75
criminology, phrenology use in, 232n37
Crummell, Alexander, 63, 230n9
Crumpler, Rebecca Davis Lee, 229n7
Cuffe, Paul, 80

Dain, Norman, 123–24
death: "The Black News-Vender" on, 80; of Black women at GLA, 168–69; of enslaved through discipline, 115; Tennyson on, 79–80; Tubman vision of Brown, 118, 126
Delany, Martin, 63, 230n9
disability studies, 15, 215n19
disability theory, 10, 213n7
Dix, Dorothea, 22, 32, 34, 225n66; asylum movement and, 121
Donaldson, Elizabeth, 8
Douglass, Frederick, 27, 64, 173; on "Heads of the Colored People" as demeaning, 75; on phrenology as scientific racism, 63; phrenology denouncement, 62–63, 74, 234n47; phrenology reading of head of, 63; J. Smith friendship with, 51; suicidal ideation of, 101; on white and Black equality, 63–64

INDEX

drapetomania, 102, 114, 226n87, 228n101; as mental disease causing slaves to run away, 38
Du Bois, W. E. B., 48, 261n16, 265n48; on color line problem, 141
Dunbar, Erica Armstrong, 119
Dunbar, Paul Lawrence, 173, 260n4
dysaesthesia aethiopis, 226n87; mental disability of slaves instead of free Blacks, 38–39

Earle, Pliny, 121, 124
Easley, E. T., 156
Eastern Lunatic Asylum (ELA): free and enslaved Blacks at, 22, 24–25; Galt administration of, 24
"Editor, The" (Smith, J.), 84–85
Edwards-Grossi, Elodie, 26, 142, 251n7
ELA. See Eastern Lunatic Asylum
Eliot, T. S., 79
emancipation: Black people enthusiasm for marriage after, 163–64, 257n80; Black people insanity increase after, 250n2; colored insane regimes of care before, 24–28, 221n33; mass lynchings and, 260n11; medicalized thought on Black mental disability after, 154–55, 255n50; Topinard on Black mental disability after, 155. See also regimes of care
Emancipation Day (1827), 83
Emerson, Ralph Waldo, 116
emotions: enslaved harm to, 108; Fugitive Slave Act and incessant fear, 1–2; Jacobs on costs of freedom to, 89; mental disability and disabling features of trauma, 8; mental illness term for health concerns of, 5; mental suffering responses of, 7–8, 214n9; slavery and trauma to, 8; J. Smith on Black people capacity to suffer, 78
enchanted universe, Chireau on, 222n34
enslaved: Boster on, 82; Combe rejection of phrenology and, 61; devastation of motherhood, 162; Fett on doctoring men and women, 90–91; Galt on less severe insanity of, 103; Harriss on unsoundness of, 114; injury or death through discipline, 115; Jacobs by Norcom, 88; physical and emotional harm to, 108; psychic wounding of, 89; sexual violence of women, 2, 95–96, 99; unreliable figures on disability of, 243n10; Weld on brutality and insanity prevalence of, 28
epilepsy: Galt on religious expression and, 123; psychiatric perspective of, 122; TLE of Tubman, 119–20
Equiano, Olaudah, 101
"Essay on Some of the Distinctive Peculiarities of the Negro Race, An" (Merrill), 42, 227nn99–100
eugenics, 157; Powell and, 251n6

"Facts Concerning Free Negroes" (Smith, J.), 55
familial separation, in slavery, 89, 96; Black women insane label and, 151; Powell belief in asylum, 163; slave narratives on, 102–4, 107
fanatic religion, psychiatric perspectives on, 124–25, 246n48
Felton, Rebecca Ann, 142, 251n4
Fett, Sharla, 28, 90–91
Fitzhugh, George, 32; on Black inferiority, 38; on paternalistic view of Black people, 37–38
Fogel, William, 73
Forten, Charlotte, 134
Forwood, W. S., 31
Foucault, Michel, 12, 204
Fowler, Lorenzo Niles, 60
Fowler, Orson Squire, 60
Frankel, Noralee, 162
Frederick Douglass' Paper: on Blacks equal access to psychiatric facilities, 27; "Heads of the Colored People" sketches in, 72

"Freedom and Slavery for Afric-Americans" (Smith, J.), 36, 47, 55
Freedom's Journal, 80
Fugitive Slave Act (1850), 52, 74; emotional experience and incessant fear from, 1–2; Jacobs on life under, 1–2, 89
"Future American, The: A Complete Race Amalgamation Likely to Occur" (Chesnutt), 176, 261n16
"Future American, The: A Stream of Dark Blood in the Veins of the Southern Whites" (Chesnutt), 176
"Future American, The: What the Race Is Likely to Become in the Process of Time" (Chesnutt), 176, 263n30

Gall, Franz Joseph, 59
Galt, John Minson, 32, 241n55; on Black insanity rates, 34; as ELA administrator, 24; on enslaved less severe insanity, 103; on religious expression and epilepsy, 123
Garnet, Henry Highland, 63, 127
Gates, Henry Louis, 51
genetic makeup and transmission, of Black people, 267n69
Georgia Lunatic Asylum (GLA), 9, 17, 139, *143*; Alice M. narrative, 143, 170; Amanda C. narrative, 143, 146–47, 162–65, 168, 170; Black femininity and insanity intersection, 4; Black patient absence of records at, 144; Black women depicted as insane, 150; Black women psychiatric incarceration at, 11–12, 140–70; elevated mortality rates for Black women at, 163; interior of operating room at, *159*; Jane G. narrative, 143, 146, 147, 151, 170; newspaper articles and asylum ledgers of, 145, 252n12; Olivia W. narrative, 143, 145–46, 151–52, 162–65, 168–70, 252n12, 256n75; Powell as superintendent of, 36, 140–41, 152–53, 156; racial hostility at, 166; view of day room at, *158*; Viney W. narrative, 143, 147, 151–52, 165, 168–70, 252n12; white women depicted as passive and fragile, 150
ghosts, Tubman belief in, 129
Gilman, Charlotte Perkins, 142
Gilman, Sander, 33, 39, 224n56
GLA. *See* Georgia Lunatic Asylum
Glasgow Emancipation Society, 52
Goldsby, Jacqueline, 14
Gonaver, Wendy, 142, 152
"Goophered Grapevine, The" (Chesnutt), 171
Gradual Emancipation Act (1799), 230n11
Grandfather Stories (Adams), 136

Harriet, the Moses of Her People (Bradford), 117, 130, 137
Harriet Tubman Home for Aged and Indigent Negroes, 4, 111, 137–39, *138*, 250n113
Harriss, Juriah, 114–15
Hartman, Saidiya, 96, 148, 238n4, 269n12
Hawthorne, Nathaniel, 116
Hayden, C. B., 32, 35, 225n72
head injury, of Tubman, 16, 114–16; at Bucktown General Store, 112–13, *113*; spiritual gifts and supernatural abilities after, 118–20, 125–28
"Heads of the Colored People, The" (Smith, J.), 52, 72, 87; biracial realities of Black people, 77; "The Black News Vendor," 73, 76–80; "The Boot-Black" in, 83; Douglass on demeaning content of, 75; on economic challenges for Black people in New York City, 73–74; "The Editor" in, 84–85; "The Inventor" in, 85; on mental disability, 73; on middle-class respectability, 75–76, 234n61; pen name of Communipaw for, 72; "The Schoolmaster" in, 85–86; "The Sexton" in, 83–84; on skilled trades people, 73; "The Washerwoman" in, 80–82
Hemming, Sally, 77

hereditary mental disease of Blacks, Powell on, 142, 156–57
heroic medicine solutions, of physicians for mental disability, 41, 218n2
Heroic Slave, The (Douglass), Crane on, 75
homeopathy, J. Smith criticism of, 232n34
Hough, Mazie, 41
House Behind the Cedars, The (Chesnutt), 176
Howe, Samuel Gridley, 121–22
Howells, William Dean, 173, 260n8

Incidents in the Life of a Slave Girl, Written by Herself (Jacobs), 3, 7, 90–92, 109–10; Child help in writing, 88; as illness narrative, 95; mental asylum as slavery metaphor, 93–97; mental disability within confinement, 98–103; motherhood and mental disability links, 103–8
Indian Removal Act, slavery expansion through, 23
inferiority, of Black people, 225n68; Fitzhugh on, 38; Jefferson on, 23, 74, 202, 219n8, 220n10; phrenology and, 61–62; Rush on, 61, 228n111
In Memoriam (Tennyson), J. Smith use of, 79–80
insanity, 4; as brain disease, 122; Camp on, 41; Galt on enslaved less severe, 103; legal consequences of, 6; physician racist theories on, 270n17; poorly defined terms of, 20; repercussions to, 10; as scientific language, 6; symptoms of, 20; Woodward on link between alcohol abuse and, 43–44
interventions, 15–18
"Inventor, The" (Smith, J.), 85

Jackson, Mattie, 103
Jacobs, Harriet, 3, 9, 17, 88, *108*, 110, 200, 204, 205; on alternative ideas about Black mental health, 90; children with Sawyer, 237n1; confinement in attic of grandmother, 89, 97–100, 104; on emotional costs of freedom, 89; historical facts about mental disability, 90; on life under Fugitive Slave Act, 1–2, 89; mental suffering of, 7, 16; Norcom enslaving of, 88; physical and sexual abuse during slavery, 2; on resistance to slavery, 97, 109; school for Black children, 242n73; slave narrative of, 13, 97; on slavery harm to Black bodymind, 87; N. Willis and C. Willis as employers of, 93
Jane G. narrative, on GLA, 143, 146, 147, 151, 170
Jarvis, Edward, 47, 223n54; on Black insanity reduction in South due to slavery, 34; on census of 1840 errors, 32–34, 47, 229n4; on civilization state belief, 34, 224n61; on high rates of mental disability in North, 34
Jefferson, Thomas: on Black people inferiority, 23, 74, 202, 219n8, 220n10; on Black people transient grief, 78; Black women sexual relationships by, 78, 236n90; comparison of Blacks to apes, 36–37; questioning of Black people capacity for feeling, 90; on scientific racism, 23, 219n8; on slavery damage to white children, 233n44
Jim Crow practices, 161
"Joe's Song," Tubman on, 130–34
Johnson, Mattie, 101
Joint Select Committee to Inquire Into the Condition of Affairs in the Late Insurrectionary States, of 1872, 166
Jones, Fred, 29
Jones, Jacqueline, 150
Judd, Bettina, 200–201

Kant, Immanuel, 219n8
kinship networks, for Black mental disability, 91
Kirkbride, Thomas, 22
Kirkbride Plan hospital blueprint, 22
Koch, Robert, 169
Kossuth, Louis, 235n73

"Lament of Tasso, The" (Byron), Jacobs use about life under slavery, 93–97, 240n21
Larson, Kate Clifford, 119–20
LeFrancois, Brenda A., 6
Legal Rights Association in New York, J. Smith establishment of, 52
Lewis, Nathaniel John, 129
"Life Among the Contrabands" (Jacobs), 242n73
Life and Times of Frederick Douglass (Douglass), 62
literature: Black feminism, 201, 269n5; of Black women, 203, 270n13; postbellum Black creative writings, 206–7
Lost Cause movement, 161
Lowry, Beverly, 113–14
lunacy, 5, 6, 19
lynching, 267n70; Chesnutt on, 176, 190, 264n37; after emancipation, 260n11; Felton on lynching, 142, 251n4

madness, 4, 5, 6
Madness in the City of Magnificent Intentions (Summers), 220n14, 221n20
madwoman in attic image, resistance signified by, 98
Magdalen Asylum, 59, 232n33
Mann, Horace, 121
maramus (severe malnutrition), Black women deaths at GLA from, 169–70, 259n117
marriage, of Black people after emancipation, 163–64, 257n80
Marrow of Tradition, The (Chesnutt), 171, 172, 174, 187, 263n30, 266n59; on Black cognitive and intellectual capabilities, 191–94; fiction as mode of social change in, 185–87; on psychological scars of post-emancipation racial violence, 188–91; vision of American future, 194–98; on Wilmington massacre, 16, 185–91
"Mars Jeem's Nightmare" chapter, in *The Conjure Woman*, 181–85

McCurley, W. S., 177
McDonald, James, 68–70
McKittrick, Katherine, 238n4
McLean Hospital (asylum), in Boston, 22
medical case studies, of J. Smith: on menstrual cycles and mental health, 57–58; New York Medical and Surgical Society rejection of, 57; on ptyalism, 57
medical degrees, of Black women, 229n7
Medical Inquiries and Observations Upon Diseases of the Mind (Rush), 21
medicalized proslavery: on Black bodyminds as prone to mental illness, 19; on Black people inherent mental capacity and lack of intelligence, 19; on slavery protection of Blacks from mental disorder, 16, 19, 153
medicalized thought, on Black mental disability, 152–53, 253n40; Chesnutt criticism of, 173–74; Easley on segregation, 156; Miller on increases after emancipation, 154–55, 255n50; pathologization of Black freedom, 160; psychiatrists on Black bodymind and slavery, 19, 153; Roberts on racial reclassifications, 161; on suicide of Blacks, 155–56, 255n55. *See also* physicians
medical model, of disability, 213n7
medical perspectives on mental disability: alcohol abuse and, 43–44; on Black freedom injurious to mental health, 40; Rush on slave owners mental health, 44–45; Weiner and Hough on, 41
menstrual cycles: mental disability and, 25, 98, 145, 157, 164, 232n29; J. Smith on mental health and, 57–58
mental asylum as slavery metaphor, in *Incidents*: irrational, disordered, absurd description of, 94; Jacobs on psychological illness through confinement, 94; Jacobs use of Byron "Lament of Tasso," 93–97, 240n21; mental suffering and, 96; moral insanity and,

95–96; Norcom use of intimidation and sexual violence, 96; sexual violence for enslaved women, 95; on social order in relation to real health outcomes, 95
mental conditions, terminology of, 219n3
mental disability, 4, 73; belief that slavery protected against, 16, 19, 31–40, 42, 47, 153; Black perspectives on, 3; census of 1840 data on, 20, 32, 47, 229n2; civilization state belief link to, 34; colored insane approach to, 9–10; disabling features of emotional and psychological traumas, 8; experiences of mental illness, distress and pain, 8; Jacobs historical facts about, 90; menstrual cycles and, 25, 57–58, 98, 145, 157, 164, 232n29; moral therapy in asylum, 20; motherhood link in *Incidents*, 102–8; from outside intervention or rupture, 6; physician heroic medicine solutions for, 41, 218n2; physicians on somatic causes of, 40, 122; Siebers on, 76; supernatural origins of, 29, 218n2, 222n49, 245n44. *See also* Black mental disability
mental disability, Chesnutt on age of black freedom, 171–72; American future vision, 194–98; on Black cognitive and intellectual capabilities, 191–94; in *The Conjure Woman*, 174, 179–85, *180*, 263n32; mad characters in fiction of, 264n37; *The Marrow of Tradition* fiction as mode of social change, 185–87; medicalized concept of, 173–74; psychological scars of post-emancipation racial violence, 188–91; racial amalgamation theory, 174, 175–79, 261n16
mental disability, Tubman and: African-derived healing traditions, 135–37; as colored insane, 111–12; Harriet Tubman Home for Aged and Indigent Negroes, 4, 111, 137–39, *138*, 250n113; psychiatric perspectives on religion and, 121–25; religious expression and, 112, 118, 130–35; sanity speculations on Tubman, 116–21, 248n79, 248n81; trans-sense and, 118–20, 125–29; Tubman head injury, 112–16, 118–20, 126–28

mental disability and intellectual thoughts, of J. Smith, 230n9; on abolition of slavery and medicine, 50–51, 52; census of 1840 and, 46–47, 54–55; Colored Orphan Asylum, 67–72; "Heads of the Colored People" sketches, 72–87, 234n61; literary works of, 48–49; medical case studies, 57–59; phrenology and, 59–67, 232n35; J. Smith background, 51–53; statistical counternarratives, 53–56
mental disability treatment: of drugs, tonics, bleeding and laxatives, 33, 218n2; with moral therapy, 21, 33, 245n45
mental disability within confinement, in *Incidents*, 101–3; Bronte and, 98; Jacobs narrative of confinement in attic, 89, 97–100, 104; madwoman in attic image, 98; McKittrick and Hartman on, 238n4; multilevel harm emphasis, 99–100
mental health: conditions, 5; Donaldson on disability-informed understanding of, 8; reformers, 2
mental healthcare, Rush and AMSAII members programs of, 22
mental illness, 5; archaic treatment of, 20; curability of, 20; pathologization of, 7; proslavery psychiatry and medical discourse on Black prone to, 19; stupidity as synonym for, 244n21
mental suffering, 4, 206; from being severed from children, 104; Black perspectives on, 3; on emotional responses, 7–8, 214n9; of Jacobs, 7, 16; mental asylum as slavery metaphor and, 96; sexual predation role in, 99
Menzies, Robert, 6
Merrill, A. P., 31, 227nn99–100; on alcohol abuse, 44; on Black bodymind, 42, 70; on race-based therapeutic interventions, 43; on slave holders violence and mental health, 44

metaphor. *See* mental asylum as slavery metaphor
Michigan Pregnancy Risk Assessment Monitoring System (MI-PRAMS) survey, 199
middle-class respectability," The Heads of the Colored People" on, 75–76, 234n61
Miller, J. F., 154–55
MI-PRAMS. *See* Michigan Pregnancy Risk Assessment Monitoring System
moral insanity, 95–96
moral therapy: activity regulation, 21; in asylum, 20; for mental disability treatment, 33, 245n45
moral treatment, of insanity, 20; on emotions, mind, and soul factors, 21; Philadelphia Quakers Friends Asylum for, 22; religious instruction in, 124; Tomes on psychiatrist understanding of, 21
Morton, Samuel, 61
motherhood: devastation of, for enslaved, 162; practice of selling children in slavery and, 104–7; psychiatric incarceration and, 162
motherhood and mental disability link, in *Incidents*, 108; Jacobs personal description of, 106; Northup *Twelve Years a Slave* depiction, 104–6, *105*; practice of selling children in slavery, 104–7; slave narratives on familial separation, 102–4
Mulcahy, Judith, 230n9
multidirectional power, in asylums, 12

narcolepsy, of Tubman, 118, 119
natal alienation, from slavery, 104
National Council of Colored People, J. Smith and Douglass formation of, 52
"Negro in Africa and America, The" (Tillinghast), 177
New York Medical and Surgical Society, rejection of J. Smith medical case studies, 57
New York State Asylum, 22, 125

nineteenth century terms, of mental illness: insanity, 5, 6, 19; lunacy, 5, 6, 19; madness, 4, 5, 6; medical and psychiatric discourse on, 17, 19–45, 215n17
Norcom, James: as apprentice of Rush, 91, 100–101; Jacobs enslaved by, 88; Jacobs rape avoidance, 237n1
Northup, Solomon, 104–6, *105*
Notes on the State of Virginia (Jefferson), 23; on slavery damaging to white children, 233n44; J. Smith on anti-negroisms in, 78

Observations on the Deranged Manifestation of the Mind (Spurzheim), 60
Observations on the Influence of Religion Upon the Health and Physical Welfare of Mankind (Brigham), 125
Olivia W. narrative, on GLA, 143, 145–46, 151–52, 162–65, 168–70, 252n12, 256n75

Painter, Nell Irvin, 16; on soul murder, 99–100
Parry, Tyler, 89
Patterson, Orlando, 104
Pennington, James C., 52, 63
Pennsylvania Hospital: Kirkbride hospital blueprint and, 22; Rush allocation of separate mental ward at, 21
perinatal mood and anxiety disorder (PMAD): medical and mental health professionals research and, 199; MI-PRAMS survey on, 199
phrenology: antislavery advocates response to, 62; Black inferiority and, 61–62; Brigham on, 60; Caldwell on Black inferiority and, 61–62; Douglass denouncement of, 62–63, 74, 234n47; L. Fowler and O. Fowler leaflets on, 60; Gall beginning of, 59; intellectual thoughts of J. Smith, 59–67, 232n35; opposition to, 59–60; public lectures on fallacy of, 65, 234n54; reading of the head of Douglass, 63; religion component of,

66–67; scientific racism and, 77; scientific study of, 65, 225n68; on skull examination for individual traits, 59; J. Smith fallacy lectures, 65, 234n54; Spurzheim and Combe popularization of, 59; use in criminology, 232n37

physicians: belief in Black mental disability and brain abnormalities, 26; on Black bodymind constitution, 41–42; on Black social vices and health conditions, 43; heroic medicine solutions for mental disability, 41, 218n2; on race and mental health, 47; racist theories on insanity, 270n17; J. Smith as chief physician at Colored Orphan Asylum, 53, 67–69; on somatic causes of mental disabilities, 41, 122

"Physician's Report," of McDonald and Proudfit, 68–71

Pickens, Theri A., 15, 90

Pinel, Philippe, 21

Plessy v. Ferguson, on segregation, 142

PMAD. *See* perinatal mood and anxiety disorder

Porter, Roy, 245n44

postbellum Black creative writings, 206–7

Powell, Theophilus O., *141*; on alcoholism, syphilis and tuberculosis as causes of insanity, 160; on care for colored insane in southern asylums, 140; emphasis on race and Black mental disability, 162; familial separation belief of, 163; as GLA superintendent, 36, 140–41, 152–53, 156; on hereditary mental disease of Blacks, 142, 156–57; on South experts on Black bodymind, 140–41; treatment protocol of asylum useful employment, 165

Price, Margaret, 5, 9

Prichard, James Cowles, 232n37

proslavery psychiatry, 16, 31–35, 226n92; on Black bodyminds as prone to mental illness, 19, 153, 202; on Black insanity prevalence in North, 32; on Black insanity reduction in South due to slavery, 32; Cartwright on Blacks inherent mental disability in body, 36; on comparison of Blacks to children, 37–38; Fitzhugh paternalistic view in, 37–38; genesis of and 1840 census, 20; scientific studies on, 65, 225n68

Proudfit, James, 68–70

psychiatric perspectives, on religion and mental disability, 121, 247n77; Black religion influence, 125; epilepsy and, 122; rational and fanatic religion discussion, 124–25, 246n48; on religious expression, 123, 125; somatic causes, 123–24

psychiatrists: on Black anatomical differences, 42; dismissive of Conjure, 31; on freedom from slavery harm to Black bodymind, 19, 153; lack of uniformity in insanity definition, 122; on mental disabilities absence of supernatural origins, 123–24; on negative impact of alcohol abuse, 43; race-specific mental health treatments, 43; religious instruction in moral treatment, 124; Summers on centering care on white people, 26–27; Tomes on moral treatment of insanity, 21

psychiatry studies, race and mental health addressed in, 239n6

psychological impact of slavery, 88–110; Black people articulation of, 2; Painter and White on, 16

ptyalism, J. Smith medical case study, 57

race and gender: asylum incarceration impacts from, 161–65; disorder construction according to, 3

Races of Europe (Ripley), 262n22

racial amalgamation, Chesnutt theory of, 174, 175–76, 179; Du Bois and barriers to, 261n16; McCurley argument against, 177

racial equality: J. Smith pursuit of, 52, 85–86; Stauffer on religious beliefs and, 231n18

racial hierarchies: Combe belief in, 61; Douglass attacks on claims of, 63
racial hostility, 166
racial reclassifications, Roberts on, 161
racial violence, Chesnutt on psychic wounding of, 16, 188–91
rational religion, 124–25, 246n48
Ray, Isaac, 32
reading practices, for book, 15; asylum case narratives, 11–12; Black-authored works, 11, 12–14; disability studies, 11, 12; examination of multiple sources, 10; Foucault on asylums relations of power, 12; Goldsby on, 13; literary works as valuable sources of evidence, 13–14; medical journals, 11–12; proslavery leanings of mainstream psychiatry, 12; white-authored medicalized documents, 10–11
Reaume, Geoffrey, 4–5, 6
Reconstruction, 4, 16, 150, 152, 175, 194, 260n11; attempts to create modern schools for Blacks, 264n44
"Reflections on the Census of 1840," in *Southern Literary Messenger*, 35–36
regimes of care for colored insane before emancipation: asylum segregation, 23, 24, 26, 27; Edwards-Grossi on, 26; at ELA, 24–25; slaveholders reluctance to treat, 26; Summers on, 25; Weld on Blacks with mental disabilities, 27–28, 221n33
religion: asylums practice of, 124; Chireau on history of supernatural and, 129; psychiatric perspectives on, 121–25; psychiatric perspectives on mental disability, 121–25, 247n77; J. Smith on, 66–67, 81; Stewart on history of, 126; Wells-Oghoghomeh as historian of, 127–28
religious expressions, 249n88; Brigham on, 125; Galt on epilepsy with, 123; Porter on, 245n44; Sernett on Tubman use of, 135; Tubman mental disability and, 112, 118, 130–35

"Report on the Diseases and Physical Peculiarities of the Negro Race" (Cartwright), 36
resistance: Jacobs slavery, 97, 109; signified by madwoman in attic image, 98; Sommerville and Synder on self-murder as, 240n32
Ripley, William, 177, 262n22
Roberts, Dorothy, 161
Ross, Araminta. *See* Tubman, Harriet
Rusert, Britt, 50, 230n10
Rush, Benjamin: on Black bodymind, 21, 219n5; on Black inferiority, 61, 228n111; Norcom as apprentice of, 91, 100–101; programs of mental healthcare, 22; on slave owners mental health, 44–45

Samuels, Ellen, 40
Sanborn, Franklin Benjamin, 116–18, 121
sanity speculations, on Tubman, 121; Black religious practices, 112, 118, 130–35; Bradford biographical sketch of, 116–18, 248n79, 248n81; brain surgery of, 120; Conrad biographic information on, 118–19; historians on symptoms and medical diagnoses, 119; Larson on TLE, 119–20; narcolepsy of Tubman, 118, 119; Sanborn biographical sketch of, 116–18, 121; Tubman spiritual gifts and supernatural visions, 118–20, 126–28
Sawyer, Samuel, 237n1
Scenes in the Life of Harriet Tubbman (Bradford), 116, 130
Schalk, Sami, 15
"Schoolmaster, The" (Smith, J.), 85–86
scientific racism, 77; Douglass on phrenology as, 63; Jefferson on, 23, 219n8; phrenology and, 77; proslavery psychiatry and, 31–40
segregation: of Black people in asylums, 10, 23, 24, 26, 27, 122, 142, 165–66, 258n107; Easley on Black mental disability and, 156; *Plessy v. Ferguson* on, 142

segregation and standards of care, at GLA: Black women death from, 168–69; Black women maramus deaths, 169–70, 259n117; Black women tuberculosis prevalence, 169–70, 259n115; housing for Black people, 168; overcrowding, poor provisions, unsanitary conditions, 168, 258n106

Segrest, Mab, 142

Sernett, Milton, 135

severe malnutrition. *See* maramus

Seward, Frederick, 128

"Sexton, The" (Smith, J.), 83–84

sexual exploitation: emotional and psychological trauma of, 8; of Jefferson with Black women, 78, 236n90; of Norcom to Jacobs, 88, 237n1

sexual violence: in asylums, 10; against Black women, 16, 166; of enslaved women, 2, 95–96, 99; Hartman on, 96

She Came to Stay (Dunbar, E.), 119

Siebers, Tobin, 76

slave narratives: abolition goal of, 97; on familial separation, 102–4, 107; intertextuality of, 93; of Jacobs, 13, 97; Parry on, 89; Pickens on, 90; suicidal ideation in, 101

slavery: Black mental capacity as justification for, 23, 225n68; common incidents during, 7; defenses of, 23; emotional and psychological trauma from, 8; family separation in, 89, 96, 102–4, 107, 151, 163; foundational histories of, 239n18; historians on psychological costs of, 16; historical studies on mind impacted by, 238n3; Indian Removal Act and expansion of, 22–23; Jacobs on psychological costs of, 92; Jacobs on resistance to, 97, 109; Jefferson on damage to white children from, 233n44; mental asylum as metaphor of, 93–97; mental suffering and emotional responses to, 7–8, 214n9; Patterson on natal alienation, 104; physical and sexual abuse during, 2, 95–96, 99; psychological cost to Black women, 88–110; psychological economy of, 2; role in American psychiatry development, 17; J. Smith born into, 51; J. Smith freedom at age 14, 51. *See also* abolition

Smith, Gerrit, 53

Smith, James McCune, 3, 9, 13, 36, 49, 70, 200, 202–3, 205, 231n26; on abolition of slavery and medicine, 48, 50–51, 52; advocating for Blacks to move to rural communities, 74; background on, 51–53; on Black bodymind, 17, 48, 53, 77–78; as Black intellectual, 47, 48; on Black mental health multifactorial elements, 50; contributions to Black newspapers, 52; Douglass friendship with, 51; as editor of *The Colored American* newspaper, 52; fluency in seven languages, 51; free under Gradual Emancipation Act, 230n11; Gates on historical significance of, 51; as highly educated, 51–52; homeopathy criticism by, 232n34; on Kossuth, 235n73; mental disability and intellectual thought of, 46–87, 230n9, 234n61; on national government imperatives, 54; racial equality pursuit, 52; Rusert on, 50; on social predictors of adverse health consequences, 71

Smith, Theophus, 28

Snyder, Terri, 240n32

social identities, medicine and psychiatry beliefs about, 40

social model, of disability, 213n7

social order, on human bondage, 19

somatic causes, of mental disabilities: Cheney on, 122; physicians on, 41, 122; religion and, 123–24

Sommerville, Diane, 240n32

soul murder, Painter on, 99–100

spiritual gifts, of Tubman, 118–20, 125–28
Spurzheim, Johann, 59, 60
statistical counternarratives, of J. Smith: debunking Calhoun statements, 54, 55; on good morals acquisition, 55; on longevity rates of southern Blacks, 55–56; on Northern Blacks literacy rates, 55; on psychiatric institutionalization of Blacks in North, 54; statistical study on free Blacks in North, 55
"Statistics of Insanity in the United States" (Jarvis), 33
Stauffer, John, 82, 230n9, 230n12, 231n18, 235n74
St. Elizabeth Hospital: acceptance of Black mentally disabled people, 25; Summers on Black experiences at, 220n14
stereotypes, of Black women, 149
Stewart, Diane, 126
Stribling, Francis T., 221n16
suicidal ideation, in slave narratives, 101
suicide, of Blacks, 155–56, 255n55, 270n17
Summers, Martin, 25, 26–27, 142, 221n20; on Black experiences at St. Elizabeth Asylum, 220n14
supernatural origins, of mental disability, 29, 125, 218n2, 222n49
syphilitic infections, 6, 160
System of Phrenology, A (Combe), 62

Tasso, Torquato, 93
Taylor, John, 233n44
Taylor, Ula, 148
Telford, Emma Paddock, 114, 138; Tubman interview with, 117–18; on Tubman spiritual gifts, 126–27
temporal lobe epilepsy (TLE), of Tubman, 119–20
Tennyson, Alfred, 79–80
terminology: of Black mental disability, 4–10; of mental conditions, 219n3
Terrell, Mary Church, 187, 265n48
Thompson, George, 80

Thoreau, Henry David, 116
Tillinghast, Joseph Alexander, 177
TLE. *See* temporal lobe epilepsy
Tomes, Nancy, 21
Topinard, Paul, 155
trans-sense, of Tubman, 125; spiritual gifts and visions, 118–20, 126–28; Tubman on ghosts, 128–29; Wells-Oghoghomeh on, 128
tuberculosis: Black women prevalence at GLA, 169–70, 259n115; Koch on, 169; Powell on insanity caused from, 160
Tubman, Harriet, 9, 13, 17–18, 110, *131*, 200, 203, 244n26; on altered mental states, 3–4; Bradford biographical sketch of, 116–18, 248n79, 248n81; Brown death vision, 118, 126; Civil War vision, 118, 127; connection to Sanborn, Mann, and Howe, 121; drapetomania of, 114; head injury of, 16, 112–16, 118–20, 126–28; on "Joe's Song," 130–34; mental disability conceptions, 111–39; organizing for abolition, 111, 121; religious expressions, 112, 118, 130–35; as skilled orator, 131–32; as spy and nurse in Civil War, 111, 136; Underground Railroad and, 111, 112, 135, 136. *See also* mental disability, Tubman and
Tuke, William, 21
Twelve Years a Slave (Northup), 104–6, *105*

Underground Railroad, 18, 52, 242n1; Tubman and, 111, 112, 135, 136

Viney W. narrative, on GLA, 143, 147, 151–52, 165, 168–70, 252n12
visions, of Tubman, 118–20, 126–28
vulgar theory of race, 176; Ripley criticism of, 177

Ward, Samuel, 63
"Washerwoman, The" (Smith, J.), 80, 82; on religion and freedom concept, 81
Washington, Booker T., 141–42, 173, 256n58
Wayward Lives (Hartman), 269n12

Weiner, Marli, 41
Weld, Theodore Dwight, 27–28, 221n33
Wells-Oghoghomeh, Alexis, 127–28
Western Lunatic Asylum, Stribling opposed to Blacks entering, 221n16
White, Deborah Gray, 16
white-authored medicalized documents, 10–11
white people: Summers on psychiatrist centering of care of, 26–27; women at GLA depicted as passive and fragile, 150
white superiority, 85
Willis, Cordelia Grinnell, 93

Willis, Nathaniel Parker, 93
Wilmington massacre (1896), 156, 266n66; Chesnutt on psychic wounding from, 16, 185–91; mob celebration and, *188*
Woodward, Samuel, 32, 34, 43–44, 121
Worcester Lunatic Asylum, Mann and establishment of, 121
Wordsworth, William, 79

Yellin, Jean Fagan, 98
York retreat (1796): as global model for mentally ill institutions, 21; Tuke opening of, 21

GPSR Authorized Representative: Easy Access System Europe, Mustamäe tee
50, 10621 Tallinn, Estonia, gpsr.requests@easproject.com

www.ingramcontent.com/pod-product-compliance
Lightning Source LLC
Chambersburg PA
CBHW022034290426
44109CB00014B/863